PUBLIC HEALTH: PRACTICES, METHODS AND POLICIES

SERVICE LEADERSHIP

TOOLS TO ASSESS KNOWLEDGE, ATTITUDE AND BEHAVIOR

PUBLIC HEALTH: PRACTICES, METHODS AND POLICIES

JOAV MERRICK - SERIES EDITOR

MEDICAL DIRECTOR, HEALTH SERVICES, DIVISION FOR INTELLECTUAL AND DEVELOPMENTAL DISABILITIES, MINISTRY OF SOCIAL AFFAIRS AND SOCIAL SERVICES, JERUSALEM, ISRAEL

Service Leadership: Tools to Assess Knowledge, Attitude and Behavior
Daniel TL Shek, Xiaoqin Zhu, Li Lin and Joav Merrick (Editors)
2019. ISBN: 978-1-53614-852-7 (Hardcover)
2019. ISBN: 978-1-53614-853-4 (e-book)

Public Health Yearbook 2017
Joav Merrick (Editor)
2018. ISBN: 978-1-53613-792-7 (Hardcover)
2018. ISBN: 978-1-53613-793-4 (e-book)

Resilience and Health: A Potent Dynamic
I Leslie Rubin and Joav Merrick (Editors)
2018. ISBN: 978-1-53613-412-4 (Hardcover)
2018. ISBN: 978-1-53613-413-1 (e-book)

Medical History: Some Perspectives Second Edition
Donald E. Greydanus and Joav Merrick, (Editors)
2018. ISBN: 978-1-53613-319-6 (Hardcover)
2018. ISBN: 978-1-53613-320-2 (e-book)

University Students: Promotion of Holistic Development in Hong Kong
Daniel TL Shek, Lu Yu and Joav Merrick (Editors)
2017. ISBN: 978-1-53612-535-1 (Hardcover)
2017. ISBN: 978-1-53612-537-5 (e-book)

Alzheimer's Disease: Awareness among Young Adults
Ronald Chow, Drew Hollenberg, Michael Borean and Joav Merrick (Editors)
2017. ISBN: 978-1-53612-456-9 (Softcover)
2017. ISBN: 978-1-53612-457-6 (e-book)

Service Leadership Education for University Students
Daniel TL Shek, Po Chung, Li Lin and Joav Merrick (Editors)
2017. ISBN: 978-1-53611-949-7 (Hardcover)
2017. ISBN: 978-1-53611-969-5 (e-book)

Leadership: Promoting Leadership and Intrapersonal Development in University Students
Daniel TL Shek, Cecilia MS Ma and Joav Merrick (Editors)
2017. ISBN: 978-1-53611-950-3 (Hardcover)
2017. ISBN: 978-1-53611-970-1 (e-book)

Caribbean Adolescents: Misuse and Abuse of Alcohol
Cecilia Hegamin-Younger and Joav Merrick (Editors)
2017. ISBN: 978-1-63485-880-9 (Hardcover)
2016. ISBN: 978-1-63485-894-6 (e-book)

Public Health: An Ecological Framework for Child Environmental Health Interventions
I. Leslie Rubin and Joav Merrick (Editors)
2017. ISBN: 978-1-53610-700-5 (Hardcover)
2017. ISBN: 978-1-53610-714-2 (e-book)

Diabetes Mellitus: A Medical History Journey
Donald E. Greydanus and Joav Merrick
2016. ISBN: 978-1-53610-094-5 (Softcover)
2016. ISBN: 978-1-53610-103-4 (e-book)

Education in Hong Kong: Service Leadership for University Students
Daniel TL Shek, Cecilia MS Ma, Li Lin and Joav Merrick (Editors)
2016. ISBN: 978-1-63484-928-9 (Hardcover)
2016. ISBN: 978-1-63484-960-9 (e-book)

Environmental Health Disparities: Costs and Benefits of Breaking the Cycle
I. Leslie Rubin and Joav Merrick (Editors)
2016. ISBN: 978-1-63484-211-2 (Hardcover)
2016. ISBN: 978-1-63484-212-9 (e-book)

Higher Education in Hong Kong: Nurturing Students to be Caring Service Leaders
Daniel TL Shek, Andrew MH Siu, Hildie Leung and Joav Merrick (Editors)
2016. ISBN: 978-1-63484-980-7 (Hardcover)
2016. ISBN: 978-1-63485-009-4 (e-book)

Measles: Epidemiology and Control of Measles in the Gweru Urban District in Zimbabwe
Tawanda Marufu, Seter Siziya, Mazyanga L. Mazaba and Joav Merrick (Editors)
2016. ISBN: 978-1-63485-559-4 (Hardcover)
2016. ISBN: 978-1-63485-573-0 (e-book)

Medical History: Some Perspectives
Donald E. Greydanus and Joav Merrick
2016. ISBN: 978-1-63484-747-6 (Hardcover)
2016. ISBN: 978-1-63484-849-7 (e-book)

Public Health: Some International Aspects
Joav Merrick (Editor)
2016. ISBN: 978-1-63484-612-7 (Hardcover)
2016. ISBN: 978-1-63484-630-1 (e-book)

Public Health: International Aspects on Environment and Health
I. Leslie Rubin and Joav Merrick (Editors)
2016. ISBN: 978-1-63484-834-3 (Hardcover)
2016. ISBN: 978-1-63484-849-7 (e-book)

Smoking and Adolescence: International Public Health Experiences
Mazyanga L. Mazaba, Seter Siziya and Joav Merrick (Editors)
2016. ISBN: 978-1-63484-311-9 (Hardcover)
2016. ISBN: 978-1-63484-312-6 (e-book)

Arbovirus: Public Health Experience from Zambia
Seter Siziya, Mazyanga L. Mazaba, and Joav Merrick (Editors)
2015. ISBN: 978-1-63463-601-8 (Hardcover)
2015. ISBN: 978-1-63463-618-6 (e-book)

Health Issues in Diverse Cultures
Cecilia Obeng, Samuel Gyasi Obeng and Joav Merrick (Editors)
2015. ISBN: 978-1-63463-613-1 (Hardcover)
2015. ISBN: 978-1-63463-619-3 (e-book)

Public Health, Social Work and Health Inequalities
Bruce D. Friedman and Joav Merrick (Editors)
2015. ISBN: 978-1-63482-838-3 (Hardcover)
2015. ISBN: 978-1-63482-850-5 (e-book)

Patient Dumping: Background, Protections, and the Mentally Ill
Tabitha E. Rivers (Editor)
2015. ISBN: 978-1-63483-726-2 (Hardcover)
2015. ISBN: 978-1-63483-727-9 (e-book)

Tomorrow's Leaders: Service Leadership and Holistic Development in Chinese University Students
Daniel TL Shek, Andrew MH Siu and Joav Merrick (Editors)
2015. ISBN: 978-1-63321-880-2 (Hardcover)
2014. ISBN: 978-1-63321-943-4 (e-book)

Environment and Public Health: Environmental Health, Law and International Perspectives
I. Leslie Rubin and Joav Merrick (Editors)
2014. ISBN: 978-1-63463-167-9 (Hardcover)
2014. ISBN: 978-1-63463-189-1 (e-book)

PUBLIC HEALTH: PRACTICES, METHODS AND POLICIES

SERVICE LEADERSHIP

TOOLS TO ASSESS KNOWLEDGE, ATTITUDE AND BEHAVIOR

DANIEL TL SHEK
XIAOQIN ZHU
LI LIN
AND
JOAV MERRICK
EDITORS

nova science publishers
New York

Library of Congress Cataloging-in-Publication Data

ISBN: 978-1-53614-852-7
Library of Congress Control Number: 2018967620

Published by Nova Science Publishers, Inc. † New York

CONTENTS

INTRODUCTION

In: Service Leadership
Editors: Daniel TL Shek, Xiaoqin Zhu, Li Lin et al.
ISBN: 978-1-53614-852-7

Chapter 1

DEVELOPMENT AND VALIDATION OF ASSESSMENT TOOLS ON SERVICE LEADERSHIP KNOWLEDGE, ATTITUDE AND BEHAVIOR

Daniel TL Shek[1-6,*], PhD, FHKPS, BBS, SBS, JP, Xiaoqin Zhu[1], PhD and Joav Merrick[6-9], MD, MMedSci, DMSc

[1]Department of Applied Social Sciences,
The Hong Kong Polytechnic University, Hong Kong, PR China
[2]Centre for Innovative Programmes for Adolescents and Families,
The Hong Kong Polytechnic University, Hong Kong, PR China
[3]Department of Social Work, East China Normal University, Shanghai, PR China
[4]Kiang Wu Nursing College of Macau, Macau, PR China
[5]Hong Kong Institute of Service Leadership and Management Limited,
Hong Kong, PR China
[6]Division of Adolescent Medicine, Department of Pediatrics,
Kentucky Children's Hospital, University of Kentucky School of Medicine,
Lexington, Kentucky, US
[7]National Institute of Child Health and Human Development, Jerusalem, Israel
[8]Department of Pediatrics, Mt Scopus Campus,
Hadassah Hebrew University Medical Center, Jerusalem, Israel
[9]Center for Healthy Development, School of Public Health,
Georgia State University, Atlanta, Georgia, US

---

* Correspondence: Daniel TL Shek, PhD, FHKPS, BBS, SBS, JP, Associate Vice President (Undergraduate Programme), Chair Professor of Applied Social Sciences and Li and Fung Professor in Service Leadership Education, Department of Applied Social Sciences, The Hong Kong Polytechnic University, Hung Hom, Hong Kong, PR China. Email: daniel.shek@polyu.edu.hk.

Abstract

How can we develop and nurture leadership in service economies? This issue is of upmost importance, because the mode of production and requirements of the leaders are different in manufacturing and service economies. While the focus in manufacturing industries is on "do things right," the focus of services economies is on "do the right things." In this book we start out with the Service Leadership Model as well as the ingredients on Service Leadership knowledge, attitude, and behaviors (i.e., skills). Second, psychometric properties of three validated measures on Service Leadership knowledge, attitude and behavior are presented. In these chapters, the internal consistency, convergent validity and factorial validity of the measures are presented. Third, the psychosocial correlates and norms associated with these three measures of Service Leadership are presented. Through these chapters, we attempt to establish the psychometric properties and norms of the scales assessing Service Leadership knowledge, attitude and behavior. Finally, user manuals for the three assessment tools are also presented. It is our humble wish that the related work and the developed assessment tools can be used in the training, personnel decisions, intervention and research contexts.

Introduction

With the growth of service industries in the global world, there is a need to ask how we can nurture leadership in service economies. This is important because the mode of production and requirements of the leaders are different in manufacturing and service economies (1). While the focus in manufacturing industries is on "do things right," the focus of services economies is on "do the right things." Besides, leadership style in service economies is often "bottom-up," which is different from the "top-down" style in manufacturing industries. In view of the unique features of service economies, we need a leadership model which can meet the needs of service economies (2).

To address the issue of service leadership in the changing economies, Dr. Po Chung (Co-founder of DHL International and Chairman Emeritus of DHL Express (Hong Kong) Ltd. and Chairman of the Hong Kong Institute of Service Leadership and Management Limited (HKI-SLAM)) proposed the Service Leadership Model. According to HKI-SLAM (3), service leadership "is about satisfying needs by consistently providing quality personal service to everyone one comes into contact with, including one's self, others, groups, communities, systems, and environments. A service leader is a ready, willing and able, on-the-spot socialized entrepreneur who possesses relevant task competencies and is judged by superiors, peers, subordinates, and followers to exhibit appropriate character strengths and a caring social disposition." The Service Leadership Model is based on Chung's seminal works on service reborn (4), 25 principles essential for service leadership (5) and 12 dimensions of one's personal brand (6).

To promote Service Leadership education in the publicly-funded universities in Hong Kong, Li and Fung Foundation provided HK$40 million to support a project on Service

Leadership Education in Hong Kong. In the eight universities funded by the University Grants Committee, researchers developed credit-bearing subjects, non-credit-bearing programs and curriculum materials. In some programs, some evaluation work was done using some tentative measures of service leadership qualities (7, 8).

Unfortunately, Service Leadership education has been hindered due to its lack of validated measures of Service Leadership knowledge, attitude and behavior. Similarly, the lack of related validated measures also hinders the development of Service Leadership research. The development of measures based on the Service Leadership Model is important for several reasons. First, as Service Leadership Model is still at its infancy and there is limited research underlying the concepts and theories of Service Leadership, validated measurement tools are vital to the future development of the model. Slavec and Drnovšek (9) argued that "effective measurement is a cornerstone of scientific research … reliable and valid measures contribute to the legitimacy and development of a research field" (p. 39). Second, the scales would allow for investigations on the determinants and outcomes of effective Service Leadership qualities, and how these qualities are related to organizational effectiveness (2). Third, assessment tools in Service Leadership are important because they can be used to examine the effectiveness of related intervention programs. For example, it would be extremely important to understand whether Service Leadership training programs really promote Service Leadership qualities in the program participants.

THREE AREAS OF IMPORTANCE

There are three areas that should be assessed as far as Service Leadership qualities are concerned. The first area is Service Leadership knowledge. Assuming that we are asked to create a credit-bearing subject on Service Leadership, we have to ask what fundamental knowledge on Service Leadership will be included. Basically, Service Leadership knowledge includes core beliefs of the Service Leadership Model (such as everybody can be a leader) and components of effective Service Leadership (competence, moral character and caring disposition). For example, as far as moral character is concerned, a service leader should appreciate the importance of morality and integrity and what constitutes an ethical leader ("know-what"). Besides, one must know the determinants of moral judgments such as motivation to act in a moral manner, moral reasoning, and reflection on one's Personal Operating System. Regarding caring disposition, one should know its components, such as empathy, love, and sensitivity to others' needs and emotions.

For attitude to Service Leadership, it basically addresses one's beliefs and feelings about Service Leadership, such as whether one agrees to the core beliefs of Service Leadership and the basic ingredients of effective service leadership. Most important of all, it is important to assess whether one has a service mindset, such as care about oneself as well as others, and to be sensitive to others' needs. Besides, whether one identifies with the importance of moral character, such as the degree of agreement with the importance of character strengths based on the Western literature and Confucian values based on Chinese philosophies.

For Service Leadership skills, an effective service leader should possess intrapersonal skills (such as resilience, emotional competence, social competence, courage and vision) as well as interpersonal skills (such as relationship building, team building and conflict resolution skills). Besides, service leaders should learn "maritime" leadership style combining both top-down and bottom-up leadership models and appreciate distributive leadership styles. As caring leaders, effective service leaders should also know the skills of developing others and mentorship abilities.

About This Book

Against the above background, there are several parts in this book. First, the Service Leadership Model as well as the ingredients on Service Leadership knowledge, attitude and behaviors (i.e., skills) are presented. Second, psychometric properties of three validated measures on Service Leadership knowledge, attitude, and behavior are presented. In these chapters, the internal consistency, convergent validity and factorial validity of the measures are presented. Third, the psychosocial correlates and norms associated with these three measures of Service Leadership are presented in three papers. Through these chapters, we attempt to establish the psychometric properties and norms of the scales assessing Service Leadership knowledge, attitude and behavior. Finally, user manuals for the three measures on Service Leadership knowledge, attitude, and behavior are also presented. It is our humble wish that the related work and the developed assessment tools can be used in the training, personnel decisions, intervention and research contexts.

Acknowledgments

This chapter is an updated version of a publication in the special issue "Development and validation of assessment tools on service leadership knowledge, attitude and behavior" edited by Daniel TL Shek, Xiaoqin Zhu and Joav Merrick published in the International Journal of Child and Adolescent Health, 2018;11(4).

REFERENCES

[1] Shek DTL, Chung PPY, Leung H. Manufacturing economy vs. service economy: Implications for service leadership. Int J Disabil Hum Dev 2015;14(3):205-15. DOI: 10.1515/ijdhd-2015-0402.

[2] Shek DTL, Chung PPY, Leung H. How unique is the service leadership model? A comparison with contemporary leadership approaches. Int J Disabil Hum Dev 2015;14(3):217-31. DOI: 10.1515/ijdhd-2015-0403.

[3] Hong Kong Institute of Service Leadership and Management (HKI-SLAM). SLAM education. 2013. 29 Sep, 2015. URL: http://hki-slam.org/index.php?r=article&catid=2&aid=16.

[4] Chung PPY. Service reborn: The knowledge, skills and attitudes of service companies. New York: Lexingford, 2012.

[5] Chung PPY, Bell AH. 25 principles of service leadership. New York: Lexingford, 2015.

[6] Chung PPY, Elfassy R. The 12 dimensions of a Service Leader. New York: Lexingford, 2016.

[7] Shek DTL, Lin L. Changes in university studetns after joining a service leadership program in China. J Leadersh Educ 2016;15(1):96-109. DOI: 1012806/V15/I1/A2.

[8] Shek DTL, Lin L, Liu TT. Service leadership education for university students in Hong Kong: Subjective outcome evaluation. Int J Disabil Hum Dev 2014;13(4):513-21. DOI: 10.1515/ijdhd-2014-0349.

[9] Slavec A, Drnovsek M. A perspective on scale development in entrepreneurship research. Econ Bus Rev 2012;14(1):39-62.

SECTION ONE: TOOLS FOR ASSESSMENT

In: Service Leadership
Editors: Daniel TL Shek, Xiaoqin Zhu, Li Lin et al.
ISBN: 978-1-53614-852-7

Chapter 2

Leadership Assessment Tools in Different Chinese Contexts

Li Lin*[1], *PhD
and Daniel TL Shek*[1-6,*], *PhD, FHKPS, BBS, SBS, JP

[1]Department of Applied Social Sciences,
The Hong Kong Polytechnic University, Hong Kong, PR China
[2]Centre for Innovative Programmes for Adolescents and Families,
The Hong Kong Polytechnic University, Hong Kong, PR China
[3]Department of Social Work, East China Normal University, Shanghai, PR China
[4]Kiang Wu Nursing College of Macau, Macau, PR China
[5]Hong Kong Institute of Service Leadership and Management Limited,
Hong Kong, PR China
[6]Division of Adolescent Medicine, Department of Pediatrics,
Kentucky Children's Hospital, University of Kentucky School of Medicine,
Lexington, Kentucky, US

Abstract

Leadership research in different Chinese contexts is growing rapidly with plentiful assessment tools emerging in the field. Using a cross-cultural study framework, this chapter provides an overview of contemporary leadership assessment tools used in different Chinese contexts. The leadership assessment tools developed by the etic approach, emic approach and combined etic-emic approach all contribute to the knowledge advancement

* Correspondence: Daniel TL Shek, PhD, FHKPS, BBS, SBS, JP, Associate Vice President (Undergraduate Programme), Chair Professor of Applied Social Sciences and Li and Fung Professor in Service Leadership Education, Department of Applied Social Sciences, The Hong Kong Polytechnic University, Hung Hom, Hong Kong, PR China. Email: daniel.shek@polyu.edu.hk.

of leadership, yet their limitations should also be noted. This chapter ends with a critique of Chinese leadership assessment tools and recommendations for future directions.

INTRODUCTION

Contemporary leadership theories commonly define leadership as a dynamic and reciprocal process in which one influences a group of people to achieve a collective goal (1, 2). Leadership has been regarded as universal human behavior that has an evolutionary function for solving adaptive problems (3, 4). However, the views toward the relationship between leadership and culture are not uniform. On the one hand, some scholars believe that there are some fundamental components of leadership shared by different cultures (5). Additionally, the growing globalization over the world makes the leadership conceptualization and practices in Western and Eastern organizations become increasingly aligned over time (6). On the other hand, some scholars believe that how people understand and practice leadership may vary across cultures (7, 8). Cultural values may define what an ideal leader is in a specific culture, which influences how people practice their leadership in the organization and develop their leadership. Depending on their theoretical perspectives, researchers used different assessment tools to measure leadership in a particular culture.

There are three approaches to the inquiry of leadership in the Chinese contexts: the etic approach, the emic approach, and the combination of etic and emic approach (7). First, researchers translated and validated the existing scales developed in Western cultures in order to test the generalizability of the existing leadership theories and models to Chinese contexts (i.e., etic approach). Second, researchers developed an indigenous leadership scale based on the Chinese leadership construct in order to capture psychological constructs that are not present in Western cultures (i.e., emic approach). Finally, researchers developed and validated a new scale based on both Western and Chinese concepts (i.e., etic-emic approach).

In this chapter, we reviewed the commonly used leadership assessment tools in Chinese contexts with reference to the related studies conducted in mainland China, Hong Kong and Taiwan. In the organizational realm, assessment tools of leadership usually measure leadership qualities including attitudes, beliefs, behavior and styles of people who take up a leadership post, using measures such as the Multifactor Leadership Questionnaire (MLQ; 9), Authentic Leadership Inventory (10), and Paternalistic Leadership Scale (11). In addition, in the realm of leadership development and education, based on the assumption that everyone has potentials and capacities to develop leadership (12), several scales have been developed to capture the leadership capacities of ordinary people regardless of their positions, such as Socially Responsible Leadership Scale (SRLS; 12) and Leadership Practices Inventory (13). This review covers leadership assessment tools for "positional" leaders and "ordinary" leaders. In particular, based on the scales reviewed, we identified the gaps and problems of the existing literature on leadership assessment tools in different Chinese contexts.

ASSESSMENT TOOLS BASED ON THE ETIC APPROACH

One of the major inquiries in Chinese leadership study is to test whether the imported assessment instruments measure the same construct across cultures. Therefore, validating the existing leadership measures developed in Western contexts is an initial step of leadership study in the Chinese academia. With validation evidence, researchers could test whether the Western leadership theories and models are applicable to Chinese contexts, and further extend the theories by examining the mechanisms underlying the effects of a certain leadership practice or investigating the conditional boundary of these effects. This approach is called etic approach.

The characteristics of etic approach are top-down and Western in origin (14). Guided by a Western leadership theory or model, researchers usually translate the assessment tools with literal adaption following a translation-back translation procedure (15). For example, Chen and Farh (16) translated the Transformational Leadership Scale developed by Podsakoff, MacKenzie, Moorman, and Fetter (17), and found it well applied in Taiwan organizations. This scale assesses six features of transformational leadership practices, including identifying and articulating a vision, providing a role model, fostering the acceptance of collective goals, expecting high performance, offering individualized support and intellectual stimulation (17). This translated version has been successfully used in many Chinese studies. For instance, Wang, Law, Hackett, Wang, and Chen (18) successfully validated the six-dimension structure via confirmatory factor analysis (CFA), and used it to examine the mediator that explained the associations between transformation leadership and positive performance and organizational citizenship behavior of followers in mainland Chinese originations. Another example is Chan and Mak's (19) study that translated the 28-item Servant Leadership Scale developed by Liden, Wayne, Zhao, and Henderson (20) to examine the moderating effect of subordinates' organizational tenure in the association between servant leadership and subordinates' trust in leader and job satisfaction in Hong Kong organizations. This scale has seven factors – emotional healing, creating value for the community, conceptual skills, empowering, helping subordinates grow and succeed, putting subordinates first, and behaving ethically with good factorial validity. Additionally, Sun and Wang (21) translated the 23-item servant leadership scale developed by Barbuto and Wheeler (22) and examined the construct of servant leadership in mainland Chinese organizations. The original scale included five dimensions – wisdom, persuasive mapping, organizational stewardship, altruistic calling, emotional healing. This translated version demonstrated satisfactory reliability and similar internal structure (i.e.,

5-factor structure) via exploratory factor analysis (EFA) and CFA, but there were slight differences in the number of items in each factor because some items were removed due to under loading.

In addition to leadership research in organizational settings, Chinese scholars also investigated leadership capacities of ordinary people, especially young people regardless of their leadership background. Therefore, similar to the case of leadership measures for positional leaders, Chinese translated versions of existing scales that assess leadership capacities are available in the literature. For example, based on the social change model, Dugan and Komives (12) developed the Socially Responsible Leadership Scale (SRLS) and its shortened version (SRLS-R2). These scales assess eight core values, including consciousness of self, congruence, commitment, courage, collaboration, common purpose, controversy with civility, and citizenship. Leung, Ha, and Yeung (23) translated the SRLS-R2 and tested it in Hong Kong university students. Results showed adequate evidence for the eight-factor structure, and the reliability for each subscale (factor) was satisfactory except for the change and controversy with civility dimensions. Additionally, Chan (24) created a Chinese version of 26-item self-reported Roets Rating Scale for Leadership (RRSL) (25) to measure three leadership capacities (i.e., leadership, ambition and desires) of Hong Kong students in grades 7-12, which showed satisfactory reliability and convergent validity with other leadership measures based on behavioral indicators reported by parents and teachers.

Because of the rapid development in psychology and organizational behavior in China, Chinese translated version of Western leadership scales are common. Besides the scales mentioned above, there are many other examples in the literature, such as the Chinese version of Authentic Leadership Questionnaire (26) translated by Qian, Lin, and Chen (27), the Chinese version of Leadership-Member Exchange Scale (LMX-MDM; 28) translated by Wang et al. (18), and the Chinese version of Ethical Leadership Scale (29) translated by Walumbwa et al. (30).

The application of Western assessment tools has made an important contribution to leadership knowledge development. Theoretically, it helps to advance the scientific understanding of general leadership process. The use of same assessment tool makes it possible to compare the findings derived from different cultures so as to identify cultural similarities and differences in the leadership process. Practically, it enables Chinese scholars to quickly catch up with the current trend of leadership research. It also facilitates the communication between Chinese scholars and Western scholars as they would have shared language. However, there are some intrinsic limitations of the etic approach (14), which constrain the development of leadership research in Chinese contexts. Primarily, these scales overlook the cultural component in leadership process (i.e., substantive limitation). For example, some cultural practices of leadership relevant to the Chinese context are not present in Western experience, and thus would not be included in the Western assessment tools. For example, the Leader-Member exchange (LMX) theory that focuses on the exchange within work domain was developed in the Western context. However, Chinese type of leader-member interaction goes beyond work issues and permeates into personal domains (31). Hence, simple reliance on Western assessment tools leaves a large gap in understanding Chinese leadership and hinders researchers from a deep inquiry into the cultural variation in the field of leadership. It also constrains the initiative of Chinese scholars to construct leadership theories and models.

ASSESSMENT TOOLS BASED ON THE EMIC APPROACH

In response to the limitations of the etic approach that transplants Western leadership measures, some Chinese scholars proposed to focus on indigenous Chinese leadership (32, 33). In contrast with the top-down orientation adopted in the etic approach, the emic approach tends to be bottom-up and to study leadership process from laypersons' perspectives. They usually construct leadership theories and leadership assessment tools according to local phenomena and experiences, and interpret the data using Chinese concepts, such as Confucian ideas.

Paternalistic leadership is an indigenous leadership style that has been well-studied in Chinese culture, which was proposed by Farh and Cheng (32) based on the Chinese history and the traditional ideologies (i.e., Confucianism and legalism). It refers to a leadership style with strong discipline and authority accompanied with fatherly benevolence and moral integrity (32). Accordingly, Cheng, Chou and Farh (11) developed the 42-item Paternalistic Leadership Scale (PLS), which includes three unique components of Chinese leadership style – authoritarianism (i.e., "very strict with his/her subordinates"), benevolence (e.g., "encourages me when I encounter difficulties in work"), and morality (e.g., "sets an example for me"). The PLS demonstrated satisfactory reliability and consistently showed a three-factor structure across Chinese societies, including Taiwan (34), mainland China (35), and Hong Kong (36). It has become the most widely used scale that measures indigenous leadership style and demonstrated validity in predicting a wide range of leadership effectiveness indicators, such as employee's trust in and satisfaction toward leaders (11), employees' performance (34), and employees' voice behaviors (37). In particular, Cheng, Chou, Wu, Huang, and Farh (38) found that paternalistic leadership demonstrated a unique effect on employees' responses above and beyond the effect of transformational leadership, which confirmed its cultural uniqueness in influencing leadership effectiveness. Furthermore, with revision on the items of morality, Cheng et al. (39) developed the Global Paternalistic Leadership Scale (GPLS), and successfully validated it across four Asian societies, including Taiwan, mainland China, Japan and South Korea.

In addition, several other scholars also attempted to construct a cultural-specific leadership style that can well describe the leadership features and predict leadership effectiveness in Chinese culture (40). For example, Wang, Xin, and Xu (41) asked the participants of senior managers to articulate the leadership behavior of their CEO, upon which they developed a CEO leadership scale to understand the CEO leadership behavior during the economic transformation of China. This scale includes six dimensions of leadership behavior, including making innovation, coordination and communication, caring about subordinates, identifying visions, demonstrating authority, and monitoring operations. These dimensions were positively related to enterprise profit and employees' attitudes (41).

The use of indigenous leadership assessment tools helps to explore and understand some culturally specific experiences in the leadership process. Indigenous leadership research makes a significant contribution to a growing body of literature documenting human behavior from a local perspective. Although many researchers are interested in developing a scale to capture Chinese specific leadership, not all of them provided adequate validation evidence. A rigorous emic approach requires evidence for the incremental validity of the indigenous scale. In other words, the indigenous construct should explain more of the leadership effectiveness than other existing scales, but this is often missing in the scale development. Furthermore, the indigenous leadership construct may not be totally specific to a certain culture. Instead, it may be a culturally specific manifestation of a general leadership concept. For example, paternalistic leadership does not only exist in Chinese culture. Indeed, it reflects a hierarchical leader-follower relationship, in which leaders are obliged to create a family-like environment and provide protection and guidance to their followers in both the work and non-work domain, and the followers are expected to show obedience and loyalty toward the leaders, which can be observed in multiple cultures (42). However, people's prototypical understanding of paternalistic leadership varies across culture. For example, Chinese people perceived typical paternalistic leadership incorporating more authoritarianism than Western people (43). Therefore, simple reliance on indigenous leadership assessment tools may fail to capture the common component in leadership shared by different cultures. It also hinders the communication between Chinese researchers and Western researchers due to a lack of shared framework. In order to advance the field of leadership, we need to address both culturally universal and specific aspects of the leadership process.

ASSESSMENT TOOLS BASED ON THE ETIC-EMIC APPROACH

In different Chinese societies, an emerging effort has been made to study leadership by using a combined etic-emic approach. Researchers usually develop a leadership assessment tool based on Western literature theories, cultural theories, indigenous concepts and local leadership experiences (44). This approach is able to link the indigenous leadership understanding with the so-called mainstream leadership understanding derived from

Western research, and provide a more comprehensive framework to understand both the culturally universal and specific components in the leadership process.

The operationalization of transformational leadership in Chinese context can exemplify this approach. Transformational leadership refers to a leadership style, in which leaders strive to inspire followers to work toward common goals through setting up a role model for followers, showing individualized consideration toward followers, stimulating cognitive transformation of the followers, and inspiring their motivation to achieve higher (45). However, Chinese researchers (44) argued that Chinese leaders may demonstrate different practices in order to reach the transformational goal due to the larger power distance between leaders and followers and stronger concern for interpersonal relationship. Thus, they asked Chinese managers to provide leadership behavior examples, upon which they worked out a new scale to measure Chinese transformational leadership. This scale contains four dimensions – moral modeling, charisma, visionary, and individualized consideration. The inclusion of moral modeling, which is missing in Bass's MLQ, shows the importance of moral modeling in Chinese people's understanding of good leadership. Additionally, in the dimension of individualized consideration, behavior of caring about the family and personal lives are included, which suggests the range of leader-follower interaction is expected to be broader than that in Western contexts.

A similar case was found in the construct of authentic leadership. There are at least two scales developed in the Chinese contexts to measure this leadership style (46, 47). Taking Wang and Chen's (46) scale as an example, they developed this scale based on the previous scales developed in the Western contexts (e.g., 48) and their qualitative studies in Chinese organizations which examined employees and leaders' views toward authentic leadership. With this scale, they found the common components of authentic leadership shared by Chinese and Western cultures, including self-consciousness and internalized moral values, and an additional Chinese component of value-behavior congruency.

The use of combined etic-emic approach to developing leadership assessment tool has several merits. First, it is grounded in a larger body of literature and more integrated view about leadership, which likely provides a more comprehensive understanding on a certain leadership construct. Second, it helps to explicate both universal and cultural aspects of leadership process. It may provide generalizability evidence for a certain leadership theory and culturally unique findings that complement the theory. Finally, with a common conceptual framework, Western and Chinese researchers can better communicate their research findings and jointly endeavor to advance the field. However, the development of this combined approach in the leadership research in Chinese contexts is still in its infancy. Much more studies are needed to show the validation evidence, especially incremental validity of these scales.

UNSOLVED QUESTIONS AND FUTURE DIRECTIONS

The history of leadership assessment tools in Chinese contexts resembles that of many psychological assessment tools such as personality assessment (14). It starts with an etic approach, an emic approach, and then a combined etic-emic approach. However, the etic approach still dominated the field of leadership, probably because of its ease of implementation. Obviously, this would hinder the contribution of Chinese experience to the leadership research and the initiative of Chinese scholars in the leadership theory construction. Emerging research has informed us that leadership is an integration of universal human nature and cultural influence (5). For example, based on a study of 62 countries and areas, the Global Leadership and Organizational Behavior Effectiveness (GLOBE) Project found that some leadership qualities are universally desirable (e.g., charismatic and value-based leadership), while others are more culturally sensitive (e.g., participative leadership; 49). Hence, to cover both universal and cultural elements of leadership, using a combined etic-emic approach to develop leadership assessment tools is an ideal direction. By doing this, researchers need to incorporate cultural variations by using samples from multiple cultural origins when developing and validating a scale (6). The current validation of Chinese original leadership scales is often limited in one single culture, and thus requires more replications.

Additionally, there is an obvious lack of leadership assessment tools for ordinary people in Chinese contexts. The majority of the leadership scales were developed in an organizational context to assess leadership qualities or practices of formal leaders or positional authorities. However, in the field of leadership development and education, more and more researchers and educators believe that everyone has the potentials and capacities that enable him/her to carry out effective leadership no matter whether he/she takes up a leadership position (12, 50). Increasing research has been conducted to understand how ordinary people develop their leadership capacities and how leadership program helps to enhance their leadership capacities (12, 51). The dearth of leadership assessment tools for ordinary people in Chinese contexts hinders the advance of research on leadership development and education as well as the improvement of leadership programs. Moreover, leadership development and education would benefit if a norm of leadership capacities can be built, so that people can know how well their leadership capacities are by referring to the norm. It is thus necessary to develop a scale that measures leadership capacities for a wide range of population in Chinese contexts.

Indeed, a leadership scale is an instrument to operationalize a leadership concept, and thus whether the initial conceptualization is clear matters. Nowadays, there are plentiful leadership theories that try to capture an effective leadership style in contemporary organizational or social settings, including, but not limited to, transformational leadership (52), authentic leadership (53), servant leadership (22), and service leadership (50). For the leadership development, theories and models are also growing, including relational leadership model (54), social change model (12), and leadership identity development model (55). It remains a big challenge for Chinese researchers to synergize different perspectives and generate a suitable theoretical model of leadership that can well explain leadership experience in Chinese contexts but also contribute to the understanding of basic leadership process. Before developing a new assessment, Chinese researchers may need to adopt an integrated or cross-cultural view to conceptualize leadership. As suggested by Komives and Dugan (1), contemporary leadership theories share three essential themes, including importance of leaders' self-awareness, morality and social responsibility in leadership, and shared leadership. Chinese leadership theory may need to integrate these three themes in the conceptualization of leadership, and develop the scales accordingly. In brief, we encourage future research to adopt an etic-emic approach in studying leadership and measuring leadership in Chinese contexts. We also call for developing reliable and valid assessment tools to measure leadership capacities of ordinary people. Addressing these unsolved questions requires a joint effort of Chinese scholars and collaboration of Western and Chinese scholars.

There are several recommendations regarding development of leadership scales in the Chinese contexts in future. First, a well-articulated conceptual model of leadership should be used. It could be a Western theory with or without adaptation, an indigenous theory derived from Chinese experience and/or theory, and integrated leadership model integrating Chinese and Western models of leadership. Second, validation is another task to be taken which includes several steps: a) development of an item pool; b) refinement of the pool by experts; c) empirical validation to ascertain the reliability and validity of the developed measures. For reliability, besides internal consistency (i.e., homogeneity of the items), there is a need to look at whether the scale is stable across time. For validity, besides examining content validity and criterion-related validities (such as concurrent validity and predictive validity), dimensionality of the measures based on the guiding conceptual model should also be tested to give support for the theory behind the measures.

ACKNOWLEDGMENTS

The validation project is financially supported by the Victor and William Fung Foundation. The preparation for this paper is supported by the Foundation and the Endowed Professorship in Service Leadership Education at The Hong Kong Polytechnic University. This chapter is an updated version of a publication in the special issue "Development and validation of assessment tools on service leadership knowledge, attitude and behavior" edited by Daniel TL Shek, Xiaoqin Zhu and Joav Merrick published in the International Journal of Child and Adolescent Health, 2018;11(4).

REFERENCES

[1] Komives SR, Dugan JP. Contemporary leadership theories. In: Couto RA, ed. Political and civic leadership: A reference handbook. Thousand Oaks, CA: Sage, 2010;1:111-20.

[2] Yukl GA. Leadership in organizations. Englewood Cliffs, NJ: Prentice Hall, 1981.

[3] Bass BM. Bass and Stogdill's handbook of leadership: Theory, research, and managerial applications. 3rd ed. New York: Free Press, 1990.

[4] Van Vugt M. Evolutionary origins of leadership and followership. Pers Soc Psychol Rev 2006;10(4):354-71.

[5] House R, Javidan M, Hanges P, Dorfman P. Understanding cultures and implicit leadership theories across the globe: An introduction to project GLOBE. J World Bus 2002;37(1):3-10.

[6] Liden RC. Leadership research in Asia: A brief assessment and suggestions for the future. Asia Pac J Manage 2012;29(2):205-12.

[7] Cao YF, Li PP. Indigenous research on Chinese leadership: Problems and suggestions. Chin J Manage 2010;7(11):1704-9. [Chinese].

[8] Fu PP, Yukl G. Perceived effectiveness of influence tactics in the United States and China. Leadersh Q 2000;11(2):251-66.

[9] Bass BM, Avolio BJ. MLQ, Multifactor Leadership Questionnaire Sampler Set: Technical report, leader form, rater form, and scoring key for MLQ Form 5x-short. Redwood City, CA: Mind Garden, 2000.

[10] Neider LL, Schriesheim CA. The authentic leadership inventory (ALI): Development and empirical tests. Leadersh Q 2011;22(6):1146-64.

[11] Farh JL, Cheng BS, Chou LF. A triad model of paternalistic leadership: Constructs and measurement. Indigenous Psychol Res Chin Soc 2000;14:3-64. [Chinese].

[12] Dugan JP, Komives SR. Influences on college students' capacities for socially responsible leadership. J Coll Stud Dev 2010;51(5):525-49.

[13] Kouzes JM, Posner BZ. Student leadership practices inventory. San Francisco, CA: Jossey-Bass, 1998.

[14] Cheung FM, van de Vijver FJ, Leong FT. Toward a new approach to the study of personality in culture. Am Psychol 2011;66(7):593-603.

[15] Brislin RW, ed. Applied cross-cultural psychology. Newbury Park, CA: Sage, 1990.

[16] Chen XP, Farh JL. The effectiveness of transactional and transformational leader behaviors in Chinese organizations: Evidence from Taiwan. Chicago, IL: 59th Annual meeting of the Academy of Management, 1999.

[17] Podsakoff PM, MacKenzie SB, Moorman RH, Fetter R. Transformational leader behaviors and their effects on followers' trust in leader, satisfaction, and organizational citizenship behaviors. Leadersh Q 1990;1(2):107-42.

[18] Wang H, Law KS, Hackett RD, Wang D, Chen ZX. Leader-member exchange as a mediator of the relationship between transformational leadership and followers' performance and organizational citizenship behavior. Acad Manage J 2005;48(3):420-32.

[19] Chan CHS, Mak WM. The impact of servant leadership and subordinates' organizational tenure on trust in leader and attitudes. Pers Rev 2014;43(2):272-87.

[20] Liden RC, Wayne SJ, Zhao H, Henderson D. Servant leadership: Development of a multidimensional measure and multi-level assessment. Leadersh Q 2008;19(2):161-77.

[21] Sun JM, Wang B. Servant leadership in China: Conceptualization and measurement. In: Mobley WH, Wang Y, Li M, eds. Advances in global leadership. Bingley, UK: Emerald Group, 2009;5:321-44.

[22] Barbuto JEJr, Wheeler DW. Scale development and construct clarification of servant leadership. Group Organ Manage 2006;31(3):300-26.

[23] Leung DYP, Ha T, Yeung L. Factor structure and reliability of the socially responsible leadership scale in a sample of Hong Kong first year undergraduate students. Hong Kong: the 5th International Technology, Education and Development Conference (INTED), 2011:202-9.

[24] Chan DW. Assessment of leadership characteristics among Chinese secondary students in Hong Kong: The development of the scaled version of the Roets Rating Scale for Leadership. In: Nata R, ed. Progress in education. New York: Nova Science, 2001;3:299-312.

[25] Roets L. Roets rating scale for leadership. Des Moines, IA: Leadership Publishers, 1986.

[26] Avolio BJ, Gardner WL, Walumbwa FO. Authentic Leadership Questionnaire. Singapore: Gallup Leadership Institute 2009.

[27] Qian J, Lin X, Chen GZX. Authentic leadership and feedback-seeking behaviour: An examination of the cultural context of mediating processes in China. J Manage Organ 2012;18(3):286-99.

[28] Liden RC, Maslyn JM. Multidimensionality of leader-member exchange: An empirical assessment through scale development. J Manage 1998;24(1):43-72.

[29] Brown ME, Trevino LK, Harrison DA. Ethical leadership: A social learning perspective for construct development and testing. Organ Behav Hum Decis Process 2005;97(2):117-34.

[30] Walumbwa FO, Mayer DM, Wang P, Wang H, Workman K, Christensen AL. Linking ethical leadership to employee performance: The roles of leader–member exchange, self-efficacy, and organizational identification. Organ Behav Hum Decis Process 2011;115(2):204-13.

[31] Law KS, Wong CS, Wang D, Wang L. Effect of supervisor–subordinate guanxi on supervisory decisions in China: An empirical investigation. Int J Hum Resour Manage 2000;11(4):751-65.

[32] Farh JL, Cheng BS. A cultural analysis of paternalistic leadership in Chinese organizations. In: Li JT, Tsui AS, Weldon E, eds. Management and organizations in the Chinese context. London: Palgrave Macmillan, 2000:84-127.

[33] Zhang X, Fu P, Xi Y, Li L, Xu L, Cao C, et al. Understanding indigenous leadership research: Explication and Chinese examples. Leadersh Q 2012;23(6):1063-79.

[34] Chen XP, Eberly MB, Chiang TJ, Farh JL, Cheng BS. Affective trust in Chinese leaders: Linking paternalistic leadership to employee performance. J Manage 2014;40(3):796-819.

[35] Wu M, Huang X, Chan SC. The influencing mechanisms of paternalistic leadership in Mainland China. Asia Pac Bus Rev 2012;18(4):631-48.

[36] Sheer VC. In search of Chinese paternalistic leadership: Conflicting evidence from samples of mainland China and Hong Kong's small family businesses. Manage Commun Q 2013;27(1):34-60.

[37] Lin CP, Lin MZ, Li YB. An empirical study on the effect of paternalistic leadership on employees' voice behaviors–the intermediary role of psychological empowerment. J Interdiscipl Math 2015;18(6):789-810.

[38] Cheng BS, Chou LF, Wu TY, Huang MP, Farh JL. Paternalistic leadership and subordinate responses: Establishing a leadership model in Chinese organizations. Asian J Soc Psychol 2004;7(1):89-117.

[39] Cheng BS, Boer D, Chou LF, Huang MP, Yoneyama S, Shim D, et al. Paternalistic leadership in four East Asian societies: Generalizability and cultural differences of the triad model. J Cross Cult Psychol 2014;45(1):82-90.

[40] Zhang ZX, Chen ZX, Ang S. Business leadership in the Chinese context: Trends, findings, and implications. Manage Organ Rev 2014;10(2):199-221.

[41] Wang H, Xin R, Xu, SY. The leadership behavior of CEO in Chinese enterprises and its influence on enterprise profit. Manage World 2006;4:87-97. [Chinese].

[42] Aycan Z. Paternalism: Towards conceptual refinement and operationalization. In: Yang KS, Hwang KK, Kim U, eds. Scientific advances an indigenous psychologies: Empirical, philosophical, and cultural contributions. London: Cambridge University Press, 2006:445-66.

[43] Aycan Z, Schyns B, Sun JM, Felfe J, Saher N. Convergence and divergence of paternalistic leadership: A cross-cultural investigation of prototypes. J Int Bus Stud 2013;44(9):962-9.

[44] Li C, Shi K. The structure and measurement of transformational leadership in China. Front Busi Res Chi 2008;2(4):571-90. [Chinese].

[45] Avolio BJ, Waldman DA, Yammarino FJ. Leading in the 1990s: The four I′ s of transformational leadership. J Eur Ind Train 1991;15(4):9-20.

[46] Wang Y, Chen WM. Study on the structural dimensions of the authentic leadership in enterprises. East Chi Econom Manage 2012;7:98-101. [Chinese].

[47] Xie, HX. The study of content and structure of authentic leadership and its relationships with other related variables. Dissertation. Guangzhou: Jinan University, 2007. [Chinese].

[48] Walumbwa FO, Avolio BJ, Gardner WL, Wernsing TS, Peterson SJ. Authentic leadership: Development and validation of a theory-based measure. J Manage 2008;34(1):89-126.

[49] Dorfman P, Javidan M, Hanges P, Dastmalchian A, House R. GLOBE: A twenty year journey into the intriguing world of culture and leadership. J World Bus 2012;47(4):504-18.

[50] Shek DTL, Chung PPY, Lin L, Leung H, Ng E. Service leadership under the service economy. In: Chin JL, Trimble JE, Garcia JE, eds. Global and culturally diverse leaders and leadership: New dimensions and challenges for business, education and society. Bingley, UK: Emerald, 2018:143-61.

[51] Shek DTL, Lin L. Changes in university students after joining a service leadership program in China. J Leadersh Educ 2016;15(1):96-109.

[52] Bass BM. Transformational leadership: Industrial, military and educational impact. Mahwah, NJ: Lawrence Erlbaum, 1998.

[53] Avolio BJ, Gardner WL. Authentic leadership development: Getting to the root of positive forms of leadership. Leadersh Q 2005;16(3):315-38.

[54] Komives SR, Lucas N, McMahon TR. Exploring leadership: For college students who want to make a difference, 2nd ed. San Francisco, CA: John Wiley, 2007.

[55] Komives SR, Longerbeam SD, Mainella F, Osteen L, Owen JE, Wagner W. Leadership identity development: Challenges in applying a developmental model. J Leadersh Educ 2009;8(1):11-47.

In: Service Leadership
Editors: Daniel TL Shek, Xiaoqin Zhu, Li Lin et al.
ISBN: 978-1-53614-852-7

Chapter 3

CONCEPTUAL BACKGROUND AND THE DEVELOPMENT OF SERVICE LEADERSHIP KNOWLEDGE SCALE

Daniel TL Shek[1-6,*], PhD, FHKPS, BBS, SBS, JP, Xiaoqin Zhu[1], PhD and Alex YF Zhu[1], PhD

[1]Department of Applied Social Sciences, The Hong Kong Polytechnic University, Hong Kong, PR China
[2]Centre for Innovative Programmes for Adolescents and Families, The Hong Kong Polytechnic University, Hong Kong, PR China
[3]Department of Social Work, East China Normal University, Shanghai, PR China,
[4]Kiang Wu Nursing College of Macau, Macau, PR China
[5]Hong Kong Institute of Service Leadership and Management Limited, Hong Kong, PR China
[6]Division of Adolescent Medicine, Department of Pediatrics, Kentucky Children's Hospital, University of Kentucky College of Medicine, Lexington, Kentucky, US

ABSTRACT

Knowledge plays a key role in shaping behavior in human beings. Leadership knowledge has been extensively studied for its contribution to productivity at both individual and organizational levels. With the service industries rooted as the key to the success of Hong

* Correspondence: Daniel TL Shek, PhD, FHKPS, BBS, SBS, JP, Associate Vice President (Undergraduate Programme), Chair Professor of Applied Social Sciences and Li and Fung Professor in Service Leadership Education, Department of Applied Social Sciences, The Hong Kong Polytechnic University, Hung Hom, Hong Kong, PR China. Email: daniel.shek@polyu.edu.hk.

Kong's economy, an appropriate service leadership knowledge framework should be developed based on the demand for leaders in the modern service economies. This chapter introduces the conceptual background of the Service Leadership Theory, and how Service Leadership Knowledge Scale was developed and validated based on the basic knowledge points under the Service Leadership Theory.

INTRODUCTION

Knowledge refers to one's awareness of an objective, related processes, and how to do something (1). It is widely believed that people's previous experience and knowledge shape not only people's judgement and attitudes but also the actual behaviors (2). For example, people's level of environmental knowledge including environmental responsibility (3) and ecological awareness (4) was found to be associated with their ecological consumer behaviors, such as consumption, reuse and willingness to pay more for ecological products. In a systematic review (5), the importance of cardiac patients' knowledge was highlighted where patients' level of knowledge about cardiac care facilitates the health behavior change such as participating in physical activities, healthier dietary habits and smoking cessation. Moreover, increasing financial knowledge was a means of increasing people's responsible credit card use behavior (6).

Given the influence of knowledge on human behaviors in many fields, numerous theorists have explored the way in which knowledge influences behavior. For example, the mediated role of attitude has been emphasized. The Knowledge-Attitude-Behavior model proposes that accumulation of knowledge can motivate changes in attitude, thus further lead to behavioral changes (7). The theory of planned behavior suggests that subjectively held information determines certain behavior (8). Besides, the process of putting knowledge into action is considered worthy of attention. In the information-motivation-behavioral skills model, knowledge and motivation jointly influence behavior to the equivalen extent throught the mediation of developing behavioral skills (9). Knowledge-to-action cycle suggests knowledge phase can influence action phase at any point, and the process of translating knowledge to behavior is an iterative cycle in which knowledge and behavior update themselves anytime through dynamic interactions (10).

INFLUENCE OF LEADERSHIP KNOWLEDGE ON LEADERSHIP BEHAVIOR

As an important form of human behavior, leadership behavior is affected by leadership knowledge as well. Leadership knowledge includes three dimensions. First, leaders have to be equipped with hard leadership knowledge, which can be defined as a series of basic knowledge concerning managing different kinds of resources in organizations, including human resources (11), information resources (12), and financial resources (13). Second, leaders are expected to have soft leadership knowledge, which can be defined as the knowledge used to establish emotional connections in a team. This form of knowledge includes how to build relationships with others, how to construct effective collaboration and how to improve management environment (14). Third, an excellent leader needs to accumulate adequate or a very high level of leadership content knowledge, which was purposed and conceptualized by Stein and Nelson (15) as the technical or academic related knowledge in the industrial field. In other words, leaders are expected to be equipped with knowledge and technical skills closely related with industries before constructing and strengthening leadership among subordinates.

Leadership knowledge serves as a unique window to look inside the science of organizational behavior and has been found to exert influence on leadership behavior at the individual and organizational levels. At the individual level, Weitz and colleagues (16) emphasized the role of leadership content knowledge and suggested that content knowledge of service providers in understanding their customers may change the directions of their behavior towards a more effective way. Similarly, Yammarino and colleagues (17) demonstrated that basic management knowledge, soft leadership knowledge like perspective-taking, creative problem solving, and social judgment skills and leadership content knowledge related with industries all positively directed management behaviors, including assessing a solution, identifying limitations, making action plans, and organizing supporting resources as input to management activities. At the behavioral outcome level, by surveying 102 teams in hotel properties in the United States, Srivastava and colleagues (18) showed that leadership content knowledge and self-efficacy positively predicted service performance.

Several theoretical proposals can be utilized to explain how leadership knowledge as a complex management input can be connected to positive management behavior and outputs at the individual level. For instance, leadership knowledge as a general cognitive capability may have positive effect on leadership behavior through the mediation of improving positive management attitude, increasing self-efficacy and strengthening administrative behavioral control, the theoretical foundation of which is supported by the model of planned behavior (19). The extended model of the planned behavior adds another two likely pathways connecting leadership knowledge to leadership behavior through self-identity and affective self-beliefs (20). Similarly, based on the theory of reasoned action, leadership knowledge can impact on leadership behavior through shaping the positive attitude and positive subjective norms (21). The similar technology model also supports the role of leadership knowledge in directing positive management behaviors (22). In this model, leadership content knowledge as an external force motivates leaders to evaluate the usefulness and feasibility of purposed management plans, which further promotes positive leadership behavior through the effect on positive behavioral intentions (22).

At the organizational level, hard leadership knowledge improves the capacity of transforming resource into productivity; soft leadership knowledge spurs the potential of team and increases the motivation of its members, while leadership content knowledge helps leaders to expose organizations to external opportunities for development (23). These mechanisms suggest a positive association between leadership knowledge and favorable organizational behavior and outcome. In line with this notion, soft leadership knowledge was proven critical to the success of organizations in terms of the performance of workers based on qualitative analysis in the study of Pearce and Manz (24). In addition, with a sample of 144 U.S. employees in a network of university libraries, it was found that leadership content knowledge positively predicted organizational citizenship behaviors (25). With a sample of 710 nurses in the South Korea, Lin and Hsiao (26) found leadership content knowledge and trust to subordinates were positively related to the organizational citizenship behaviors. Similarly, with a sample of industrial companies from four innovative industries in Spain, hard leadership knowledge and leadership content knowledge were found to promote organizational behavior and innovation through the effect of positive management practice (27).

As shown, a majority of pervious empirical studies connecting different types of leadership knowledge and leadership behavior (and behavioral outcomes) actively examined the role of leadership content knowledge, and only a very small part of them aimed to investigate the importance of soft leadership knowledge. With the global transformation in economic structure from the manufacture economy to the service economy, the framework of leadership knowledge needs to be redefined. It needs to be transformed from a framework focusing on hard leadership knowledge and leadership content knowledge, which best responded to the production and cooperative mode in the manufacture economy, to the one emphasizing on soft leadership knowledge, which can maximize the effectiveness and quality of service in the service economy. When specifying the leadership in modern service economy, Chung and Elfassy (28) proposed the Service Leadership Theory, which displays 12 dimensions of positive attributes an effective service leader should be equipped with. Under the framework of the Service Leadership Theory, the basic knowledge points are summarized and presented in section below.

SERVICE LEADERSHIP KNOWLEDGE

Based on Service Leadership Theory, service leadership knowledge can be summarized in six domains. These domains are "general description of Service Leadership Theory," "three realms of service leadership," "everyone can be a leader," "Principle $E = MC^2$," "manufacturing versus service economies in contemporary world," and "distinction of Service Leadership Theory and other leadership theories." Knowledge points in these six domains are briefly outlined below.

General description of service leadership theory

Unlike the old paradigm of leadership where the relationship is hierarchical and the leader only places orders to those who are in lower positions for self-serving purpose, Service Leadership Theory emphasizes the importance of satisfying not only the needs of oneself but also others and the systems such as community, society, and environments (29). The traditional concept of "leader" is signified with power and pride, and the leader is likely to be served by others instead of the opposite. To an extreme extent, the leaders might use their power to scarify others' needs and benefits to fulfill their own needs. Such action is considered as unethical. In order to be an ethical service leader, one should work with others with care, value their wellness and benefits as much as oneself, and encourage to transcend self-interest to serve others and the system. According to Shek and colleagues (30), good service leaders are those who influence their subordinates with good personal qualities such as being caring and genuine, rather than manipulating others.

Three realms of service leadership

Noteworthy, service leadership emphasizes not only personal interest and achievement, but also the intention to fulfill the needs of others and the systems. The three realms including self, other, and the system of service leadership indicate the importance for a person to manage himself or herself before leading others. Chung (31) suggested that before a person becoming a competent service leader, one should focus on improving his or her intrapersonal competence. It is believed that "a leader is unable to optimize his or her ability to lead others well unless he or she is healthy in mind, body, and spirit." In other words, one's ability to lead oneself is one of the best indicators of his or her capacity to lead others (32). Such concept shares similar value to a Confucianism thought in Daxue, which points out that if people are able to regulate the standpoint of showing love for others, interpersonal harmony and social stability will follow (33).

Everyone can be a leader

In traditional beliefs, a leader normally carries a superior, talented, and competent image. Only these leaders in high positions need to be equipped with leadership capability (34). Conversely, Service Leadership Theory believes that everyone has his or her strengths; hence, has the potential to lead. There are a wide variety of service transaction, ranging from self-serving personal achievement at work to complex service such as managing a team. Everyone has the potential to utilize his or her skills and strengths and become a leader in the collaborative process. It is important to be open-minded to see every person's potential. With such beliefs, service leaders will serve and lead in a humble and respectful manner, which can help them fully utilize their followers' skills, enhance their performance, and nurture the followers to become service leaders as well.

Principle $E = MC^2$

According to Chung and Elfassy (28), effective service leadership (E) is a function of one's moral character (M), competencies (C), and caring disposition (C) (i.e., $E = MC^2$). It is believed that effective service leaders should demonstrate good leadership competence, interpersonal competence, intrapersonal competence, as well as domain-specific knowledge in order to guide their leadership practice (30). Moral character emphasizes the importance to serve others with integrity and moral values while taking the lead. Caring disposition emphasizes one's sincerity to learn and to meet the needs of others. It is believed that a caring leader will not sacrifice the needs and benefits of others to fulfill one's own.

Although it is emphasized that the three determinants are equally important, morality and integrity appear to be essential features of effective leaders in the service industry. It is believed that the subordinates as well as service-receivers have difficulties trusting a person who lies, breaks promise, and neglects the feelings and needs of others, regardless of his or her actual work performance. These qualities are particularly important in certain industries such as counseling and nursing, where the nature of the service relies heavily on the interpersonal relationship. In addition, effective leaders serve not only clients but everyone in life, including one's self, peers, subordinates, followers, and surroundings. Good leaders should always be "ready," "willing," and "able" to serve. They are continuously being evaluated by superiors, peers, subordinates, and all other service-receivers. Hence, instead of merely being skillful and knowledgeable, service leaders should demonstrate character strengths, moral character, leadership competency, and caring social disposition in order to perform effectively.

Manufacturing versus service economies in contemporary world

Traditional leadership education emphasizes the importance of knowledge and skills in the field. Such concept applies very well in industrialized societies, when the operation system required hands-on skills. However, in recent decades, the manufacturing industry is gradually replaced by the rapidly growing service industry, especially in Hong Kong. As a result, skills are no longer the only quality that makes one a competent leader. It is suggested that the new concept of effective leadership focuses on whether one is moral and caring to followers and service recipients, as the basic concept is that the person himself/herself is considered as the "service" (34).

Distinction of service leadership theory and other leadership theories

Different from other leadership theories, Service Leadership Theory puts great emphasis on the "collaborative service-focused" attitude and behavior. In addition, Service Leadership Theory purposes seven core beliefs, including 1) service means serving "oneself, others, and systems"; 2) "everyone can be a leader"; 3) "leadership effectiveness is dependent on possessing relevant situational task competences plus being judged by superiors, peers, and subordinates as possessing character and exhibiting care"; 4) "leaders should ethically improving one's competences, abilities, and willingness to help satisfy the needs of others"; 5) "high quality personal service should be consistently provided to everyone that one comes into contact with, including oneself"; 6) "service leadership is the world's oldest, most competitive, and longest surviving business model"; and 7) "high-paying, high status positions and management promotions will go to people who have domain specific knowledge and skills plus service leadership competences, character, and care" (30, 31).

Development of the Service Leadership Knowledge Scale

A validated service leadership knowledge assessment tool is indispensable to measure and investigate the influence of service leadership knowledge. Moreover, it is also a key to evaluate participants' knowledge gain through service leadership education. In view of the lack of such validated scales, the research team at The Hong Kong Polytechnic University (PolyU) conducted a project entitled "Development and validation of measures based on the service leadership model," which entailed the construction and validation of a knowledge scale aimed at "capturing the essential knowledge points of service leadership in a format of multiple-choice questions" (30, p. 164). Accordingly, the Long-Form Service Leadership Knowledge Scale (i.e., SLK-LF-200), which comprises 200 multiple-choice items covering fundamental service leadership knowledge points as outlined above (also see Table 2 for the domains and several sample items). Each item has a "correct" answer with one point whereas participants get zero point if they answer incorrectly. By adopting an objective method, the Service Leadership Knowledge Scale could reliably and validly show one's knowledge level (35). Through several validation studies as outlined below, the trimmed versions of the knowledge scale were also created which were shown to be valid and reliable.

Table 1. Literature review on measures of leadership and service leadership

Steps	Details
Step 1: Literature Review on leadership knowledge measures, particularly in different Chinese contexts	Examples of references: – Chan, D. W. (2007). Leadership competencies among Chinese gifted students in Hong Kong: The connection with emotional intelligence and successful intelligence. *Roeper Review, 29*(3), 183-189. – Chiaburu, D. S., Huang, J. L., Hutchins, H. M., & Gardner, R. G. (2014). Trainees' perceived knowledge gain unrelated to the training domain: the joint action of impression management and motives. *International Journal of Training and Development, 18*, 37–52. – Farh, J.-L., & Cheng, B.-S. (2000). A cultural analysis of Paternalistic Leadership in Chinese organizations. In J. T. Li, A. S. Tsui, & E. Weldon, (Eds.), *Management and organizations in the Chinese Context* (pp. 84-127). London: Palgrave. – Peng, J., Liu, Y., Lu, H., Liu, Y., & Wu, W. (2014). Emotional leadership: Conceptualization, measurement, development and model construction. *Advances in Psychological Science, 22*(11), 1757-1769. – Sitzmann, T., Ely, K., Brown, K. G., & Bauer, K. N. (2010). Self-assessment of knowledge: A cognitive learning or affective measure? *Academy of Management Learning & Education, 9*, 169–191. – Stedman, N. L., Rutherford, T. A., Rosser, M. H., & Elbert, C. (2009). When leadership counts: Engaging youth through the Washington Leadership Conference. *Journal of Agricultural Education, 50*, 92–104.
Step 2: Literature Review on Service Leadership	Examples of references: – Chung, P. P. Y., & Elfassy, R. (2016). *The 12 dimensions of a Service Leader* (1st ed.). New York, NY: Lexingford Publishing. – Shek, D. T. L., Chung, P. P. Y., Lin, L., Leung, H., & Ng, E. C. W. (2018). Service Leadership under the Service Economy. In J. L. Chin, J. E. Trimble & J. E. Garcia (Eds.), *Global and culturally diverse leaders and leadership: New dimensions and challenges for business, education and society* (pp. 143–161). Bingley: Emerald Publishing. – Shek, D. T. L., & Leung, H. (2015). Service Leadership qualities in university students through the lens of student well-being. In D. T. L. Shek & P. P. Y. Chung (Eds.), *Promoting Service Leadership qualities in university students* (pp. 1-16). Singapore: Springer. – Shek, D. T. L., & Lin, L. (2017). Validation of the Service Leadership knowledge scale: Criterion-related validity. In D. T. L. Shek, P. P. Y. Chung, L. Lin & J. Merrick (Eds.), *Service Leadership education for university students* (pp. 189–204). New York, NY: Nova Sciences. – Shek, D. T. L., Lin, L., Leung, H., Yu, L., Ma, C. M. S., & Li, X. (2017). Development and validation of the Service Leadership knowledge scale in a Chinese context. In D. T. L. Shek, P. P. Y. Chung, L. Lin & J. Merrick (Eds.), *Service Leadership Education for University Students* (pp. 163–188). New York, NY: Nova Sciences. – Shek, D. T. L., Sun, R. C. F., & Liu, T. T. (2015). Evolution and realms of Service Leadership and leadership models. *International Journal on Disability and Human Development, 14*(3), 243-254.

Content validation

The SLK-LF-200 was subjected to a content validation study administered by the research team at PolyU (30). Four experts who were highly familiar with and involved in the development of the service leadership curriculum framework rated the 200 items based on three criteria, namely, i) relevance, ii) clarity, and iii) representativeness. The individual (I-CVI) and average scale content validation index (S-CVI/ave) based on experts' ratings on the three abovementioned criteria were employed to reflect the content validity of the scale. Both the I-CVI and S-CVI/ave metrics corroborated the meritorious content validity of the SLK-LF-200 on both the item and the scale levels (30).

Criterion-related validation

The SLK-LF-200 was administered in the 2014-15 academic year involving 161 PolyU students (36). The experimental group included 67 students who had taken credit-bearing training in service leadership before, while those who received no such training at the time of testing served as the control (N= 94). Results of the independent samples t-tests indicated that the experimental group scored significantly higher (i.e., all *t*s > 2.46, *p*s < .05) in all seven component scores so as the total score (computed by summing all 200 items), indicating the criterion-related validity of the SLK-LF-200. Furthermore, analyses on the individual item highlighted that the experimental group performed significantly better on 63 of those items (i.e., all χ^2s > 2.46, *p*s <. 05). These 63 items were subjected to a screening procedure conducted by the first author of this paper, leading to the deletion of 13 items after consideration of item redundancy and face validity. Consequently, 50 items (see Table 2 for the sample items) were retained to form the short version of Service Leadership Knowledge Scale (i.e., SLK-SF-50).

Large-scale validation

The SLK-SF-50 was administered in a large-scale validation study involving 4,486 undergraduates recruited from eight government-funded universities in Hong Kong. Initial reliability analyses suggested the removal of ten items with (i.e., < 0.30) item-total correlations. As a result, a single-factor, shortened 40-item solution (i.e., SLK-SF-40) was subjected to the Confirmatory Factor Analysis (CFA) using the robust weighted least squares (WLSMV) estimator. The goodness-of-fit indices underscored the excellent fit of this proposed solution with the data (see Table 3 for details). The SLK-SF-40 also demonstrated excellent internal consistency ($\alpha = 0.94$, mean inter-item correlations = 0.28) and robust convergent validity, with the latter evidenced by the positive correlation between SLK-SF-40 and the list of theoretically-relevant constructs such as Servant Leadership (37) and Moral Self-concept (38). Taken as a whole, this large-scale, joint-institution validation study underlined the adequacy of SLK-SF-40 (see Table 3 for the sample items) as a reliable, valid, and robust measurement tool in examining people's mastery of fundamental knowledge points on the Service Leadership Theory.

Table 2. Initial Development of the Long-Form (SLK-LF-200) and Short-Forms (SLK-SF-50 and SLK-SF-40) Service Leadership Knowledge Scale

Steps	Details
Step 3: Development of the item pool (200 items) with reference to the main proposed domains	Seven key domains were conceptualized to be subsumed under the original, 200-item Long-form Service Leadership Knowledge Scale (SLK-LF-200). These include: General description of Service Leadership; Three realms of Service Leadership; Everyone can be a leader; Principle $E = MC^2$; Manufacturing vs. service economies and current societal status; Distinction of Service Leadership and other leadership theories; Other knowledge points in SLAM curriculum framework. Three sample items are featured in the following: 2. According to the SLAM model, competence,________, and ________ affect employees' loyalty and commitment. [Domain 1] A) fame; character; B) intelligence; care; C) intelligence; character; D) character; care (Correct answer: D); 27. Self-serving effort entails improving one's ________ in helping to satisfy others' needs. [Domain 2] A) fame; B) wealth; C) authority and power; D) competencies, abilities and willingness (Correct answer: D); 149. Which of the below is typically a desired behavioral attribute of employees in a manufacturing economy? [Domain 5] A) Flexible; B) Creative; C) Controllable; D) Unpredictable (Correct answer: C).
Step 4: Initial validation of the original scale (i.e., SLK-LF-200; 200 items)	The SLK-LF-200 was tested in a criterion-related validation study involving 161 PolyU students conducted in semester 2 of the 2014/15 academic year. Of those 161 participants 67 took the Service Leadership course before while the rest (N= 94) did not. Findings revealed that the former significantly performed better than the latter on 63 items of the SLK-LF-200. The first author of this paper commissioned a screening procedure on these 63 items, resulting in the removal of 13 items out of duplicity or face validity concern. Ultimately, a one-factor, 50-item short-form of Service Leadership Knowledge Scale (SLK-SF-50) was retained for the main study. See below for two sample items.
Step 5: Development of scale used in the main survey (i.e., SLK-SF-50; 50 items) and the major domains	*Single-factor, SLK-SF-50* 35. The two dimensions of social cognition include ________ and________ . A) warmth; talent; B) warmth; competence; C) popularity; talent; D) popularity; competence (Correct answer: B) 43. The manufacturing economy emphasizes ________ . A) Capital assets; B) Human assets; C) Financial assets; D) Social assets (Correct answer: A)

Note. All sample items were slightly re-worded to avoid familiarity effect.

Table 3. Refined scales based on exploratory factor analyses and confirmatory factor analyses

Steps	Details
Step 6: Refined scale based on exploratory factor analyses	N/A. No EFA was carried out.
Step 7: Refined scale based on confirmatory factor analyses (i.e., SLK-SF-40)	The whole working sample (N= 4,486) was utilized to validate the 50-item SLK-SF-50. Initial reliability analyses informed the deletion of 10 items due to low (i.e., < 0.30) item-total correlations. The resultant hypothesized one-factor, 40-item solution (i.e., SLK-SF-40) was accordingly subjected to CFA using the robust weighted least squares (WLSMV) estimator. The findings revealed the excellent fit of the SLK-SF-40 (i.e., CFI = 0.984; NNFI = 0.985; RMSEA = 0.029) to the data. The SLK-SF-40 also demonstrated excellent internal consistency (α = 0.94, mean inter-item correlations = 0.28) as well as strong convergent validity (i.e., positive and significant correlations with all external criterion scales as well as other Service Leadership scales under validation). The SLK-SF-40 was accordingly accepted as the finalized solution. Three sample items are shown as follows: 8. A manager under the service economy wants to hire someone. Based on the Service Leadership model, which of the following advice would you give him/her? A) Hire for qualifications, train for character B) Hire for character, train for skills C) Hire for attitude, train for character D) Hire for efficiency, train for mindset (Correct answer: B); 22. In the four options below, which one belongs to an attribute of the intelligent quotient (IQ)? A) Raw power B) Attractiveness C) Sexual Orientation D) Problem-solving skills (Correct answer: D) 37. Which of the following statements is inconsistent with the concept of "respect"? A) Showing off one's strength B) Accepting and appreciating differences C) Accepting and appreciating oneself D) Serving as a key element in nurturing authentic relationship (Correct answer: A)

Note. All sample items were slightly re-worded to avoid familiarity effect.

ACKNOWLEDGMENTS

The validation project is financially supported by the Victor and William Fung Foundation. The preparation for this paper is supported by the Foundation and the Endowed

Professorship in Service Leadership Education at The Hong Kong Polytechnic University. This chapter is an updated version of a publication in the special issue "Development and validation of assessment tools on service leadership knowledge, attitude and behavior" edited by Daniel TL Shek, Xiaoqin Zhu and Joav Merrick published in the International Journal of Child and Adolescent Health, 2018;11(4).

REFERENCES

[1] Worsley A. Nutrition knowledge and food consumption: Can nutrition knowledge change food behaviour? Asia Pac J Clin Nutr 2002;11(Suppl):579-85.
[2] Ferguson MJ, Bargh JA. How social perception can automatically influence behavior. Trends Cogn Sci 2004;8:33-9.
[3] Stone G, Barnes JH, Montgomery C. Ecoscale: A scale for the measurement of environmentally responsible consumers. Psychol Mark 1995;12:595-612.
[4] Fraj-Andrés E, Martínez-Salinas E. Impact of environmental knowledge on ecological consumer behaviour: An empirical analysis. J Int Consum Mark 2007;19:73-102.
[5] De Melo Ghisi GL, Abdallah F, Grace SL, Thomas S, Oh P. A systematic review of patient education in cardiac patients: Do they increase knowledge and promote health behavior change? Patient Educ Couns 2014;95:160-74.
[6] Robb CA, Woodyard A. Financial knowledge and best practice behavior. J Financ Couns Plan 2011;22:60-70.
[7] Baranowski T, Cullen KW, Nicklas T, Thompson D, Baranowski J. Are current health behavioral change models helpful in guiding prevention of weight gain efforts? Obesity 2003;11(Suppl):23-43.
[8] Ajzen I, Fishbein M. Understanding attitudes and predicting social behaviour. Englewood Cliffs, NJ: Prentice-Hall, 1980.
[9] Fisher JD, Fisher WA, Williams SS, Malloy TE. Empirical tests of an information-motivation-behavioral skills model of AIDS-preventive behavior with gay men and heterosexual university students. Health Psychol 1994;13:238-50.
[10] Straus SE, Tetroe J, Graham I. Defining knowledge translation. Can Med Assoc J 2009;181:165-8.
[11] Ogunyomi P, Bruning NS. Human resource management and organizational performance of small and medium enterprises (SMEs) in Nigeria. Int J Hum Resour Manage 2016;27:612-34.
[12] Caldwell C, Ndalamba KK. Human resource professionals as strategic leaders - A behavioral opportunity for improving information management. J Values-Based Leadersh 2017;10:1-9.
[13] Finkler SA, Smith DL, Calabrese TD, Purtell RM. Introduction to financial management. In: Finkler SA, Smith DL, Calabrese TD, Purtell RM, eds. Financial management for public, health, and not-for-profit organizations. Washington, DC: CQ Press, 2016.
[14] Scamardo M, Harnden SC. A manager coaching group model: Applying leadership knowledge. J Workplace Behav Health 2007;22:127-43.
[15] Stein MK, Nelson BS. Leadership content knowledge. Educ Eval Policy Anal 2003;25:423-48.
[16] Weitz BA, Sujan H, Sujan M. Knowledge, motivation, and adaptive behavior: A framework for improving selling effectiveness. J Mark 1986;50:174-91.
[17] Yammarino FJ, Dionne SD, Schriesheim CA, Dansereau F. Authentic leadership and positive organizational behavior: A meso, multi-level perspective. Leadersh Q 2008;19:693-707.
[18] Srivastava A, Bartol KM, Locke EA. Empowering leadership in management teams: Effects on knowledge sharing, efficacy, and performance. Acad Manage J 2006;49:1239-51.

[19] Ajzen I. Perceived behavioral control, self-efficacy, locus of control, and the theory of planned behavior. J Appl Soc Psychol 2002;32:665-83.
[20] Conner M, Armitage CJ. Extending the theory of planned behavior: A review and avenues for further research. J Appl Soc Psychol 1998;28:1429-64.
[21] Madden TJ, Ellen PS, Ajzen I. A comparison of the theory of planned behavior and the theory of reasoned action. Pers Soc Psychol Bull 1992;18:3-9.
[22] Mathieson K. Predicting user intentions: comparing the technology acceptance model with the theory of planned behavior. Inf Syst Res 1991;2:173-91.
[23] Kelloway EK, Barling J. Knowledge work as organizational behavior. Int J Manage Rev 2000;2:287-304.
[24] Pearce CL, Manz CC. The new silver bullets of leadership: The importance of self- and shared leadership in knowledge work. Organ Dyn 2005;34:130-40.
[25] Bettencourt LA, Gwinner KP, Meuter ML. A comparison of attitude, personality, and knowledge predictors of service-oriented organizational citizenship behaviors. J Appl Psychol 2001;86:29-41.
[26] Lin RSJ, Hsiao JK. The relationships between transformational leadership, knowledge sharing, trust and organizational citizenship behavior. Int J Innovat Manage Techol 2014;5:171-4.
[27] Donate MJ, de Pablo JDS. The role of knowledge-oriented leadership in knowledge management practices and innovation. J Bus Res 2015;68:360-70.
[28] Chung PPY, Elfassy R. The 12 dimensions of a service leader. Grandville, MI: Lexingford, 2016.
[29] Shek DTL, Li X. The role of a caring disposition in service leadership. Int J Disabil Hum Dev 2015;14:319–32.
[30] Shek DTL, Lin L, Leung H, Yu L, Ma CMS, Li X. Development and validation of the service leadership knowledge scale in a Chinese context. In: Shek DTL, Chung PPY, Lin L, Merrick J, eds. Service leadership education for university students. New York: Nova Science, 2017:163-88.
[31] Chung PPY. Service reborn. New York: Lexingford, 2012.
[32] Shek DTL, Chung PPY, Leung H. How unique is the service leadership model? A comparison with contemporary leadership approaches. Int J Disabil Hum Dev 2015;14:217–31.
[33] Sun CTL. Themes in Chinese psychology. Singapore: Cengage Learning, 2013.
[34] Shek DTL, Lin L. Intrapersonal competencies and service leadership. Int J Disabil Hum Dev 2015;14:255–63.
[35] Schrader PG, Lawless KA. The knowledge, attitudes, and behaviors approach how to evaluate performance and learning in complex environments. Perform Improv 2004;43:8-15.
[36] Shek DTL, Lin L. Validation of the service leadership knowledge scale: Criterion-related validity. In: Shek DTL, Chung PPY, Lin L, Merrick J, eds. Service leadership education for university students. New York: Nova Science, 2017:189-204.
[37] Wong PTP, Page D. Servant leadership: An opponent-process model and the revised servant leadership profile. Virginia Beach, VA: Regent University, 2003.
[38] Cheng CHK. The Chinese Adolescent Self-Esteem Scales: A user manual. Hong Kong: City University of Hong Kong Press, 2005.

In: Service Leadership
Editors: Daniel TL Shek, Xiaoqin Zhu, Li Lin et al.
ISBN: 978-1-53614-852-7

Chapter 4

DEVELOPMENT OF THE ATTITUDE TO SERVICE LEADERSHIP SCALE IN HONG KONG

Cecilia MS Ma[1,*], PhD,
Daniel TL Shek[1-6], PhD, FHKPS, BBS, SBS, JP
and Yanto Chandra[7], PhD

[1]Department of Applied Social Sciences, The Hong Kong Polytechnic University, Hong Kong, PR China
[2]Centre for Innovative Programmes for Adolescents and Families, The Hong Kong Polytechnic University, Hong Kong, PR China
[3]Department of Social Work, East China Normal University, Shanghai, PR China
[4]Kiang Wu Nursing College of Macau, Macau, PR China
[5]Hong Kong Institute of Service Leadership and Management Limited, Hong Kong, PR China
[6]Division of Adolescent Medicine, Department of Pediatrics, Kentucky Children's Hospital, University of Kentucky School of Medicine, Lexington, Kentucky, US
[7]Department of Public Policy, City University of Hong Kong, Hong Kong, PR China

ABSTRACT

Attitude is an important component of leadership qualities. Leaders who believe in the potential of the followers would allow more room for followers to make decisions. Leaders who believe in the importance of moral character would uphold moral principles in their

---

* Correspondence: Cecilia MS Ma, PhD, Department of Applied Social Sciences, The Hong Kong Polytechnic University, Hong Kong, PR China. Email: cecilia.ma@polyu.edu.hk.

work. With the gradual decline of manufacturing industries and the rise of service industries, there is a need to nurture leaders who can effectively lead in the challenging environment of service economies. In particular, fostering positive attitudes is an important task to be achieved. Unfortunately, measures of service leadership qualities are almost non-existent in the scientific leadership literature. In this chapter, the theory and concepts surrounding attitudes towards Service Leadership are outlined. The different steps underlying the development of the Service Leadership Attitude Scale are also described, including literature review, item development, initial validation and main survey.

INTRODUCTION

The 21st century has undergone paradigm shifts in the concepts, framework and application of leadership (1). Hence, the traditional economic theory, which is based on the industrial paradigm, might not be applicable to the service world (2). With the rapid evolution in information and communication technology, personalized services have become increasingly important. In fact, service has become the major economic sector in most developed nations. For example, service industry accounts for almost 80% of the economy in the United Kingdom and the United States (3). In 2013, about 93% of the Gross Domestic Product in Hong Kong was comprised of a wide range of services, such as hotel and food services, banking and insurance, and professional and business services (4).

According to Shek, Chung and Leung (5), there are differences between manufacturing economy and service economy in terms of leadership qualities. For example, while leadership in manufacturing economy is more top-down, it is more bottom-up in service economy. Besides, service leaders need to be more sensitive to different needs and expectations of the customers (6). Moving from a manufacture-oriented economy to a service-oriented economy means that the leaders need to be more responsive to customers' needs in the knowledge-intensive market (7).

THE NATURE OF SERVICE LEADERSHIP

With the rise of the service economy, customers have become part of the organizational system (8). The increased diversity of customer backgrounds has imposed variability in the service provider-customer (supplier-customer) relationship (9) and led to a greater level of organizational uncertainty (7). Hence, identifying and satisfying the needs of customers have become an integral cost of the firm (10). In particular, emphasis on consumer experiences of services has become a key differentiator in this highly competitive world (11). Leaders have to manage their organization effectively in order to stay ahead in the highly competitive market. Researchers proposed the use of "customer-centered" service-related competence models, which focus on the leadership behaviors and skills of Service Leadership to promote the quality of service.

Based on his experience in the service industries, Chung (12) proposed the Service Leadership Theory which posited that it is important to identify effective leadership competencies in the face of the competitive business environment. Under the framework of the Hong Kong Institute of Service Leadership and Management (SLAM), service leaders aim at "providing quality personal service to everyone one comes into contact with, including one's self, others, groups, communities, systems, and environments" (12, p. 5). Compared with the conventional leadership theories (e.g., authentic leadership, transformation leadership), Service Leadership focuses on changing the followers' beliefs and perceptions about themselves and promoting followers' positive behavior (13-15).

There are several unique characteristics of Service Leadership. First, meeting others' needs is a unique feature of Service Leadership. The major premise of the Service Leadership Theory is that leaders promote positive organizational outcomes by satisfying the followers' needs and facilitating their development. Through this empowering process, followers feel more attracted to their service leaders, see them as role models and thereby recognize their optimal level of performance. This is different from the leader-oriented and hierarchical nature of the previous leadership theories (5). The de-emphasis of the hierarchical nature of leadership allows employees to act proactively and initiate changes from the bottom-up in order to address the needs at work (16). Through this changing authority process, employees perceive themselves as part of the organization and feel that they have autonomy to exercise their personal judgment with greater job responsibilities, resulting in increasing job satisfaction and organizational commitment (17, 18). Research studies show that adaptive employees reported better well-being (19, 20), a higher level of proactive skills (21) and greater organizational identification (16).

Second, development of followers' competence is another unique feature of the Service Leadership Theory. Effective leaders motivate others to excel themselves through achieving the organizational goals (22). Service leaders encourage the followers to take challenges and to develop personal accountability. In order to differentiate themselves from others who are competitive and to keep staying ahead in the market, leaders seek ways to provide high-quality service for their customers (23, 24). Providing high-quality service thus becomes a prerequisite for organizational success.

Third, high-quality service is provided when the service leaders possess effective intrapersonal and interpersonal competencies (5, 25, 26). Effective service leaders should have high intrapersonal competencies in four areas, namely intelligence quotient (IQ), adversity quotient (AQ), emotional quotient (EQ) and spiritual quotient (SQ). IQ refers to the ability to critically analyze a problem and to search for innovative ways to solve the problem. AQ is defined as the ability to accept and overcome the difficulties by bouncing back from the challenges. EQ refers to the ability to understand one's own and others' emotions and to manage one's emotions when interacting with others. SQ refers to the ability to share the vision and mission with the followers and to solve problems by utilizing spiritual resources. Moreover, service leaders should have good interpersonal competencies so that they can communicate and work effectively with people of diverse backgrounds (27).

Fourth, moral character is an important attribute of effective service leaders. In particular, honesty and integrity are two major characteristics of a highly effective leadership (28). Service leaders respond with trust and respect and express a strong preference for followers' needs over their own needs (29). Ethical leaders are fully aware of the effects of their behavior on the development of the followers. They are always aware of their own moral values, perspectives and behaviors and transform their followers into moral agents (30). Acting as change agents, service leaders transform followers into moral agents by behaving morally, developing a moral identity and creating ethical atmosphere (31). Babalola et al. (32) highlighted the importance of ethical leadership in promoting followers' ability to handle conflicting situations. Empirical evidence (14, 33, 34) has shown the link between ethical leadership and followers' morality (i.e., moral identity, moral emotions, moral behaviors, and organizational commitment).

Fifth, effective service leaders must put the interests of the followers first. More specifically, the focus on helping and serving others is the central tenet of Service Leadership (35). Service leaders show a genuine concern for the followers' welfare and focus on personalized care in creating an atmosphere that promotes the effectiveness of the team (29). They serve as role models for intellectual stimulation and inspirational motivation (25). Under this warm and supportive environment, employees feel secured and are encouraged to explore innovative solutions in their work and to share their thoughts with their leaders (36).

Sixth, self-improvement is an important attribute of an effective service leader. Effective service leaders constantly evaluate their behavior and performance through reflection (37). Self-reflection helps individuals to rethink or restructure their assumptions that underlie their own actions, beliefs and behaviors (38). The significance of critical reflection has been demonstrated (39, 40). Self-development is one of the significant competencies in the service industry (37, 41). Customized service is characterized by complexity and utilization of specialized knowledge and skills (42, 43). Effective service leaders are likely to rethink their own working performance, are more aware of others' needs and feel more motivated to promote personal growth. Reflection helps the individuals in personal growth and continuous improvement of leadership skills and knowledge. They are more willing to make changes and seek resources in order to adapt to the uncertain environment (37). This leads to positive influence on the employees through the empowerment process (44, 45). Employees become more welcome for changes and actively engage in continuous personal and professional development (46, 47).

Finally, the notion of "everyone can be a leader" is a defining characteristic of Service Leadership. In contrast to the concept of "elitist leadership" (i.e., only those who are talented can be leaders), the Service Leadership Theory emphasizes the notion that "everybody can be a leader." This notion suggests that everybody has potential to be a leader and the key is training and opportunities for development. This humanistic assumption is very empowering in nature, providing much space for development for the leaders and followers.

ASSESSMENT OF ATTITUDE TO LEADERSHIP

Facing the ever-changing business environment, new organization learning processes and informational activities have been rapidly increasing (2). Leaders are expected to acknowledge individual differences and tailor their service to meet individual needs (15). Yukl (48) argued that effective leadership may largely depend on the contexts (49). The contemporary leadership theories often focus on how leaders' characteristics and behaviors influence the followers and organizational outcomes (50). As such, some researchers began to study the factors related to effective leadership from the followers' perspective (17, 51-53). In leadership research, attitude towards the leader refers to the degree of favorability one perceives a leader (54). Wielkiewicz et al. (55) highlighted the importance of understanding of leadership development from the followers' perspective.

Recently, researchers have developed measurement tools to assess attitudes to leadership. For example, Wielkiewicz (56) developed the Leadership Attitudes and Beliefs Scale (LABS-III) which assessed both hierarchical thinking and systematic thinking about leadership. The scale has two dimensions with 14 items per subscale. This scale has been used to assess college students' attitude towards leadership (55, 57, 58). Also, the Operating Room Management Attitudes Questionnaire (ORMAQ; 59, 60) was used to measure the attitudes towards six areas of leadership: assertiveness, teamwork, communication, leadership structure, awareness of personal limitations, and organizational issues. This scale has been tested in the fields of aviation (61) and medicine (59) but no factor analysis (e.g., confirmatory factor analysis) has been conducted.

Besides, the attitude towards service has been studied (23, 62, 63). For example, customers' perception of service quality is an assessment of overall service excellence (23) and subjective evaluation of service quality has a close relationship with customer satisfaction (64). Literature on service quality suggests that employees' attitude towards leaders are essential to determine customer satisfaction (65). Parasuraman et al. (23) developed a 22-item tool assessing five dimensions of service quality, namely tangibles, reliabilities, responsiveness, assurance and empathy, and found support for the reliability and factor structure of the scale.

Unfortunately, although there are some measures assessing the attitude to service quality, existing scales for measuring the attitude towards Service Leadership are relatively scarce. For example, Wu (66) developed three items (e.g., "My service provider offers a larger choice of services for customers"; "My service provider satisfies customers' different needs with more diversified service"; "My service provider offers services of great variety") to assess Service Leadership and tested its impact on loyalty and brand equity via structural equation modeling which showed support for the reliability and validity of this construct. However, the coverage of these items on leadership qualities is not in-depth. In fact, despite the fact that service is playing an important role in the global economy, research on service development has lagged behind compared with the research on the manufacturing industry (67). More research in this area can be helpful for the employers to understand which type of leadership style is the most suitable and appropriate in terms of the organizational and follower outcomes. Studying the attitudes of Service Leadership from employees' perspective is important because leaders need to create a positive atmosphere and accountability for employees so that organizational outcomes of interest (e.g., performance, satisfaction, leadership) can be achieved. Hence, psychometrically sound instruments would help researchers and practitioners understand individuals' attitudes towards Service Leadership.

Service is a process of applying one's knowledge and skills for the benefit of employees or customers (68). Empirical findings showed that followers' attitudes toward leadership were positively related to follower positive outcomes, such as teamwork performance (62), job satisfaction (69) and organizational performance (70). The establishment of psychometrically sound instruments will definitely increase our understanding of effective leadership in the service industry. Given the emergence of service-oriented economy which stresses the importance of intangible products, such as experiences and the quality of the goods, more research is warranted for helping us better understand effective leadership in this area.

Besides developing scales on Service Leadership, testing the psychometric properties of the developed scales is an important step. While the majority of research has mostly focused on assessing convergent/divergent validity (23) and content validity (71), little is known about the factor structure of the existing scales. More specifically, exploratory factor analysis has been commonly conducted when testing the factor structure (23, 56). Although Service Leadership is perceived as a multidimensional concept (5, 25), a unidimensional tool has been employed (66). Clearly, more research should be conducted to test the generalizability of the Service Leadership Attitude Scale in different contexts and populations.

DEVELOPMENT OF THE SERVICE LEADERSHIP ATTITUDE SCALE

In Hong Kong, service industries account for nearly 93% of the GDP. Despite the importance of service industries, there is a gap in the development of Service Leadership in Hong Kong. In view of this deficiency, the Victor and William Fung Foundation made a donation of HK$40 million to support the Service Leadership Education initiative with the participation of the eight institutions supported by the University Grants Committee. In each university, curriculum materials and subjects on Service Leadership were developed. With this good foundation, one unresolved question is on the availability of objective measures of Service Leadership knowledge, attitude and skills.

With further funding from the Victor and William Fung Foundation, the eight universities collaborated to develop scales on the Service Leadership knowledge, attitude and skills. As mentioned above, the Service Leadership Attitude Scale was developed within this context. As far as the Service Leadership Attitude Scale is concerned, several steps were involved:

Step 1: Literature review on attitudes to leadership measures, particularly in different Chinese contexts
Step 2: Literature review on Service Leadership
Step 3: Development of the item pool (132 items) with reference to the main proposed domains
Step 4: Initial validation of the original scale (132 items)
Step 5: Development of scale used in the main survey (73 items) and the major domains
Step 6: Refined scale based on exploratory factor analyses in the main survey (46 items)
Step 7: Refined scale based on confirmatory factor analyses (46 items)

The details of different steps are outlined in Table 1-3. To assess the attitude to Service Leadership, Shek and colleagues (71) developed the 132-item long-form Service Leadership Attitude Scale (i.e., SLA-LF-132) and conducted the initial content validity test of the scale. This scale measures various aspects of service leadership, including service orientation, the belief that everyone can be a leader, leadership competence, moral character, caring disposition, and commitment to continuous improvement. The content validity of the scale has been established by the high content validity of the individual items and the overall questionnaires.

In this book, the findings on the psychometric properties of the Service Leadership Attitude Scale based on exploratory factor analyses are reported. We hope that from this book, it can be seen that the Service Leadership Attitude Scale possesses good psychometric properties and therefore can be used in research, assessment, education, evaluation and personnel decision contexts.

Table 1. Literature review on measures of leadership and service leadership

Steps	Details
Step 1: Literature review on attitudes to leadership measures, particularly in different Chinese contexts	Examples of references: – Casimir, G., & Waldman, D. A. (2007). A cross cultural comparison of the importance of leadership traits for effective low-level and high-level leaders: Australia and China. *International Journal of Cross Cultural Management, 7*(1), 47-60. – Chan, K. Y., & Drasgow, F. (2001). Toward a theory of individual differences and leadership: Understanding the motivation to lead. *Journal of Applied Psychology, 86*(3), 481-498. – Cheng, B. S., Boer, D., Chou, L. F., Huang, M. P., Yoneyama, S., Shim, D., ... & Tsai, C. Y. (2014). Paternalistic leadership in four East Asian societies: Generalizability and cultural differences of the triad model. *Journal of Cross-Cultural Psychology, 45*(1), 82-90. – Ho, J., & Nesbit, P. L. (2009). A refinement and extension of the self-leadership scale for the Chinese context. *Journal of Managerial Psychology, 24*(5), 450-476. – Lan, X. M., & Chong, W. Y. (2015). The mediating role of psychological empowerment between transformational leadership and employee work attitudes. *Procedia-Social and Behavioral Sciences, 172*, 184-191. – Liden, R. C., Wayne, S. J., Zhao, H., & Henderson, D. (2008). Servant leadership: Development of a multi-dimensional measure and multi-level assessment. *The Leadership Quarterly, 19*(2), 161-177. – Ling, W., Chia, R. C., & Fang, L. (2000). Chinese implicit leadership theory. *The Journal of Social Psychology, 140*(6), 729-739. – Spreitzer, G. M., Perttula, K. H., & Xin, K. (2005). Traditionality matters: An examination of the effectiveness of transformational leadership in the United States and Taiwan. *Journal of Organizational Behavior, 26*(3), 205-227.
Step 2: Literature review on Service Leadership	Examples of references: – Shek, D. T. L., & Li, X. (2015). The role of a caring disposition in service leadership. *International Journal on Disability and Human Development, 14*(4), 319-332. – Shek, D. T. L., & Lin, L. (2015a). Leadership and mentorship: Service leaders as mentors of the followers. *International Journal on Disability and Human Development, 14*, 351-359. doi: 10.1515/ijdhd-2015-0456 – Shek, D. T. L., & Lin, L. (2015b). Intrapersonal competences and service leadership. *International Journal on Disability and Human Development, 14*(3), 255-263. – Shek, D. T. L., Lin, L., Leung, H., Yu, L., Ma, C. M. S., & Li, X. (2017). Content validation of the service leadership attitudes scale. In D. T. L. Shek, P. P. Y. Chung, L. Lin, & J. Merrick (Eds.), *Service leadership education for university students* (pp. 205-225). New York: Nova Sciences. – Shek, D. T. L., Ma, C. M. S., & Liu, T. T. (2015). Adolescent developmental assets and service leadership. *International Journal on Disability and Human Development, 14*(3), 275-283. – Shek, D. T. L., Ma, C. M. S., Liu, T. T., & Siu, A. M. H. (2015). The role of self-leadership in service leadership. *International Journal on Disability and Human Development, 14*, 343-350. doi: 10.1515/ijdhd-2015-0455 – Shek, D. T. L., Yu, L., & Siu, A. M. H. (2015). Interpersonal competence and service leadership. *International Journal on Disability and Human Development, 14*, 265-274. doi: 10.1515/ijdhd-2015-0407

Table 2. Initial development of the Long-Form (SLA-LF-132) and Short-Form (SLA-SF-73) Service Leadership Attitude Scale

Steps	Details
Step 3: Development of the item pool (132 items) with reference to the main proposed domains	Eight domains were proposed in 132-item long-form Service Leadership Attitude Scale (SLA-LF-132) including: [1] Service Orientation (e.g., Good leaders serve without expecting any rewards), [2] Everyone can be a leader (e.g., Only the elites can lead, reverse-item), [3] Distributed Leadership (e.g., Good leaders are open to challenges and criticism), [4] Employability (e.g., Lucrative leadership positions go to people who are eager and able to serve others), [5] Personalized Service (e.g., Sensitivity towards people's specific needs is an important trait for any leaders), [6] Attitudes towards Service (e.g., Service providers find it intrinsically enjoyable to render good-quality service), [7] Principle "$E = MC^2$" (e.g., Moral character: Good leaders do not break promises; Competence: Good leaders make convincing arguments; Caring disposition: Good leaders are forgiving.), and [8] Commitment to Continuous Improvement (e.g., One can devleop his/her ability to lead).
Step 4: Initial validation of the original scale (i.e., SLA-LF-132; 132 items)	The SLA-LF-132 was subjected to a quasi-experimental validation study in semester 1 of the 2016/17 academic year. A total of 208 PolyU students took the pre-test while 190 did the post-test. An exploratory factor analysis (EFA) was performed on 200 sets of pre-test questionnaires. Results of the EFA informed the retention of a 5-factor, 73-item solution (i.e., SLA-SF-73) which recorded good reliability and a significant and positive correlation with the short-form Service Leadership Knowledge Scale (SLK-SF-50). See below for the five factors extracted and two sample items for each factor.
Step 5: Development of scale used in the main survey (i.e., SLA-SF-73; 73 items) and the major domains	*Factor 1: Attitudes towards service and competences* 1. Good leaders serve with a genuine heart. 20. Good leaders can handle stressful situations calmly. *Factor 2: Attitudes towards moral character and caring disposition* 29. A good leader should be people-oriented. 39. Good leaders always tell the truth. *Factor 3: Attitudes towards self-reflection* 64. A good leader is self-restraint. 68. Genuine leaders are aware of their own strengths and weaknesses. *Factor 4: Everyone can be a leader* 5. Not everyone is able to lead others. (reverse-item) 6. Only the "best of the best" can lead. (reverse-item) *Factor 5: Implicit theory of leadership* 62. Leadership competence is not something that can be changed through learning. (reverse-item) 63. The ability to lead is inborn and not changeable. (reverse-item)

Note. All sample items were slightly re-worded to avoid familiarity effect.

Table 3. Refined scales based on exploratory factor analyses and confirmatory factor analyses

Steps	Details
Step 6: Refined scale based on exploratory factor analyses (i.e., SLA-SF-46E)	Nine items, which were demonstrated to possess low item-total correlation (i.e., <0.25), were dropped before the ensuing principal component analysis (PCA). Accordingly, the PCA was performed on the remaining 64 items of the SLA-SF-73 using a subset (N = 2,246) of the total sample (N = 4,486), resulting in a 7-factor structure demonstrated to be stable. Upon removing 18 items with loadings below 0.50, a 7-factor, 46-item solution (i.e., SLA-SF-46E) was retained to be subjected to CFA utilizing the other subset (N = 2,240). The SLA-SF-46E recorded excellent internal consistency and strong convergent validity, with the latter evidenced by its positive and significant correlations with the external criterion scales as well as other Service Leadership scales under validation. The seven factors of SLA-SF-46E include: Vision and competence (Factor 1), People Orientation (Factor 2), Caring Disposition (Factor 3), Ethical Role Model (Factor 4), Social Competence (Factor 5), Self-Reflection and Self-Understanding (Factor 6), and Positive Views about Human Beings (Factor 7). Three sample items are featured below: 28. Good leaders do not give in easily amidst adversity. (Factor 1) 38. Good leaders closely examine their thoughts and behaviors. (Factor 6) 41. Everyone has what it takes to be a leader. (Factor 7)
Step 7: Refined scale based on confirmatory factor analyses (i.e., SLA-SF-46)	The 7-factor SLA-SF-46E was subjected to CFA utilizing the Maximum Likelihood (ML) estimator, which showed acceptable fit to the data (i.e., CFI = 0.91; NNFI = 0.90; RMSEA = 0.048). Analyses were based on re-incorporating a previously removed seven-item subscale (from the PCA, due to low item-total correlations) back to the main factor structure. The 8-factor, 53-item factorial structure was subjected to CFA, whereby the fit indices (i.e., CFI = 0.87; NNFI = 0.86; RMSEA = 0.053) suggested an unsatisfactory fit. Inspection of the modification indices (MI) informed the removal of 7 items, due to their extreme MIs with multiple items on the same factor. The CFA was re-run on this 8-factor, 46-item structure where results suggested a much improved fit (i.e., CFI = 0.90; NNFI = 0.90; RMSEA = 0.054). Inspection of MIs revealed four pairs of parameters showing extreme covariance. After incorporating the correlation between errors for these four pairs of parameters, the findings corroborated the reasonable fit of this modified structure (i.e., CFI = 0.93; NNFI = 0.92; RMSEA = 0.041). This modified 8-factor, 46-item solution was accordingly accepted as the finalized solution (i.e., SLA-SF-46). The SLA-SF-46 comprises an *identical factor structure* and *labeling as the SLA-SF-46E,* with the addition of the eighth factor entitled "Unchangeable and Dark Human Nature". Two sample items of this factor were shown below: 43. One's ability to lead is inborn and hardly changeable (reverse-item). 45. People need to be checked to ensure they work as required (reverse-item). The SLA-SF-46 and the subscales showed good reliability and convergent validity, with the latter evidenced by the positive and significant associations with the external criterion scales and other Service Leadership scales.

Note. All sample items were slightly re-worded to minimize familiarity effect.

ACKNOWLEDGMENTS

The validation project is financially supported by the Victor and William Fung Foundation. The preparation for this paper is supported by the Foundation and the Endowed Professorship in Service Leadership Education at The Hong Kong Polytechnic University. This chapter is an updated version of a publication in the special issue "Development and validation of assessment tools on service leadership knowledge, attitude and behavior" edited by Daniel TL Shek, Xiaoqin Zhu and Joav Merrick published in the International Journal of Child and Adolescent Health, 2018;11(4).

REFERENCES

[1] White RF. Toward an integrated theory of leadership. Polit Life Sci 2011;30(1):116-21.
[2] Bandt JD. The concept of labour and competence requirements in a service economy. Serv Ind J 1999;19(1):1-17.
[3] The World Bank. Service, value added (% of GDP). URL: https://data.worldbank.org/indicator/NV.SRV.TETC.ZS.
[4] Hong Kong Information Services Department. Hong Kong as a service economy, 2016. Available at: https://www.gov.hk/en/about/abouthk/factsheets/docs/service_economy.pdf.
[5] Shek DTL, Chung PPY, Leung H. Manufacturing economy vs. service economy: Implications for service leadership. Int J Disabil Hum Dev 2015;14(3):205-15.
[6] Orsingher C, Valentini S, De Angelis M. A meta-analysis of satisfaction with complaint handling in services. J Acad Market Sci 2010;38(2):169-86.
[7] Chowdhury S, Miles G. Customer-induced uncertainty in predicting organizational design: Empirical evidence challenging the service versus manufacturing dichotomy. J Bus Res 2006;59:121-9.
[8] Hoffer Gittell J. Coordinating mechanisms in care provider groups: Relational coordination as a mediator and input uncertainty as a moderator of performance effects. Manage Sci 2002;48(11):1408-26.
[9] Skaggs BC, Youndt M. Strategic positioning, human capital, and performance in service organizations: A customer interaction approach. Strategy Manage J 2004;25(1):85-99.
[10] Keaveney SM. Customer switching behavior in service industries: An exploratory study. J Mark 1995;59(2):71-82.
[11] Zeithaml VA, Berry LL, Parasumaran A. The behavioral consequences of service quality. J Mark 1996;60(2):31-46.
[12] Chung PPY. Hong Kong Institute of Service Leadership and Management curriculum framework. Hong Kong: Hong Kong Institute of Service Leadership and Management, 2011.
[13] Avolio BJ, Walumbwa FO, Weber TJ. Leadership: Current theories, research, and future directions. Annu Rev Psychol 2009;60:421-49.
[14] Brown ME, Treviño LK, Harrison DA. Ethical leadership: A social learning perspective for construct development and testing. Organ Behav Hum Decis Process 2005;97:117-34.
[15] Bass BM. Leadership and performance beyond expectations. New York: Free Press, 1985.
[16] Wang HJ, Demerouti E, Le Blanc P. Transformational leadership, adaptability, and job crafting: The moderating role of organizational identification. J Vocat Behav 2017;100:185-95.

[17] Neubert MJ, Hunter EM, Tolentino RC. A servant leader and their stakeholders: When does organizational structure enhance a leader's influence? Leadersh Q 2016;27(6):896-910.
[18] Brunetto Y, Farr-Wharton R, Shacklock K. Supervisor-subordinate communication relationships, role ambiguity, autonomy and affective commitment for nurses. Contemp Nurse 2011;39(2):227-39.
[19] Petrou P, Demerouti E, Schaufeli WB. Job crafting in changing organizations: Antecedents and implications for exhaustion and performance. J Occup Health Psychol 2015;20(4):470-80.
[20] Maggiori C, Johnston CS, Krings F, Massoudi K, Rossier J. The role of career adaptability and work conditions on general and professional well-being. J Vocat Behav 2013;83(3):437-49.
[21] Taber BJ, Blankemeyer M. Future work self and career adaptability in the prediction of proactive career behaviors. J Vocat Behav 2015;86:20-7.
[22] Burns JM. Leadership. New York: Harper Row, 1978.
[23] Parasuraman A, Zeithaml VA, Berry LL. SERVQUAL: A multiple-item scale for measuring consumer perceptions of service quality. J Retailing 1988;64(1):12-40.
[24] Rudie MJ, Wansley HB. The Merrill Lynch quality program. In: Bloch TM, Upah GD, Zeithaml VA, eds. Services marketing in a changing environment. Chicago, IL: American Marketing Association, 1985:7-9.
[25] Chung PPY. Service reborn. New York: Lexington Publishing, 2012.
[26] Shek DTL, Yu L, Siu AMH. Interpersonal competence and service leadership. Int J Disabil Hum Dev 2015;14(3):265-74.
[27] Shek DTL, Lin L. Intrapersonal competencies and service leadership. Int J Disabil Hum Dev 2015;14(3):255-63.
[28] Den Hartog DN, House RJ, Hanges PJ, Ruiz-Quintanilla SA, Dorfman PW, Globe-Associates. Culture specific and cross culturally generalizable implicit leadership theories: Are attributes of charismatic/transformational leadership universally endorsed? Leadersh Q 1999;10(2):219-56.
[29] Shek DTL, Lin L. Core beliefs in the service leadership model proposed by the Hong Kong Institute of Service Leadership and Management. Int J Disabil Hum Dev 2015;14(3):233-42.
[30] Avolio BJ, Gardner WL. Authentic leadership development: Getting to the root of positive forms of leadership. Leadersh Q 2005;16(3):315-38.
[31] Zhu W, Avolio BJ, Riggio RE, Sosik JJ. The effect of authentic transformational leadership on follower and group ethics. Leadersh Q 2011;22(5):801-17.
[32] Babalola MT, Stouten J, Euwema MC, Ovadje F. The relation between ethical leadership and workplace conflicts: The mediating role of employee resolution efficacy. J Manage 2016. doi:http://dx.doi.org/10.1177/0149206316638163.
[33] Den Hartog DN, De Hoogh AHB. Empowering behavior and leader fairness and integrity: Studying perceptions of ethical leader behavior from a levels-of-analysis perspective. Eur J Work Organ Psychol 2009;18(2):199-230.
[34] Walumbwa FO, Hartnell CA, Misati E. Does ethical leadership enhance group learning behavior? Examining the mediating influence of group ethical conduct, justice climate, and peer justice. J Bus Res 2017;72:14-23.
[35] Chung PPY. Distinguishing characteristics of service leadership and management education. Hong Kong Institute of Service Leadership and Management Limited, 2010. URL: http://hki-slam.org/index.php?r=article&catid=2&aid=29.
[36] Hirak R, Peng AC, Carmeli A, Schaubroeck JM. Linking leader inclusiveness to work unit performance: The importance of psychological safety and learning from failures. Leadersh Q 2012;23(1):107-17.
[37] Testa MR, Sipe L. Service-leadership competencies for hospitality and tourism management. Int J Hosp Manag 2012;31(3):648-58.
[38] Watt M, Lawson M. Using a meta-analysis activity to make critical reflection explicit in teacher education. Teach Teach Educ 2009;25(5):609-16.

[39] Ash SL, Clayton PH. Generating, deepening, and documenting learning: The power of critical reflection in applied learning. J Appl Learn High Educ 2009;1(1):25-48.
[40] Runhaar P, Sanders K, Yang H. Stimulating teachers' reflection and feedback asking: An interplay of self-efficacy, learning goal orientation, and transformational leadership. Teach Teach Educ 2010;26(5):1154-61.
[41] Kay C, Russette J. Hospitality-management competencies: Identifying managers' essential skills. Cornell Hotel Restaur Adm Q 2000;41(2):52-63.
[42] BizEd. Top 4 CEO. AACSB International, 2016. URL: https://bized.aacsb.edu/articles/2016/07/top-four-ceo-concerns.
[43] De Brentani U, Ragot E. Developing new business-to-business professional services: What factors impact performance? Ind Mark Manage 1996;25(6):517-30.
[44] Houghton JD, Yoho SK. Toward a contingency model of leadership and psychological empowerment: When should self-leadership be encouraged? J Leadersh Organ Stud 2005;11(4):65-83.
[45] Manz CC, Sims HP Jr. The new super leadership: Leading others to lead themselves. San Francisco, CA: Berrett-Koehler, 2001.
[46] Vecchio RP, Justin JE, Pearce CL. Empowering leadership: An examination of mediating mechanisms within a hierarchical structure. Leadersh Q 2010;21(3):530-42.
[47] Amundsen S, Martinsen ØL. Empowering leadership: Construct clarification, conceptualization, and validation of a new scale. Leadersh Q 2014;25(3):487-511.
[48] Yukl GA. Leadership in organizations, 6th ed. Englewood Cliffs, NJ: Prentice Hall, 2006.
[49] Avolio BJ. Promoting more integrative strategies for leadership theory-building. Am Psychol 2007;62(1):25-33.
[50] Hollander EP. Leadership, followership, self, and others. Leadersh Q 1992;3(1):43-54.
[51] Meindl JR. The romance of leadership as a follower-centric theory: A social constructionist approach. Leadersh Q 1995;6(3):329-41.
[52] Dasborough MT, Ashkanasy NM, Tee EYJ, Tse HHM. What goes around comes around: How meso-level negative emotional contagion can ultimately determine organizational attitudes toward leaders. Leadersh Q 2009;20(4):571-85.
[53] Kalshoven K, Den Hartog DN, De Hoogh AHB. Ethical leadership at work questionnaires (ELW): Development and validation of a multidimensional measure. Leadersh Q 2011;22(1):51-69.
[54] Lee A, Martin R, Thomas G, Guillaume Y, Maio GR. Conceptualizing leadership perceptions as attitudes: Using attitude theory to further understand the leadership process. Leadersh Q 2015;26(6):910-34.
[55] Wielkiewicz RM, Prom CL, Loos S. Relationships of the leadership attitudes and beliefs scale with student types, study habits, life-long learning, and GPA. Coll Stud J 2005;39(1):31-44.
[56] Wielkiewicz RM. The Leadership Attitudes and Beliefs Scale: An instrument for evaluating college students' thinking about leadership and organizations. J Coll Stud Dev 2000;41(3):335-47.
[57] Wielkiewicz RM, Fischer DV, Stelzner SP, Overland M, Sinner AM. Leadership attitudes and beliefs of incoming first-year college students: A multi-institutional study of gender differences. J Leadersh Educ 2012;11(2):1-25.
[58] Fischer DV, Overland M, Adams L. Leadership attitudes and beliefs of incoming first-year college students. J Leadersh Educ 2010;9(1):1-16.
[59] Flin R, Fletcher G, McGeorge P, Sutherland A, Patey R. Anaesthetists' attitudes to teamwork and safety. Anaesthesia 2003;58(3):233-42.
[60] Helmreich RL. Cockpit management attitudes. Hum Factors 1984;26(5):583-9.
[61] Crichton M. Attitudes to teamwork, leadership, and stress in oil industry drilling teams. Saf Sci 2005;43(9):679-96.
[62] Berry LL. Retail businesses are service businesses. J Retailing 1986;62(1):3-6.

[63] Olshavsky RW. Perceived quality in consumer decision making: An integrated theoretical perspective. In: Jacoby J, Olson J, eds. Perceived quality. Lexington, MA: Lexington, 1985.
[64] Momparler A, Carmona P, Lassala, C. Quality of consulting services and consulting fees. J Bus Res 2015;68(7):1458-62.
[65] Hays JM, Hill AV. A preliminary investigation of the relationships between employee motivation/vision, service learning, and perceived service quality. J Oper Manage 2001;19(3):335-49.
[66] Wu CW. The study of service innovation for digiservice on loyalty. J Bus Res 2014;67(5):819-24.
[67] Hauser J, Tellis GJ, Griffin A. Research on innovation: A review and agenda for marketing science. Mark Sci 2006;25(6):687-717.
[68] Hidalgo A, D'Alvano L. Service innovation: Inward and outward related activities and cooperation mode. J Bus Res 2014;67(5):698-703.
[69] Dewettinck K, Van Ameijde M. Linking leadership empowerment behaviour to employee attitudes and behavioural intentions: Testing the mediating role of psychological empowerment. Pers Rev 2011;40(3):284-305.
[70] O'Dea A, Flin R. Site managers and safety leadership in the offshore oil and gas industry. Saf Sci 2001;37(1):39-57.
[71] Shek DTL, Lin L, Leung H, Yu L, Ma CMS, Li X. Content validation of the service leadership attitude scale. In: Shek DTL, Chung PPY, Lin L, Merrick J, eds. Service leadership education for university students. New York: Nova Science, 2017:205-25.

In: Service Leadership ISBN: 978-1-53614-852-7
Editors: Daniel TL Shek, Xiaoqin Zhu, Li Lin et al.

Chapter 5

Development of Service Leadership Behavior Scale: Background and Conceptual Model

Daniel TL Shek*[1-6,*]*, PhD, FHKPS, BBS, SBS, JP,
Xiaoqin Zhu*[1]*, PhD and Kin-Man Chan*[7]*, PhD
[1]Department of Applied Social Sciences, The Hong Kong Polytechnic University, Hong Kong, PR China,
[2]Centre for Innovative Programmes for Adolescents and Families, The Hong Kong Polytechnic University, Hong Kong, PR China,
[3]Department of Social Work, East China Normal University, Shanghai, PR China,
[4]Kiang Wu Nursing College of Macau, Macau, PR China,
[5]Hong Kong Institute of Service Leadership and Management Limited, Hong Kong, PR China,
[6]Division of Adolescent Medicine, Department of Pediatrics, Kentucky Children's Hospital, University of Kentucky School of Medicine, Lexington, Kentucky, US
[7]Department of Sociology, The Chinese University of Hong Kong, Hong Kong, PR China

Abstract

The growth of the service economy in the contemporary world calls for a shift in the requirement of leadership qualities as compared to the manufacturing economy. However, contemporary leadership approaches and associated leadership behavior scales fail to fully encompass the required leadership qualities in the service economy. To satisfy the emerging needs of service economy which is predominant in Hong Kong, the Service

[*] Correspondence: Associate Vice President (Undergraduate Programme), Chair Professor of Applied Social Sciences and Li and Fung Professor in Service Leadership Education, Department of Applied Social Sciences, The Hong Kong Polytechnic University, Hung Hom, Hong Kong, PR China. E-mail: daniel.shek@polyu.edu.hk.

Leadership Model has been proposed by the Hong Kong Institute of Service Leadership and Management Limited. To objectively assess service leadership behavior, the Service Leadership Behavior Scale (SLB) was developed. This chapter presents the background of the development of the Service Leadership Model, outlines its unique features as the theoretical foundation of the SLB, documents the content of the initial SLB (i.e., SLB-LF-97) regarding its four key domains, and summarizes the findings surrounding the validation studies on the SLB.

INTRODUCTION

Leadership has a long history as a universal human behavior that has evolved to solve adaptive challenges throughout history (1). In the contemporary world, leadership is still indispensable for almost every aspect of human life to function effectively in different areas, such as the economic, professional, military, religious, and political fields. Traditionally, leadership is conceived as a dynamic process in which a leader exerts influence on a group to work enthusiastically towards a collective goal (2, 3). However, traditional leadership theories are no longer able to encapsulate the contemporary leadership needs due to the substantial change in economic structure over the world.

During the past few decades, along with the growing globalization and technological innovation, the structure of global economy has transformed from an industrial to a postindustrial mode, which is characterized by the expansion of service industries and the shrinking of manufacturing industries (4). For example, from 2000 to 2016, the share of the services sector (e.g., trades, financial, personal services, etc.) in Gross Domestic Product (GDP) has increased from 64.9% to 69.3% in Japan, from 87.3 to 92.2 in Hong Kong, and from 39.8% to 51.6% in mainland China (5). The manufacturing economy makes tangible goods from tangible raw materials through standardized procedures, which involve little human interactions or employees' personal input. In such circumstance, leadership is usually task-oriented and the top-down leadership style with highly centralized decision-making and minimal empowerment of followers appears to be adaptive due to its high standardization in mass production process (6). In contrast, the service economy produces intangible services through personalized interactions between service providers and recipients, which call for distributed leadership and "service leaders" who are service-oriented and people-oriented (6).

A number of leadership scholars came to realize the emerging requirements of service-oriented economy and regarded leadership as a relational process between leader and followers instead of merely focusing on the leader (7). In fact, different leadership models have been proposed in the postindustrial era to highlight adaptive leadership styles as well as vital qualities associated with each style. For example, the transformational leadership theory highlights ethical behavior and willingness to change of an effective transformational leader, who demonstrates idealized influence, inspirational motivation, personalized consideration, and intellectual stimulation (8). Similarly, servant leadership theory primarily focuses on the leader's motivation to serve others and give priority to others' needs rather than their own (9). Based on these leadership models, a considerable number of instruments have also been developed to measure leadership qualities in terms of knowledge, attitude, skill or behavior. For example, Multifactor Leadership Questionnaire (10) and Transformational Leadership Scale (11) are two examples of widely used leadership behavior scales.

Apart from these endeavors, some scholars have explicitly highlighted the importance of people skills (or interpersonal competence) in determining leadership effectiveness, such as communication and teamwork, which are also highly desired by contemporary employers (12). Additionally, shared decision-making has been gradually adopted in organizations and new assessment tools have been developed to capture effective empowering leader behaviors (13). Furthermore, there is a growing tendency to emphasize the ethical parts of leadership and value moral behaviors and qualities such as integrity, trust, honesty and caring (14, 15).

The above-mentioned developments in leadership literature have deepened our understanding of the leadership requirements in a postindustrial age. Unfortunately, these advances are not adequate to satisfy the needs of service economy. Particularly, there are still three problems need to be addressed. First, previous leadership theories or related studies stressed some of the requirements for an effective "service leader", such as interpersonal competence or ethical concerns. In other words, there is a lack of holistic leadership framework which can fully encompass required leadership qualities in service economy. Second, the existing leadership behavior scales developed based on previous theories are not able to comprehensively assess effective leadership behaviors in service economy. For instance, transformational leadership scales primarily assess a leader's skills in satisfying the needs of followers and the organization by motivating and stimulating the followers as well as demonstrating ethical behaviors as a role model (11, 16). However, other constructs desired in service economy such as a leader's people skills and caring characteristics were not included. Third, as mentioned above, the service industry is of dominance in Hong Kong and growing rapidly in mainland China. However, little effort has been devoted to delineating what an ideal "service leader" is with specific reference to the Chinese culture. Most important of all, leadership assessment tools including behavior scales that are tailor-made for Chinese people are also missing. This issue is particularly relevant when we consider the possibility that culture values may shape one's understanding of leadership which lead to particular ideal leadership practices in a specific culture (17, 18). Indeed, some scholars have advocated for considering cultural settings and traditional Chinese wisdom in studying contemporary leadership practices in China (19).

To address these issues, Chung (20) proposed the notion of "servicc leadership" which is conceived as "satisfying needs by consistently providing quality personal service to everyone one comes into contact with, including one's self, others, groups, communities, systems, and environments" (20). Based on this notion, the Service Leadership Model was developed as a theoretical foundation to guide service leadership education in Hong Kong (21, 22). Moreover, based on the Service Leadership Model, service leadership scales were tentatively developed for the purpose of assessing service leadership qualities and evaluating the effectiveness of service leadership education (23-25). This chapter will focus on one of the service leadership assessment instruments, namely "Service Leadership Behavior Scale" (SLB). In following sections, we will briefly introduce several distinguishing features of the Service Leadership Model, based on which the item pool of the SLB was constructed. Second, the work surrounding the development and validation of the SLB will be outlined as well.

UNIQUE FEATURES OF THE SERVICE LEADERSHIP MODEL

The notion of service leadership incorporates and goes beyond the propositions of the extant leadership theories in the postindustrial era by adopting the strengths of previous theories and adding new arguments that are seldom mentioned in other leadership approaches. In other words, service leadership theory shares some commonalities with other classic leadership approaches, while it has its own distinct features (6). In particular, the uniqueness of the Service Leadership Model is manifested in its seven core beliefs, which systematically address what is effective service leadership as well as its determinants. As the seven core beliefs have been presented elsewhere in details (22), we briefly highlight several notable ideas of the Service Leadership Model, which reflect the paradigm shift in leadership mindset and serve as the principal references of the development of SLB.

First, the Service Leadership Model strongly emphasizes service orientation. Instead of treating leadership as a means of achieving personal and organizational success, the Service Leadership Model holds that leadership is "a service aimed at ethically satisfying the needs of self, others, groups, communities, systems, and environments" (22). The underlying belief is that people evolved service propensities as an outcome of natural selection, so that both serving others and being served by others are inherent tendencies hard-wired into human minds (26). Therefore, leadership prioritizing service can reach the hearts of people and thus satisfy the needs of others and the leaders themselves.

Second, in strong contrast to traditional conception of leadership that leaders were "great men and women" (27), the Service Leadership Model contends that "every day, every human occupies a position of leadership and possess the potential to improve his or her leadership quality and effectiveness" (22). Primarily, the notion of "everyone can be a leader" enhances confidence in every individual and encourages all employees to contribute to decision-making, constituting a timely response to the needs of distributed leadership in service economy. Besides, to take a leading role effectively whenever is necessary, one should take initiatives and be well-prepared by continuously improving one's abilities and willingness to provide high-quality service. Therefore, self-leadership by means of actively engaging in self-reflection, self-management, and self-improvement is regarded as indispensable for one to achieve leadership success.

Table 1. Literature review on measures of leadership behavior and service leadership

Steps	Details
Step 1: Literature Review on leadership behavior measures, particularly in different Chinese contexts	Example of references: - Aycan, Z., Schyns, B., Sun, J. M., Felfe, J., & Saher, N. (2013). Convergence and divergence of paternalistic leadership: A cross-cultural investigation of prototypes. *Journal of International Business Studies, 44*(9), 962-969. - Chan, SCH., & Mak, W. M. (2014). The impact of servant leadership and subordinates' organizational tenure on trust in leader and attitudes. *Personnel Review, 43*(2), 272-287. - Chen, X. P., Eberly, M. B., Chiang, T. J., Farh, J. L., & Cheng, B. S. (2014). Affective trust in Chinese leaders linking paternalistic leadership to employee performance. *Journal of Management, 40*(3), 796-819. - Cheng, B. S., Chou, L. F. & Farh, J. L. (2000). A triad model of Paternalistic Leadership: The constructs and measurement. *Indigenous Psychological Research in Chinese Societies, 14*, 3-64. (in Chinese) - Li, C., Shi, K. (2005). The Structure and Measurement of Transformational Leadership in China. *Frontiers Bus Res China, 2*(4), 571-590. - Qian, J., Lin, X., & Chen, G. Z. X. (2012). Authentic leadership and feedback-seeking behaviour: An examination of the cultural context of mediating processes in China. *Journal of Management & Organization, 18*(3), 286-299. - Sun, J. M. & Wang, B. (2009). Servant leadership in China: Conceptualization and measurement. *In:* Mobley WH, Wang Y, Li M, eds. *Advances in global leadership.* Bingley: Emerald Group, *5:*321-344. - Sheer, V. C. (2013). In search of Chinese paternalistic leadership: Conflicting evidence from samples of mainland China and Hong Kong's small family businesses. *Management Communication Quarterly, 27*(1), 34-60. - Wang, Y. & Chen, W. M. (2012). Study on the Structural Dimensions of the Authentic Leadership in Enterprises. *East China Economic Management, 7*, 98–101. (In Chinese)
Step 2: Literature Review on Service Leadership	Example of references: - Chung, P. P. Y. (2012). *Service reborn: The knowledge, skills and attitudes of service companies.* New York, NY: Lexingford Publishing. - Chung, P. P. Y. & Bell A. H. (2015). *The 25 Principles of Service Leadership.* New York, NY: Lexingford Publishing. - Shek, D. T. L., Chung, P. P. Y., & Leung, H. (2015). How unique is the service leadership model? A comparison with contemporary leadership approaches. *International Journal on Disability and Human Development, 14*(3), 217-231. - Shek, D. T. L., Chung, P. P. Y., & Leung, H. (2015). Manufacturing economy vs. service economy: Implications for service leadership. *International Journal on Disability and Human Development, 14*(3), 205-215. - Shek, D. T. L., & Lin, L. (2015). Core beliefs in the service leadership model proposed by the Hong Kong Institute of Service Leadership and Management. *International Journal on Disability and Human Development, 14*(3), 233-242. - Shek, D. T. L., Sun, R. C. F., & Liu, T. T. (2015). Character strengths in Chinese philosophies: Relevance to service leadership. *International Journal on Disability and Human Development, 14*(4), 309-318. - Shek, D. T. L., & Yu, L. (2015). Character strengths and service leadership. International *Journal on Disability and Human Development, 14* (4), 299-307.

Third, it is believed that "leadership effectiveness is dependent on possessing relevant situational task competencies plus being judged by superiors, peers, and subordinates as possessing character and exhibiting care" (22). To elaborate, the Service Leadership Model places equal importance on the three fundamental determinants in defining effective service leadership (*E*), namely *m*oral character (*M*), *c*ompetence (*C*), and *c*aring disposition (C) (i.e., $E = MC^2$). By covering a wide range of personal qualities in multiple dimensions, this framework extends beyond conventional leadership theories focusing on leadership skills and establishes a more holistic model to explain how these characteristics jointly contribute to effective leadership in service economy.

Finally, the Service Leadership Model incorporates the Chinese traditional values and integrates the philosophy of Buddhism, Confucianism, and Taoism, aiming to "help East meet West" (28). Concerning the notion of "thinking globally while acting locally", one can argue that when participating in leadership in the Chinese communities, in addition to the universally preferred leadership qualities such as problem-solving and efficiency, an effective leader should also be aware of and demonstrate the qualities historically valued in the Chinese culture such as the ability to maintain harmony and have constant self-reflection.

THE SERVICE LEADERSHIP BEHAVIOR SCALE (SLB)

With reference to the unique propositions of the Service Leadership Model, the research team at The Hong Kong Polytechnic University (PolyU), one of the eight universities funded by the University Grants Committee (UGC) in Hong Kong, developed a long-form of SLB (SLB-LF-97) which consists of 97 items (see Table 1 for the list of related references). With each of the 97 items describing a specific leadership behavior desired in service economy, the SLB-LF-97 covers a wide range of constructs emphasized in the Service Leadership Model. Specifically, the content of the SLB-LF-97 can be subsumed to the following four key domains (see Table 2 for example items).

The first domain is "service provision" (4 items), which measures behaviors related to providing individualized service to others, going beyond one's own interest, and being sensitive to others' unique needs. These behaviors are indicative of a leader's service mindset as well as automatic and genuine manifestation of care for others' needs.

The second domain is related to the Principle "$E = MC^2$", which further includes three aspects: "competence" (38 items), "character" (14 items), and "caring disposition" (15 items). As a key determinant of effective service leadership, leadership competence in service economy has broad requirements including intrapersonal competencies (29) and interpersonal competencies (30). More specifically, the SLB-LF-97 covers four types of intrapersonal competencies underlying effective leadership behaviors. First, 7 items are pertinent to intelligence quotient (IQ) which is manifested in problem-solving capacities, analytical abilities, independent and critical thinking, logical reasoning, and agile mindset. Second, 5 items measure emotional quotient (EQ), which serves as one of the most significant non-intellectual contributors to the success of personal life and career (31). Behaviors pertaining to EQ in the SLB-LF-97 includes understanding, recognizing and managing emotions of oneself and others. Third, 4 items are on the adversity quotient (AQ), which reflects one's ability not only to withstand loss, misfortune, or other types of adversity but also to rebound stronger than before (32). AQ is conceptually similar to the idea of resilience and possessing AQ is deemed vital to one's leadership quality (29). The last type of intrapersonal competencies covered in the SLB-LF-97 is spiritual quotient (SQ), which is closely related to meaning, purpose and values in one's life (33). In the SLB-LF-97, 3 items assess the extent to which one can utilize meaning, faith, and other spiritual resources to solve problems.

Regarding interpersonal competencies, scholars have proposed a five-dimensional framework including "initiating relationships", "self-disclosure", "asserting displeasure with others' actions", "providing emotional support", and "managing interpersonal conflict" (34). These five dimensions have been further adapted and enriched based on Chinese culture and philosophy. Specifically, an effective service leader should be people-oriented ("yi ren wei ben" – people as the central focus) and able to maintain positive social relationships with others. In addition, a good service leader is expected to demonstrate good communication skills in order to build collaborative relationships with teammates and assert one's personal thoughts and feelings when having conflicts with others. Apart from maintaining healthy social relationships, a competent service leader with adequate interpersonal competencies would also appreciate different opinions ("he er bu tong" – peace within diversity) and resolve interpersonal conflicts in a constructive way. As such, six revised components concerning one's ability dealing with interpersonal competencies are intrinsic to the SLB-LF-97: "passionate about people" (2 items); "positive social relationships" (5 items); "assertiveness" (3 items); "collaboration and cooperation with people" (2 items); "conflict resolution" (3 items); and "communication skills" (4 items).

"Character" (14 items) is another aspect under the second domain in the SLB-LF-97, which is also one of the three principle determinants for effective service leadership (35). Drawing on the groundwork of defining universally valued character strengths (e.g., integrity and humility) in Western societies (36) and also taking into account traditional Chinese virtues such as benevolence ("ren"), affection ("ai"), and forgiveness ("shu") (37), the SLB-LF-97 synthesizes strengths of character in both cultures and operationalizes the virtues of an effective service leader using "integrity" (5 items), "humility" (4 items), "fairness" (3 items), and "acting as an ethical role model" (2 items).

The last aspect of the second domain is "caring" (15 items). A caring service leader is supposed to show concern to others as well as to oneself (38). By referring to the Chinese culture, the SLB-LF-97 measures one's caring disposition from two aspects: the qualities of concern ("guan xin") including "empathy" (3 items) and "compassion" (3 items); and the qualities of providing care ("zhao gu") for others in terms of "loving others" (3 items), "supporting others" (3 items), and "developing others" (3 items).

Table 2. Initial development of the Long-Form (SLB-LF-97) and Short-Form (SLB-SF-65) Service Leadership Behavior Scale

Steps	Details
Step 3: Development of the item pool (97 items) with reference to the main proposed domains	Four domains were proposed to be subsumed under the 97-item long-form Service Leadership Behavior Scale (SLB-LF-97) including: [1] **Service Provision** (e.g., I work for the best interests of others instead of just for my own benefit), [2] **Principle "E = MC^2" included three aspects** (e.g., **Moral character**: I am aware of my weaknesses; **Competence**: I am able to argue logically; **Caring disposition**: I show kindness to those whom I had conflict with before.), [3] **Commitment to Continuous Improvement** (e.g., I am self-disciplined), and [4] **Distributed Leadership** (e.g., I respect others' ideas and suggestions).
Step 4: Initial validation of the original scale (i.e., SLB-LF-97)	The SLB-LF-97 was subjected to a validation study involving 231 PolyU students in November 2016. Results of the exploratory factor analysis (EFA) informed the retention of 65 items, forming the trimmed version of the scale (i.e., SLB-SF-65). The SLB-SF-65, alongside its twelve factors (see the list below), overall demonstrated good internal consistency and robust convergent validity. See the paper by Shek, Ma, and Lin in this book.
Step 5: Development of scale used in the main survey (i.e., SLB-SF-65) and the major domains	**Factor 1: Problem-Solving** 6. I am capable of independent thinking. **Factor 2: Self-leadership and Life-long Learning** 47. I spare no effort in achieving my goal. **Factor 3: Non-cognitive Intrapersonal Competences** 10. I am often aware of my emotions. **Factor 4: Distributed Leadership** 65. I hold others' ideas and suggestions in high regard. **Factor 5. Integrity** 31. Others often see me as a reliable person. **Factor 6. Care Provision** 44. I do not miss any chances to help others grow. **Factor 7. Concern** 36. I have no problem sharing my weaknesses with others. **Factor 8. Self-Reflection** 54. I often reflect on my expertise and shortcomings. **Factor 9. Service Provision** 3. I serve others based on their specific needs **Factor 10. Positive Social Relationship** 28. I am capable of developing a rapport with others. **Factor 11. Communication Skills** 24. I am adept at working with others. **Factor 12. Fairness** 35. Treating those around me equally is what I always do.

Note. All sample items were slightly re-worded to avoid familiarity effect.

Table 3. Refined scales based on exploratory factor analyses and confirmatory factor analyses

Steps	Details
Step 6: Refined scale based on exploratory factor analyses (i.e., SLB-SF-48)	Utilizing a subsample (N = 2,246) of the whole dataset (N = 4,486), a principal component analysis (PCA) was performed on the SLB-SF-65. Findings of the PCA suggested that six factors can be extracted with 48 items (loadings above 0.50) retained for the trimmed scale (i.e., SLB-SF-48). The SLB-SF-48 was revealed to be a stable factorial structure and internally consistent. The SLB-SF-48 was also correlated positively and significantly to other external criterion scales and other Service Leadership scales under validation, thereby corroborating its convergent validity. The six factors, each of which forms a subscale, include: [1] **Self-improvement and Self-reflection** (e.g., I have a habit of reflecting my work and life), [2] **People and Principles Orientation** (e.g., I allow others to decide how to get things done), [3] **Resilience** (e.g., I have a sense of purpose in my life which helps me cope with stressful situations), [4] **Social Competence** (e.g., I can maintain positive relationships with others), [5] **Problem-Solving** (e.g., I am good at analyzing problems that I come across), and [6] **Mentorship** (e.g., I can facilitate other's growth by mentoring them). Details can be found in the paper by Shek and Ma in this book.
Step 7: Refined scale based on confirmatory factor analyses (i.e., SLB-SF-38)	The SLB-SF-48 was subjected to CFA on the other subsample (N = 2,240) using the Maximum Likelihood (ML) estimator. The results overall suggested that the fit was unsatisfactory (i.e., CFI = 0.86; NNFI: 0.86; RMSEA = 0.061). Ten items with extreme modification indices (over 40.0) with multiple items on the same factor were removed. The resultant 38-item structure was again subjected to CFA. Findings revealed a considerably better fit (i.e., CFI = 0.90; NNFI: 0.89; RMSEA = 0.056). Furthermore, three pairs of parameters showed particularly large covariance. Accordingly, the correlation between errors was incorporated for these three pairs of parameters. Results of the CFA performed on this modified 38-item solution (i.e., SLB-SF-38) demonstrated that the model fit adequately (i.e., CFI = 0.92; NNFI = 0.91; RMSEA = 0.055) with the data. **The SLB-SF-38, which shared the *same factorial structure* and *labeling as SLB-SF-48*, was accepted as the final solution.** The SLB-SF-38 and the six subscales recorded good internal consistency and were shown to be positively and significantly associated with all external criterion scales. The SLB-SF-38, inclusive of the subscales, also correlated significantly and positively to other Service Leadership scales, further supporting its convergent validity.

Note. All sample items were slightly re-worded to avoid familiarity effect.

The third domain is "commitment to continuous improvement". As aforementioned, one of the key features of the Service Leadership Model is its emphasis on the need for continuous improvement, through which everyone can be a leader at a certain time (39). Besides, only through continuous professional and personal improvement could one be well prepared to serve oneself as well as others. Therefore, effective service leaders should put self-development efforts "aimed at ethically improving one's competencies, abilities, and willingness to help satisfy the needs of others" (22) in terms of promoting self-leadership (5 items), engaging in constant self-reflection (4 items), and committing to life-long learning (4 items).

"Distributed leadership" is the last domain, which also represents a timely response to the belief that "every day, every human occupies a position of leadership and possesses the potential to improve his leadership quality and effectiveness" (22). Distributed leadership in the service economy has two attributes. First, leaders encourage every team member to voice out and take initiatives and empower them to contribute to decision-making of a team. Second, leaders would trust and respect their followers by recognizing their views and trusting their abilities. As such, the domain of "distributed leadership" in the SLB-LF-97 includes three elements: "shared decision-making" (5 items), "empowerment of teammates" (4 items), and "trust and respect" (4 items).

The SLB-LF-97 is developed as a component of the scale development project supported by the Victor and William Fung Foundation. Several validation studies have been carried out to streamline the scale and provide evidence for its reliability and validity (see Table 2 and Table 3). It is worth noting that two papers based on the validation studies are included in this book and other related papers are under preparation. To show a full picture of the development of the Service Leadership Behavior Scale, the section below will briefly outline findings of these validation studies.

Validation of Service Leadership Behavior Scale (SLB)

First, an initial validation study involving 231 PolyU students was conducted to refine the original scale, i.e., SLB-LF-97. Based on the results of the exploratory factor analysis (EFA), 65 out of the 97 items were retained, forming the short form of the scale (i.e., SLB-SF-65). In addition, the SLB-SF-65 alongside its 12 sub-scales (e.g., "problem-solving", "self-leadership and life-long Learning", and "distributed leadership".) demonstrated good internal consistency and robust convergent validity, as indicated by the significant positive correlations with several theoretically linked constructs such as moral self-concept and leadership efficacy. A paper by Shek, Ma, and Lin documenting the psychometric properties of the SLB-SF-65 is included in this book.

Second, using the refined SLB-SF-65, a large-scale validation project was jointly carried out in the eight UGC-funded universities in Hong Kong including PolyU, with the adoption of both exploratory factor analyses (EFA) and confirmatory factor analyses (CFA). Utilizing a subsample (N = 2,246) of the whole dataset (N = 4,486), the EFA revealed a six-factor solution with 48 items (loadings above 0.50) being retained. These 48 items formed the trimmed scale (i.e., SLB-SF-48) as well as the six subscales named as "self-improvement and self-reflection", "people and principles orientation", "resilience", "social competence", "problem-solving", and "mentorship". The SLB-SF-48 was also found to have good reliability and convergent validity. Details of this study and findings of EFA can be found in another paper by Shek and Ma in this issue as well.

Third, the SLB-SF-48 was further subjected to CFA using the other subsample (N = 2,240). After removing 10 items with extreme modification indices (over 40.0), the resultant 38-item structure demonstrated acceptable model fit. Thus, the 38-item scale (i.e., SLB-SF-38), which shared the same 6-factor structure and labelling as SLB-SF-48, was accepted as the final solution. Likewise, the SLB-SF-38 and its six subscales showed good internal consistency and convergent validity. An article presenting the CFA and related findings is under preparation. Information on the related analyses can be seen in the User Manual.

Generally speaking, a well-developed and validated leadership behavior scale regarding service leadership is essential for educators and researchers to empirically evaluate individuals' service leadership qualities and assess their changes after service leadership education. By doing so, the Service Leadership Model as well as its associated propositions such as the principle "$E = MC^2$" can be further validated as well. As such, the development as well as the validation studies for the Service Leadership Behavior Scale not only provide a pioneering assessment tool for contemporary service leadership education, but also represent an important progress in the journal of consolidating the Service Leadership Model.

ACKNOWLEDGMENTS

The validation project is financially supported by the Victor and William Fung Foundation. The preparation for this paper is supported by the Foundation and the Endowed Professorship in Service Leadership Education at The Hong Kong Polytechnic University. This chapter is an updated version of a publication in the special issue "Development and validation of assessment tools on service leadership knowledge, attitude and behavior" edited by Daniel TL Shek, Xiaoqin Zhu and Joav Merrick published in the International Journal of Child and Adolescent Health, 2018;11(4).

REFERENCES

[1] King AJ, Johnson DDP, Van Vugt M. The origins and evolution of leadership. Curr Biol 2009;19(19):R911-6.
[2] Cyert RM. Defining leadership and explicating the process. Nonprofit Manage Leadersh 1990;1(1):29–38.
[3] Northouse PG. Leadership: Theory and practice. 5th ed. Thosand Oaks, CA: Sage, 2010.

[4] Shek DTL, Chung PPY, Leung H. Manufacturing economy vs. service economy: Implications for service leadership. Int J Disabil Hum Dev 2015;14(3):205–15. DOI: 10.1515/ijdhd-2015-0402.
[5] The World Bank. Services, etc., value added (% of GDP), 2016. URL: https://data.worldbank.org/indicator/NV.SRV.TOTL.ZS.
[6] Shek DTL, Chung PPY, Lin L, Leung H, Ng E. Service leadership under the service economy. In: Chin JL, Trimble JE, Garcia JE, eds. Global and culturally diverse leaders and leadership: New dimensions and challenges for business, education and society. Bingley, UK: Emerald Publishing, 2018:143–61.
[7] Bass BM, Bass R. The bass handbook of leadership: Theory, research, and managerial applications, 4th ed. New York: Free Press, 2008.
[8] Bass BM, Avolio BJ. Transformational leadership: A response to critiques. In: Chemers MM, Ayman R, eds. Leadership theory and research: Perspectives and directions. San Diego, CA: Academic Press, 1993:49–80.
[9] Greenleaf RK. The servant as leader. Indianapolis, IN: The Robert K Greenleaf Center, 1970.
[10] Avolio BJ, Bass BM, Zhu FWW. Multifactor leadership questionnaire: Manual and sampler set. 3rd ed. Redwood City, CA: Mind Garden, 2004.
[11] Podsakoff PM, MacKenzie SB, Bommer WH. Transformational leader behaviors and substitutes for leadership as determinants of employee satisfaction, commitment, trust, and organizational citizenship behaviors. J Manage 1996;22(2):259–98.
[12] Osmani M, Weerakkody V, Hindi NM, et al. Identifying the trends and impact of graduate attributes on employability: A literature review. Tert Educ Manag 2015;21(4):367–79. DOI: 10.1080/13583883.2015.1114139.
[13] Arnold JA, Arad S, Rhoades JA, Drasgow F. The empowering leadership questionnaire: The construction and validation of a new scale for measuring leader behaviors. J Organ Behav 2000;21(3):249–69.
[14] Brown ME, Treviño LK. Ethical leadership: A review and future directions. Leadersh Q 2006;17(6):595–616.
[15] Parris DL, Peachey JW. A systematic literature review of servant leadership theory in organizational contexts. J Bus Ethics 2013;113(3):377–93. DOI: 10.1007/s10551-012-1322-6.
[16] Zhang W, Wang H, Pearce CL. Consideration for future consequences as an antecedent of transformational leadership behavior: The moderating effects of perceived dynamic work environment. Leadersh Q 2014;25(2):329-43. DOI: 10.1016/j.leaqua.2013.09.002.
[17] Fu PP, Yukl G. Perceived effectiveness of influence tactics in the United States and China. Leadersh Q 2000;11(2):251-66. DOI: 10.1016/S1048-9843(00)00039-4.
[18] Wong K-C. Chinese culture and leadership. Int J Leadersh Educ 2001;4(4):309-19. DOI: 10.1080/13603120110077990.
[19] Ma L, Tsui AS. Traditional Chinese philosophies and contemporary leadership. Leadersh Q 2015;26(1):13-24. DOI: 10.1016/j.leaqua.2014.11.008.
[20] Chung PPY. Hong Kong Institute of Service Leadership and Management curriculum framework. Hong Kong: Hong Kong Institute of Service Leadership and Management 2011. URL: http://hki-slam.org/index.php?r=article&catid=1&aid=11.
[21] Shek DTL, Chung PPY, eds. Promoting service leadership qualities in university students: The case of Hong Kong. Singapore: Springer; 2015.
[22] Shek DTL, Lin L. Core beliefs in the service leadership model proposed by the Hong Kong Institute of Service Leadership and Management. Int J Disabil Hum Dev 2015;14(3):233-42. DOI: 10.1515/ijdhd-2015-0404.
[23] Shek DTL, Lin L, Leung H, Zhu X. The impact of an intensive service leadership course in mainland China: Objective outcome evaluation. Int J Child Adolesc Health 2017;10(1):63-71.
[24] Shek DTL, Lin L. Changes in university students after joining a service leadership program in China. J Leadersh Educ 2016;15(1):96-109. DOI: 1012806/V15/I1/A2.
[25] Shek DTL, Lin L, Liu TT. Service leadership education for university students in Hong Kong: Subjective outcome evaluation. Int J Disabil Hum Dev 2014;13(4):513-21. DOI: 10.1515/ijdhd-2014-0349.
[26] Shek DTL, Sun RCF, Liu TT. Evolution and realms of service leadership and leadership models. Int J Disabil Hum Dev 2015;14(3):243–54. DOI: 10.1515/ijdhd-2015-0405.
[27] Rost JC. Leadership for the twenty-first century. Westport, CT: Praeger, 1993.

[28] Chung PPY. Service reborn: The knowledge, skills and attitudes of service companies. New York: Lexingford, 2012.
[29] Shek DTL, Lin L. Intrapersonal competencies and service leadership. Int J Disabil Hum Dev 2015;14(3):255-63. DOI: 10.1515/ijdhd-2015-0406.
[30] Shek DTL, Yu L, Siu AMH. Interpersonal competence and service leadership. Int J Disabil Hum Dev 2015;14(3):265-74. DOI: DOI 10.1515/ijdhd-2015-0407.
[31] Mayer JD, Salovey P, Caruso DR. Emotional Intelligence: Theory, findings, and implications. Psychol Inq 2004;15(3):197–215. DOI: 10.1207/s15327965pli1503_02.
[32] Stoltz PG. Adversity quotient: Turning obstacles into opportunities. Hoboken, NJ: John Wiley, 1997.
[33] Zohar D, Marshall I. Spiritual intelligence: The ultimate intelligence. London: Bloomsbury, 2012.
[34] Buhrmester D, Furman W, Wittenberg MT, Reis HT. Five domains of interpersonal competence in peer relationships. J Pers Soc Psychol 1988;55(6):991-1008. DOI: 10.1037/0022-3514.55.6.991.
[35] Shek DTL, Yu L. Character strengths and service leadership. Int J Disabil Hum Dev 2015;14(4):299-307. DOI: 10.1515/ijdhd-2015-0451.
[36] Park N, Peterson C, Seligman MEP. Character strengths in fifty-four nations and the fifty US states. J Posit Psychol 2006;1(3):118-29. DOI: 10.1080/17439760600619567.
[37] Shek DTL, Sun RCF, Liu TT. Character strengths in Chinese philosophies: Relevance to service leadership. Int J Disabil Hum Dev 2015;14(4):309-18. DOI: 10.1515/ijdhd-2015-0452.
[38] Shek DTL, Li X. The role of a caring disposition in service leadership. Int J Disabil Hum Dev 2015;14(4):319-32. DOI: 10.1515/ijdhd-2015-0453.
[39] Shek DTL, Chung PPY, Leung H. How unique is the service leadership model? A comparison with contemporary leadership approaches. Int J Disabil Hum Dev 2015;14(3):217-31. DOI: 10.1515/ijdhd-2015-0403.

In: Service Leadership
Editors: Daniel TL Shek, Xiaoqin Zhu, Li Lin et al.
ISBN: 978-1-53614-852-7

Chapter 6

PSYCHOMETRIC PROPERTIES OF THE SERVICE LEADERSHIP BEHAVIOR SCALE: PRELIMINARY FINDINGS

Daniel TL Shek[1-6,*], PhD, FHKPS, BBS, SBS, JP, Lawrence K Ma[1], PhD, Li Lin[1], PhD and Hildie Leung[1], PhD

[1]Department of Applied Social Sciences, The Hong Kong Polytechnic University, Hong Kong, PR China,
[2]Centre for Innovative Programmes for Adolescents and Families, The Hong Kong Polytechnic University, Hong Kong, PR China,
[3]Department of Social Work, East China Normal University, Shanghai, PR China,
[4]Kiang Wu Nursing College of Macau, Macau, PR China,
[5]Hong Kong Institute of Service Leadership and Management Limited, Hong Kong, PR China
[6]Division of Adolescent Medicine, Department of Pediatrics, Kentucky Children's Hospital, University of Kentucky School of Medicine, Lexington, Kentucky, US

ABSTRACT

Using a sample of 231 students recruited from The Hong Kong Polytechnic University (PolyU), this paper reports the findings of a validation study for the 97-item long-form of the Service Leadership Behavior Scale (SLB-LF-97), which was specifically designed to

---

[*] Correspondence: Daniel TL Shek, PhD, FHKPS, BBS, SBS, JP, Associate Vice President (Undergraduate Programme), Chair Professor of Applied Social Sciences and Li and Fung Professor in Service Leadership Education, Department of Applied Social Sciences, The Hong Kong Polytechnic University, Hung Hom, Hong Kong, PR China. E-mail: daniel.shek@polyu.edu.hk.

measure the behavioral characteristics of a quality Service Leader. Results showed that the SLB-LF-97 had high internal consistency and convergent validity. Exploratory factor analysis revealed that 12 factors were extracted from the data, with 65 items retained to form the short-form of the inventory (SLB-SF-65). Both the long-form (SLB-LF-97) and the short-form (SLB-SF-65) of the scale showed excellent internal consistency, with the latter demonstrating robust convergent validity as shown by its significant positive correlation with several theoretically linked constructs.

INTRODUCTION

Regarding the transformation of manufacturing-driven to service-driven and knowledge-based economies typical of advanced capitalist societies (1-3), Hong Kong has undergone the most complete and swift transition, despite the absence of any strategic political planning (4). As such, Po Chung, Chairman of the Hong Kong Service Leadership and Management Limited (HKI-SLAM), strongly advocated the necessity to teach undergraduates in Hong Kong about effective leadership in a service economy which is vital to their career aspirations as well as personal growth (3, 5). Indeed, the HKI-SLAM is committed to the development of sustainable Service Leadership education (i.e., SLAM curriculum framework) tailored to tertiary institutions in Hong Kong (6, 7).

Against such a background, a multi-year project entitled the "Fung Service Leadership Education Initiative (FSLEI)" was implemented in eight local universities funded by the University Grants Committee (UGC). The FSLEI was conceived with the financial support of the Victor and William Fung Foundation and the collaborative effort of the HKI-SLAM and the UGC. Under the FSLEI, each participating institution independently designs curriculum materials and programs on Service Leadership based on the SLAM curriculum framework (6-8). Particularly, Chung (9, 10) contended that there are three fundamental building blocks of effective Service Leadership (**E**), namely, *competence* (**C_1**; "Expertise" dimension), *moral character* (**M**; "Moral" dimension), and *caring disposition* (**C_2**; "Compassion" dimension). Besides, the seven Core Beliefs [i.e., CBs 1 to 7] pertaining to Service Leadership and Management outlined by HKI-SLAM (11) also underlie the theoretical foundation of Service Leadership education under the FSLEI (7).

With the purpose of filling the research gap on the evaluation of leadership education (8, 12), as well as facilitating the objective assessment of qualities of an effective Service Leader (13), the research team at The Hong Kong Polytechnic University (PolyU) embarked on a project entitled "Development and validation of measures based on the Service Leadership model (i.e., "The Project" hereafter)" (14). Through the construction and validation of three scales on attitude, behavior, and knowledge which constitute the three defining attributes of an effective Service Leader (12), Shek and colleagues (14) developed three related assessment tools. The present paper reports the findings of a validation study of the long-form of Service Leadership Behavior Scale (SLB-LF-97).

Table 1. Four sample items of the SLB-LF-97

Items	Very Dissimilar to Me	Moderately Dissimilar to Me	Slightly Dissimilar to Me	Slightly Similar to Me	Moderately Similar to Me	Very Similar To Me
10. I can make convincing arguments.	1	2	3	4	5	6
18. I draw meaning from undesirable experience.	1	2	3	4	5	6
58. I find it hard to think from other people's perspectives. (Reverse-item)	1	2	3	4	5	6
89. I usually do not let others participate in the decision-making process. (Reverse-item)	1	2	3	4	5	6

Note. These sample items were slightly modified out of copyright concern.

Designed to examine the "kind of behavioral qualities a Service Leader should demonstrate" (14), the SLB-LF-97 comprises 97 English items developed based on the SLAM curriculum framework, 25 principles of Service Leadership (9), 12 dimensions of a Service Leader (10), and other relevant publications from the leadership and management literature (15-17). Each item describes a specific leadership behavior related to the Service Leadership model. Participants were asked to use a six-point Likert scale (1: very dissimilar to me; 6: very similar to me) to evaluate whether each statement appropriately describes one's behavior in a situation which warrants his/her leadership (see Table 1 for the sample items). Resembling Yukl's (18) proposed a hierarchical taxonomy of leadership behaviors, the SLB-LF-97 covered a wide range of component behaviors subsumed under four "metacategories". These "metacategories" included, i) service provision, ii) principle **E** (effective leadership) = $\mathbf{MC^2}$ (Moral character * Competence * Caring disposition), iii) commitment to continuous improvement, and iv) distributed leadership.

The SLB-LF-97 was also examined in a content validation study which is described in detail in another paper under preparation. While it is crucial in scale development to examine content validity, which informs how each item represents the construct being measured (19), it is equally important to establish the convergent validity of the measure, which can be derived from "correlations with measures purporting to measure related constructs" (20, p. 179), as well as internal consistency for the measurement tool under validation. Hence, as a preliminary step paving the way for the main study, the present study utilized a sample of 231 PolyU students to examine the reliability, factorial validity, and convergent validity of the SLB-LF-97.

OUR STUDY

A total of 231 students at The Hong Kong Polytechnic University (PolyU) completed the questionnaire used in the present study via an online survey platform. Seventeen questionnaires were excluded from the working sample due to concern about response quality. Amongst the 214 valid questionnaires, 60 (28.0%) were male respondents while 154 (72.0%) were female respondents. Most participants (55.1%) were aged 20 to 24 years (mean age: 20.0 years, SD: 1.86). The majority of respondents had previous work experience (86.0%), had taken one (or more) credit-bearing Service Leadership course(s) at PolyU (52.9%), and received other prior leadership training (32.2%). Taken as a whole, 76.6 % of respondents claimed to possess "some" or "a lot of" knowledge about Service Leadership. Finally, 49.5% were admitted to PolyU based on performance on the Hong Kong Diploma of Secondary Education Examination (HKDSE). Details regarding other basic demographics of the sample are featured in Table 2.

Table 2. Demographic information for the current working sample (N= 214)

Demographic variables		N= 214
Gender	Male	60 (28.0%)
	Female	154 (72.0%)
Age group	15 to 19 years	92 (43.0%)
	20 to 24 years	118 (55.1%)
	25 to 29 years	4 (1.9%)
Year commencing on one's undergraduate study	2016	103 (48.1%)
	2015	52 (24.3%)
	2014	23 (10.7%)
	2013	30 (14.0%)
	2012 or before	6 (2.8%)
Faculty	Faculty of Applied Science and Textiles	17 (7.9%)
	Faculty of Business	36 (16.8%)
	Faculty of Construction and Environment	27 (12.6%)
	Faculty of Engineering	60 (28.0%)
	Faculty of Health and Social Sciences	47 (22.0%)
	Faculty of Humanities	3 (1.4%)
	School of Design	1 (0.5%)
	School of Hotel and Tourism Management	22 (10.3%)
	Others	1 (0.5%)
Number of credit-bearing Service Leadership (SL) courses taken*	0	101 (47.2%)
	1	105 (49.1%)
	2	7 (3.3%)
	3	1 (0.5%)
	4	0 (0%)
Participated in the non-credit bearing "Silk Road Youth Leadership Programme"	Yes	3 (1.4%)
	No	211 (98.6%)
Other leadership training or workshops taken?	Yes	69 (32.2%)
	No	145 (67.8%)
Previous work experience	Yes	184 (86.0%)
	No	30 (14.0%)

Demographic variables		N= 214
Self-proclaimed SL knowledge	No knowledge	11 (5.1%)
	Little knowledge	39 (18.2%)
	Some knowledge	128 (59.8%)
	A lot of knowledge	36 (16.8%)
	All the knowledge	0 (0%)
Leadership position ever taken?	Yes	152 (71.0%)
	No	62 (29.0%)
Entrance Exam	Hong Kong Diploma of Secondary Education Examination (HKDSE)	106 (49.5%)
	Hong Kong Advanced Level Examination (HKALE)	4 (1.9%)
	National College Entrance Examination (NCEE) in mainland China	21 (9.8%)
	Associate Degree/Higher Diploma in Hong Kong	35 (16.4%)
	Others (e.g., SAT, Cambridge International Examinations)	48 (22.4%)
Grade Point Average**	Average Grade Point Average (GPA) out of 4.50 (SD)	3.1 (0.5)
Time of completion	Average time (in minutes) taken to complete the survey (SD)	25.0 (6.7)

Note. * The list of credit-bearing SL courses offered by PolyU included i) APSS 1L01 Tomorrow's Leaders, ii) APSS 1A22 Promotion of Leadership Qualities in University Students. iii) APSS 1A21/1A21 M Service Leadership, and iv) APSS 2S09 Service Leadership through Serving Children and Families with Special Needs.

** As the present study was conducted in November 2016, this average GPA metric was computed based only on the responses given by 111 students who did NOT start their undergraduate study at PolyU in 2016.

Procedures

The study was conducted in a computer lab with each student seated in a separate cubicle. Participants were instructed to access the electronic survey implemented via the mySurvey@PolyU electronic survey system. The rationale of the study, instructions on how to participate, the principles of voluntary participation and withdrawal, and the pledge of data confidentiality were detailed in the invitation documents and on the e-survey. It was emphasized during the invitation and before the start that 30 minutes would be required for students to conscientiously complete the whole questionnaire. Each respondent was offered for his/her participation a supermarket gift voucher valued at HK$50 (USD$6.40) and an opportunity to win an iPad Air 2 via a lucky draw. Participants indicated whether they consented to join the study (or to withdraw) on the opening page.

We used time of completion as a proxy for gauging participants' seriousness in completing the survey. Specifically, we regarded responses submitted within half of our suggested time (i.e., 30 minutes) as invalid. Accordingly, 17 cases with a completion time below 15 (mean: 13.3, SD: 2.6) minutes were deleted, resulting in 214 valid cases.

Instruments

The present e-survey consists of items of the long-form of the Service Leadership Behavior Scale (i.e., the 97-item SLB-LF-97). As part of the project entitled "Development and validation of measures based on the Service Leadership model" (14), the SLB-LF-97 was developed based on the SLAM curriculum framework, 25 principles of Service Leadership (9), 12 dimensions of a Service Leader (10), and other published papers from the leadership literature (e.g., 17, 21). The SLB-LF-97 is in English with a six-point Likert scale (1: very dissimilar; 6: very similar). Each item describes a certain leadership behavior whereby participants rate how each description resembles their own behaviors when they assume leadership roles in formal (e.g., workplace) or informal (e.g., family) contexts. Four sample items are illustrated in Table 1.

To assess the convergent validity of the SLB-LF-97, six additional measures based on the personality and leadership literature were administered alongside the SLB-LF-97. These validated criterion inventories included the Revised Servant Leadership Profile (RSLP; 20 items), the Paternal Leadership Scale (PTL; 5 items), the Leadership Attitude and Belief Scale (LABS; 28 items), the Interpersonal Reactivity Index (IRI; 14 items), the Moral Self-Concept Scale (MSC; 8 items), and the Leadership Efficacy Scale (LEF; 8 items). There were also a few closed-ended and open-ended items probing into the demographics of the respondents.

1. **Revised Servant Leadership Profile (RSLP):** The RSLP was developed by Wong and Page (22) as a self-assessment tool which assesses *Servant Leadership* as a multifactorial construct. Of the eight factors outlined in Wong and Page's (22) revised model of *Servant Leadership*, 20 items from five factors considered relevant to the SLAM framework were included in the present study. These five factors included *Empowering and developing others* (5 items), *Serving others* (7 items), *Open, participatory leadership* (2 items), *Inspiring leadership* (2 items), and *Courageous leadership* (4 items). The RSLP operates on a seven-point Likert scale, with a higher composite score denoting a higher propensity to exhibit *Servant Leadership* behaviors. The RSLP was demonstrated to possess excellent internal consistency ($\alpha = 0.93$; mean inter-item correlations = 0.42).
2. **Paternalistic Leadership Scale (PTL):** Developed by Aycan and associates (23), the PTL (5 items) measures *Paternalism* as a leadership style epitomized by a strong sense of hierarchy combined with a fatherly benevolence and moral integrity bestowed upon followers (24, 25). Items were rated on a six-point Likert scale, with a higher score illustrating a greater alignment with the mentality of a paternalistic leader. Reliability analyses underlined the acceptable internal consistency of PTL in the current study ($\alpha = 0.79$; mean inter-item correlations = 0.43).

3. **Leadership Attitude and Belief Scale (LABS):** Developed by Wielkiewicz (17) as a measure of college students' "attitudes and beliefs about regarding the nature of leadership" (p. 337), the LABS is formed of two independent dimensions probing into two distinct thinking styles regarding what leadership should be about. They includedthe *Systemic Thinking Scale* (ST; 14 items) which examines people's construal of leadership as a distributed and decentralized process, as opposed to the *Hierarchical Thinking Scale* (HT; 14 items) which assesses individuals' interpretation of leadership as involving centralization and hierarchies. Items were rated on a five-point Likert scale, with higher scale scores reflecting a greater likelihood to adopt a certain construal of the nature of leadership. Both ST ($\alpha = 0.84$; mean inter-item correlations = 0.28) and HT ($\alpha = 0.83$; mean inter-item correlations = 0.26) recorded meritorious reliability in the present study.
4. **Interpersonal Reactivity Index (IRI):** As a cross-culturally validated assessment tool (see 26-28), the IRI comprises four subscales with each assessing a dimension of empathy (29). Subscales *Perspective Taking* (PT; 7 items) and *Empathic Concern* (EC; 7 items) were adopted in this study. Participants rated the 14 items on a five-point Likert scale, with higher subscale and composite scores indicating higher empathy, which constitutes the roots of compassion as a key dimension of a Service Leader (10). Cronbach's alpha for subscales PT and EC and the composite IRI score were 0.66, 0.67, and 0.73, respectively.
5. **Moral Self-Concept (MSC):** As a subscale under the Chinese Adolescent Self-Esteem Scales (30), the MSC specifically examines students' self-evaluation on areas including i) *Conduct and virtues*, ii) *Self-control and discipline*, and iii) *Altruism*. Participants rated the eight items using a seven-point Likert scale, with a higher composite score representing the respondent's perceived significance of *morality* to oneself, which is a fundamental attribute of leadership effectiveness according to the SLAM curriculum framework (11). The MSC was shown to possess a good internal consistency in the present study ($\alpha = 0.88$; mean inter-item correlations = 0.49).
6. **Leadership Efficacy Scale (LEF):** Developed by Murphy (31), the 8-item LEF constitutes a self-report inventory in which respondents rate their self-perceived capacity to lead. The LEF operates on a five-point Likert scale, with a higher scoreindicative of one's "level of confidence in the knowledge, skills, and abilities associated with leading others" (32, p. 669). Reliability assessment again highlighted a good internal consistency of the LEF ($\alpha = 0.84$; mean inter-item correlations = 0.41).

Data analysis plan

To explore the dimensionality of SLB-LF-97, we performed the exploratory factor analysis (EFA) in this validation study. Specifically, the present EFA was conducted using the principal axis analysis (PAA) with Promax rotation (kappa = 4). Tabachnick and Fidell (33) argued that PAA should be preferred for studies which attempted to reach an uncontaminated theoretical solution and were designed on the basis of several underlying theoretical constructs. Both these criteria matched well with the objectives and nature of the present study. SPSS statistics version 24.0 (IBM) was used to perform descriptive analyses as well as internal consistency, convergent validity, and factorial validity.

Factorial validity analyses

Owing to the large number of survey items involved, we adopted the Minimum Average Partials (MAP) (34) to determine the number of factors to extract a priori as to avoid the issue of over-extraction (35). The MAP, which involves "comparison of systematic and unsystematic variance remaining in a correlation matrix after each factor is extracted" (36, p. 108), has been shown in a simulation study to be the most accurate amongst a host of alternative extraction methods (36). The MAP was administered using the SPSS R-Menu V 2.0 (see 35).

With the purpose of simplifying and enhancing the interpretability of the final factorial solution, we applied two exclusion criteria to help downsize the scale. First, double-loaded items were removed (37). Second, only non- double-loaded items that are of substantive importance (i.e., highest loadings $\geq |0.40|$) to a factor were retained (see 19). Table 3 details the post-rotation factor loadings of each item and other relevant statistics.

Reliability and convergent validity analyses

We referred to the Cronbach's alpha values and mean inter-item correlations as indicators of internal consistency of the scale and the factors derived (i.e., subscales). As regards the assessment of convergent validity, the composite scores calculated by averaging participants' responses of both the scale and subscales were correlated with the six concurrently administered external criterion measures. Specifically, we hypothesized a positive and significant association between the behavior scale (and the subscales) and the i) RSLP (i.e., Hypothesis 1), ii) LEF (i.e., Hypothesis 2), iii) MSC (i.e., Hypothesis 3), and iv) IRI (i.e., Hypothesis 4), considering that *Servant Leadership, leadership efficacy, morality,* and *empathy,* respectively are all constructs theorized to underline the behavioral standard of a bona fide Service Leader (9, 10).

Furthermore, as the SLAM framework is catered to service economies which are characterized by *distributed leadership* and *decentralization* rather than *absolute control* and *centralization* (38), we expected a positive correlation between the behavior scale with the *Systemic Thinking Scale* (i.e., Hypothesis 5) while a negative association with the *Hierarchical Thinking Scale* (i.e., Hypothesis 6). Finally, while paternalistic leadership is characterized by a strong sense of hierarchy which contradicts the SLAM framework

Table 3. Factor loadings of the SLB-LF-97 (N = 214)

			Factors extracted												
	M	SD	1	2	3	4	5	6	7	8	9	10	11	12	13	Retained?
SLB-01	4.51	1.04	-0.01	-0.05	0.00	-0.16	-0.11	-0.04	-0.02	0.04	**0.77**	-0.02	0.06	0.09	0.15	Yes
SLB-02	4.28	1.05	-0.03	0.00	-0.03	-0.15	-0.04	0.09	0.01	0.05	**0.81**	-0.14	-0.10	0.12	0.18	Yes
SLB-03	4.76	0.79	0.15	0.16	-0.13	-0.10	0.15	-0.13	0.17	-0.20	**0.64**	0.01	-0.17	0.07	0.14	Yes
SLB-04	4.69	0.93	0.25	0.12	-0.11	-0.05	0.11	-0.02	0.11	0.06	0.38	-0.19	0.13	-0.01	0.48	No
SLB-05	4.59	0.92	**0.59**	0.09	0.16	0.01	0.08	0.07	0.00	-0.02	0.04	-0.18	-0.01	0.06	0.17	Yes
SLB-06	4.21	0.96	**0.63**	0.15	0.19	-0.01	-0.05	0.11	0.02	-0.13	-0.10	-0.11	0.02	0.08	0.04	Yes
SLB-07	4.66	0.98	**0.75**	-0.07	0.03	0.01	0.04	-0.09	0.00	0.07	-0.02	0.01	0.13	0.00	0.08	Yes
SLB-08	4.66	0.95	**0.83**	-0.01	-0.05	0.02	0.01	0.00	0.01	0.00	0.09	-0.15	0.17	-0.05	0.10	Yes
SLB-09	4.63	0.96	**0.69**	-0.13	-0.02	0.06	0.03	-0.08	-0.10	0.17	0.12	0.16	0.12	-0.16	-0.01	Yes
SLB-10	4.47	1.01	**0.66**	-0.01	0.00	-0.02	0.03	0.02	-0.03	0.10	0.04	0.22	0.07	-0.06	-0.04	Yes
SLB-11	4.27	0.92	**0.48**	0.08	0.35	-0.05	0.08	0.16	-0.06	-0.10	-0.20	-0.07	0.04	0.08	-0.01	No
SLB-12	4.87	0.93	-0.02	0.02	**0.54**	0.27	0.05	-0.16	-0.02	0.04	0.03	0.03	-0.05	-0.20	0.11	Yes
SLB-13	4.71	0.92	0.09	-0.03	0.34	0.12	0.05	-0.12	-0.21	0.10	0.20	0.04	0.21	-0.15	0.53	No
SLB-14	4.22	1.14	0.02	-0.07	**0.73**	0.22	-0.24	-0.16	-0.19	-0.19	0.09	0.09	0.10	0.21	0.01	Yes
SLB-15	4.36	1.05	-0.10	-0.01	0.42	-0.04	-0.05	0.01	-0.03	-0.02	0.14	0.19	0.36	-0.09	0.10	No
SLB-16	4.30	1.13	0.09	-0.04	**0.84**	0.20	0.09	-0.11	-0.06	-0.03	-0.15	-0.12	-0.12	0.15	0.02	Yes
SLB-17	4.51	1.07	0.03	-0.07	**0.55**	-0.08	-0.04	-0.01	0.18	0.19	-0.12	-0.14	0.27	0.08	0.09	Yes
SLB-18	4.42	0.95	0.01	-0.08	**0.42**	-0.08	-0.06	0.12	0.19	0.29	-0.04	0.01	0.13	0.03	0.02	Yes
SLB-19	4.60	0.88	0.04	0.05	**0.48**	-0.18	-0.07	0.11	0.03	0.08	0.19	0.00	0.05	0.05	0.01	Yes
SLB-20	4.42	1.07	0.05	0.24	**0.58**	-0.15	-0.05	0.02	0.11	0.13	0.07	0.06	-0.15	-0.07	0.09	Yes
SLB-21	4.29	1.11	-0.02	0.31	**0.50**	-0.13	0.05	0.03	0.10	0.09	0.04	0.02	-0.21	-0.03	-0.14	Yes
SLB-22	4.42	1.07	0.12	-0.07	**0.80**	0.02	0.03	-0.10	-0.17	-0.05	-0.06	0.02	-0.11	0.05	0.01	Yes
SLB-23	4.42	1.11	-0.01	0.06	**0.60**	-0.13	-0.01	-0.08	0.19	-0.01	-0.09	0.05	0.16	0.03	0.03	Yes
SLB-24	4.44	0.81	0.04	-0.21	0.12	-0.08	0.19	0.17	0.21	-0.05	0.26	0.25	-0.09	0.07	0.01	No
SLB-25	4.66	0.82	0.01	-0.25	0.17	-0.05	0.03	0.16	0.36	0.04	0.24	0.28	0.01	0.04	-0.08	No
SLB-26	4.91	0.82	0.09	0.07	-0.05	-0.05	-0.01	0.06	0.12	-0.11	-0.10	**0.77**	0.18	-0.09	-0.07	Yes
SLB-27	4.86	0.89	-0.09	0.13	0.03	0.04	0.19	0.02	-0.08	-0.17	-0.09	**0.67**	0.12	-0.01	0.01	Yes
SLB-28	4.93	0.84	-0.07	-0.06	0.01	0.10	0.10	-0.10	-0.06	0.14	-0.13	**0.77**	0.11	0.01	-0.09	Yes
SLB-29	5.00	0.93	-0.14	0.00	-0.18	-0.12	**0.49**	-0.03	-0.10	0.14	0.22	0.28	-0.01	0.10	-0.05	Yes
SLB-30	4.87	0.89	-0.11	0.04	0.01	0.12	0.19	-0.07	-0.17	0.08	0.26	0.21	-0.02	0.32	0.14	No

Table 3. (Continued)

	M	SD	Factors extracted													Retained?
			1	2	3	4	5	6	7	8	9	10	11	12	13	
SLB-31	4.60	0.85	0.25	-0.11	0.02	0.33	0.07	-0.08	0.12	0.02	-0.02	-0.05	0.38	-0.11	-0.07	No
SLB-32	4.50	0.96	0.33	-0.16	0.16	-0.03	0.10	0.08	0.11	-0.17	0.10	0.16	0.04	0.01	-0.14	No
SLB-33	2.80	1.18	0.14	0.20	-0.05	-0.09	0.14	-0.27	-0.07	-0.08	-0.11	0.18	-0.10	-0.04	-0.29	No
SLB-34	4.60	0.89	-0.08	0.10	0.03	0.02	-0.05	0.15	0.07	-0.11	-0.06	0.23	**0.44**	0.05	0.18	Yes
SLB-35	4.63	0.86	-0.17	0.11	0.00	-0.09	0.17	0.28	-0.01	-0.10	0.03	0.28	0.27	0.04	0.15	No
SLB-36	4.55	0.98	-0.06	-0.01	-0.04	0.14	0.39	0.26	-0.04	-0.09	-0.08	0.13	0.07	-0.12	-0.04	No
SLB-37	4.50	0.91	0.09	0.00	0.25	0.06	0.36	0.18	-0.18	-0.03	0.01	0.04	0.20	-0.12	-0.12	No
SLB-38	4.76	0.84	0.06	0.11	-0.05	0.31	0.04	0.28	-0.21	-0.14	0.25	-0.04	0.25	-0.06	-0.05	No
SLB-39	4.35	1.09	0.17	-0.04	-0.05	-0.05	-0.08	0.23	0.01	-0.03	-0.06	0.14	**0.67**	0.04	0.14	Yes
SLB-40	4.40	1.08	0.30	-0.06	-0.15	0.04	-0.10	0.25	-0.06	0.08	-0.17	0.17	**0.62**	0.05	0.04	Yes
SLB-41	4.64	0.92	0.12	0.03	0.04	0.03	0.12	0.06	-0.15	-0.01	0.05	-0.02	**0.49**	0.03	0.08	Yes
SLB-42	5.03	1.10	-0.12	0.16	0.12	0.24	0.33	-0.17	-0.03	-0.11	-0.08	0.11	0.03	0.07	0.08	No
SLB-43	4.50	0.93	0.20	0.05	0.08	0.14	**0.45**	0.03	0.00	-0.02	-0.08	-0.08	0.09	0.06	0.00	Yes
SLB-44	4.95	0.90	0.13	0.12	0.03	0.04	**0.81**	-0.03	0.00	0.01	-0.16	-0.05	-0.16	0.06	-0.02	Yes
SLB-45	4.97	0.85	0.05	-0.01	-0.08	-0.04	**0.77**	-0.04	0.00	0.08	-0.01	0.04	-0.07	0.21	0.00	Yes
SLB-46	5.05	0.88	0.18	0.11	-0.14	-0.04	**0.60**	-0.14	-0.03	0.01	-0.01	0.07	0.21	0.27	-0.02	Yes
SLB-47	4.71	1.01	-0.05	0.00	0.07	0.12	0.23	0.21	-0.11	0.02	0.23	-0.11	-0.06	**0.44**	0.01	Yes
SLB-48	4.39	1.06	0.00	-0.06	0.10	0.03	0.18	0.17	-0.09	0.04	0.07	-0.02	0.01	**0.68**	-0.08	Yes
SLB-49	4.66	0.91	0.02	0.08	0.09	-0.02	0.11	0.13	-0.03	0.06	0.12	-0.08	0.19	**0.43**	-0.08	Yes
SLB-50	4.39	1.08	-0.08	-0.18	0.10	0.07	0.15	0.17	-0.11	0.16	0.12	0.00	0.04	**0.60**	-0.08	Yes
SLB-51	5.04	0.82	0.04	-0.05	-0.12	0.28	0.19	0.03	0.31	0.11	0.04	-0.01	-0.13	-0.04	-0.02	No
SLB-52	4.27	1.20	0.02	0.03	-0.16	0.04	-0.13	0.13	**0.61**	-0.18	0.13	-0.13	0.04	-0.12	-0.11	Yes
SLB-53	5.04	0.90	0.02	0.24	0.06	0.14	-0.06	-0.05	0.24	-0.06	**0.51**	-0.19	-0.03	0.00	-0.17	Yes
SLB-54	4.82	0.82	-0.08	0.28	-0.03	0.30	0.08	-0.19	0.25	0.09	0.16	-0.02	-0.01	0.04	-0.27	No
SLB-55	4.10	1.03	-0.02	0.06	-0.01	0.08	-0.03	0.13	0.18	0.01	0.05	0.06	0.22	0.24	0.01	No
SLB-56	4.39	0.94	-0.02	0.00	0.09	0.03	-0.14	0.27	0.02	0.10	0.24	0.06	0.21	0.23	0.03	No
SLB-57	5.19	0.80	-0.05	0.04	0.16	0.18	**0.41**	0.04	0.14	-0.16	0.20	-0.08	-0.02	-0.04	0.11	Yes
SLB-58	4.25	1.20	0.08	-0.09	0.01	0.43	-0.04	-0.37	-0.04	0.15	0.25	0.14	-0.05	-0.17	0.20	No
SLB-59	4.56	0.92	0.12	0.01	0.01	0.15	0.01	0.03	0.25	0.03	0.02	0.12	0.06	-0.11	0.38	No
SLB-60	4.70	0.80	0.16	-0.05	-0.10	-0.02	0.20	0.37	0.40	-0.05	0.00	0.07	-0.19	-0.02	0.22	No

			Factors extracted												
	M	SD	1	2	3	4	5	6	7	8	9	10	11	12	13	Retained?
SLB-61	4.87	0.89	0.05	-0.04	0.06	0.06	-0.08	0.07	**0.64**	0.09	0.01	0.14	-0.21	-0.12	0.11	Yes
SLB-62	4.58	1.04	-0.05	-0.17	0.07	0.06	0.17	0.21	**0.48**	0.01	-0.08	-0.07	0.14	-0.07	0.12	Yes
SLB-63	4.48	0.99	0.00	-0.01	0.02	0.36	-0.23	0.37	0.01	0.00	0.06	0.08	-0.01	0.09	-0.04	No
SLB-64	4.58	1.02	0.12	-0.09	-0.15	0.23	0.19	0.38	0.04	-0.11	0.14	0.01	-0.06	0.19	0.03	No
SLB-65	3.79	1.35	0.11	-0.01	0.11	0.05	-0.23	-0.12	0.16	-0.15	0.13	0.34	-0.13	0.20	-0.05	No
SLB-66	4.75	0.84	-0.14	-0.02	-0.05	0.12	0.30	**0.42**	0.09	0.00	0.14	-0.06	0.03	-0.02	0.19	Yes
SLB-67	4.82	0.82	-0.13	0.07	-0.01	0.23	0.21	**0.43**	-0.03	0.06	-0.01	-0.05	0.03	-0.01	0.19	Yes
SLB-68	4.81	0.95	-0.07	0.10	0.07	0.05	0.29	0.22	0.28	-0.10	-0.06	0.00	0.13	-0.11	0.16	No
SLB-69	4.46	0.98	0.10	0.17	-0.10	-0.05	-0.12	**0.58**	0.06	0.00	-0.01	0.06	0.24	-0.01	0.12	Yes
SLB-70	4.14	1.04	-0.03	0.07	-0.03	-0.09	-0.05	**0.66**	0.17	0.07	-0.02	-0.06	0.18	0.06	-0.04	Yes
SLB-71	4.21	1.09	-0.14	0.09	-0.11	-0.11	0.03	**0.64**	0.08	-0.03	0.12	-0.01	0.16	0.07	0.00	Yes
SLB-72	4.45	1.07	-0.07	**0.71**	0.23	-0.08	0.18	-0.16	-0.16	-0.04	-0.07	0.08	0.05	0.01	-0.01	Yes
SLB-73	4.88	0.89	-0.01	**0.91**	-0.10	-0.07	0.08	-0.03	-0.01	-0.04	0.08	-0.09	-0.02	-0.10	0.04	Yes
SLB-74	4.94	0.86	-0.10	**0.58**	0.05	0.10	-0.17	0.08	-0.04	0.18	0.24	-0.05	-0.03	-0.12	0.21	Yes
SLB-75	4.68	1.00	-0.09	**0.77**	0.03	-0.03	0.18	0.00	-0.07	-0.02	-0.06	0.02	0.04	-0.05	-0.05	Yes
SLB-76	4.64	1.02	0.09	**0.48**	-0.05	-0.19	0.12	-0.21	0.19	0.23	0.00	0.10	0.20	-0.02	-0.15	Yes
SLB-77	4.92	0.94	0.05	0.23	-0.08	0.03	0.08	0.11	-0.17	**0.69**	-0.01	0.01	-0.05	0.01	0.09	Yes
SLB-78	5.00	0.93	0.08	0.00	-0.04	0.15	-0.12	0.09	-0.06	**0.79**	-0.02	0.01	-0.11	0.08	0.07	Yes
SLB-79	4.81	0.97	-0.02	0.04	0.16	-0.09	0.02	-0.05	-0.07	**0.80**	0.01	-0.08	0.05	0.10	0.08	Yes
SLB-80	4.80	0.95	0.01	0.04	-0.08	0.09	0.09	-0.06	0.09	**0.72**	0.01	-0.10	0.09	0.02	0.00	Yes
SLB-81	5.10	0.79	0.10	**0.52**	0.00	0.15	-0.11	0.19	0.05	0.07	-0.02	0.07	-0.06	-0.03	-0.15	Yes
SLB-82	5.08	0.83	0.05	**0.46**	-0.12	0.08	0.03	0.16	-0.02	0.27	-0.10	0.16	-0.03	0.04	-0.03	Yes
SLB-83	4.90	0.86	0.12	**0.48**	-0.04	0.23	-0.12	0.21	0.01	0.02	-0.03	0.05	-0.01	-0.03	-0.05	Yes
SLB-84	4.88	0.89	0.09	**0.48**	-0.10	0.23	-0.06	0.22	-0.09	0.14	-0.09	0.04	-0.09	0.07	-0.03	Yes
SLB-85	4.51	0.95	0.00	0.03	0.10	0.16	0.04	**0.40**	0.05	0.02	-0.05	0.15	-0.09	0.18	-0.10	Yes
SLB-86	5.11	0.79	-0.02	-0.05	0.07	**0.62**	0.12	0.12	-0.06	0.09	-0.04	-0.01	-0.03	0.10	-0.04	Yes
SLB-87	4.44	0.98	0.00	0.04	0.15	**0.65**	0.10	0.06	0.06	0.01	-0.20	-0.05	-0.10	0.04	-0.18	Yes
SLB-88	3.74	1.33	-0.09	-0.09	0.02	0.38	0.19	0.08	0.17	0.12	-0.19	-0.08	-0.06	-0.14	0.00	No
SLB-90	4.67	0.91	-0.07	-0.04	-0.04	**0.50**	-0.09	-0.25	0.33	-0.01	-0.06	-0.10	0.25	0.14	0.04	No
SLB-91	4.82	0.79	0.01	0.21	0.05	**0.59**	-0.16	-0.19	0.06	-0.11	-0.06	0.05	0.10	0.10	0.15	Yes
SLB-92	4.44	0.98	0.16	-0.03	-0.09	**0.54**	-0.02	-0.04	0.12	-0.02	-0.09	0.01	0.15	0.02	0.14	Yes
SLB-93	3.74	1.33	-0.13	0.08	0.08	0.13	-0.03	**-0.44**	0.12	-0.03	0.07	0.02	-0.04	-0.09	0.01	Yes
SLB-94	4.66	0.78	-0.01	0.07	0.09	0.32	-0.13	0.28	0.10	0.06	-0.14	0.03	0.03	0.02	0.13	No

Table 3. (Continued)

	M	SD	Factors extracted 1	2	3	4	5	6	7	8	9	10	11	12	13	Retained?
SLB-95	5.16	0.78	-0.02	-0.04	-0.03	**<u>0.64</u>**	0.16	-0.08	0.15	0.06	-0.16	0.13	-0.02	0.04	0.10	Yes
SLB-96	4.78	0.95	-0.20	0.01	-0.03	0.37	0.03	-0.14	0.58	-0.02	-0.13	-0.01	0.11	0.08	0.04	No
SLB-97	4.63	1.14	-0.06	-0.03	0.01	0.20	0.04	-0.56	0.56	0.01	0.12	0.16	-0.07	0.04	0.02	No
Eigenvalues	27.53	5.00	3.86	2.79	2.75	2.52	2.19	2.09	1.84	1.77	1.73	1.59	1.52[a]			
Variance explained (%)			28.68	5.21	4.02	2.90	2.86	2.63	2.28	2.18	1.91	1.84	1.80	1.66	1.58[a]	
Total variance (%)[b]															57.97[b]	
S1	4.54	0.78														
S2	4.84	0.68	0.47													
S3	4.50	0.71	0.52	0.51												
S4	4.89	0.62	0.32	0.52	0.46											
S5	4.94	0.65	0.41	0.59	0.49	0.54										
S6	4.38	0.63	0.32	0.59	0.48	0.54	0.57									
S7	4.57	0.79	0.14	0.29	0.30	0.32	0.31	0.46								
S8	4.88	0.81	0.43	0.63	0.43	0.35	0.39	0.39	0.21							
S9	4.65	0.70	0.21	0.36	0.35	0.33	0.43	0.46	0.38	0.28						
S10	4.90	0.74	0.34	0.44	0.45	0.43	0.50	0.49	0.31	0.24	0.29					
S11	4.50	0.80	0.49	0.49	0.52	0.41	0.52	0.54	0.32	0.30	0.27	0.57				
S12	4.54	0.85	0.31	0.51	0.54	0.51	0.62	0.57	0.29	0.41	0.48	0.37	0.48			
SLB-LF-97	4.62	0.48	0.60	0.77	0.76	0.71	0.77	0.77	0.51	0.58	0.57	0.65	0.71	0.73		
SLB-SF-65	4.66	0.51	0.64	0.81	0.78	0.68	0.77	0.77	0.47	0.63	0.55	0.63	0.71	0.73		

Note. N = 214. M: mean scores; SD: standard deviation. Bold and underlined values are the highest loadings by a variable which are retained for subsequent analyses. Item SLB-89 was excluded here due to its unacceptable individual measure of sampling adequacy in the initial PAA (i.e., anti-image correlations diagonals <. 0.50). Sixty-five items were retained to form the short-form of the behavior scale (SLB-SF-65) which were subjected to a large-scale validation study involving 4,486 Hong Kong undergraduates.

[a]Item SLB-13, the only sufficiently-loaded (loading ≥ |0.40|) item on Component 13, was removed together with the component. [b]As component 13 only contained one item and was subsequently removed from the final solution, the total variance was computed by the summation of variance explained by the remaining twelve components. SLB-LF-97: 97-item Service Leadership Behavior Scale- Long-Form; SLB-SF-65: 12-factor, 65-item version of SLB-SF-65. S1: Subscale 1 (6 items, *Problem-Solving*); S2: Subscale 2 (9 items, *Self-leadership and Life-long Learning*); S3: Subscale 3 (10 items, *Non-cognitive Intrapersonal Competences*); S4: Subscale 4 (5 items, *Distributed Leadership*); S5: Subscale 5 (6 items; *Integrity*); S6: Subscale 6 (7 items, *Caring Behavior*); S7: Subscale 7 (3 items, *Compassion*); S8: Subscale 8 (4 items, *Self-reflection*); S9: Subscale 9 (4 items, *Service Provision*); S10: Subscale 10 (3 items, *Positive Social Relationship*); S11: Subscale 11 (4 items, *Communication Skills*); S12: Subscale 12 (4 items, *Fairness*). All correlation coefficients are statistically significant at p <.001 (two-tailed).

(7, 38), it also emphasizes leaders' exhibition of benevolence and integrity which correspond to the fundamentals of Service Leadership education (39). As a result, a positive while mild correlation between the behavior scale (and the subscales) and the *Paternalistic Leadership Scale* (PTL) was predicted (i.e., Hypothesis 7).

OUR FINDINGS

Results of the MAP showed that the squared average partial correlation was at a minimum (0.00821) upon the extraction of the thirteenth factor, suggesting that thirteen factors should be retained (40). Item 89 was deleted due to its poor (i.e., anti-image correlations diagonals below 0.50) individual measure of sampling adequacy (19). Accordingly, the PAA was re-administered on the remaining 96 items specifying the extraction of thirteen factors. Each item's factor loadings, eigenvalues, the percentage of variance explained by each factor, and the correlations amongst the different factors are presented in table 3.

Applying the two exclusion criteria as abovementioned, nine double-loaded items were first eliminated. This was followed by the removal of 21 insufficiently-loaded items. Item 13, the only item loaded sufficiently on the thirteenth factor (see Table 3), was deleted as well. Ultimately, the resultant 65-item, twelve-factor solution—which accounted for 57.97% of the total variance—formed the short-form of the Service Leadership Behavior Scale (SLB-SF-65). The twelve factors, each of which forms a subscale, were accordingly named "Problem-Solving" (items 5 to 10), "Self-leadership and Life-long Learning" (items 72 to 76, 81 to 84), "Non-cognitive Intrapersonal Competences" (items 12, 14, 16 to 23), "Distributed Leadership" (items 86, 87, 91, 92, 95), "Integrity" (items 29, 43 to 46, 57), "Caring Behavior" (items 66, 67, 69 to 71, 85, 93), "Compassion" (items 52, 61, 62), "Self-reflection" (items 77 to 80), "Service Provision" (items 1 to 3, 53), "Positive Social Relationship" (items 26 to 28), "Communication Skills" (items 34, 39 to 41), and "Fairness" (items 47 to 50).

Reliability of the total scale and subscales

As detailed in Table 4, both long-form (SLB-LF-97) and short-form (SLB-SF-65) of the behavior scale showed excellent internal consistency (all α values $\geq .95$, mean inter-item correlations $> .20$) in the whole sample ($N = 214$) and across two subsamples split based on participants' gender. All subscales, except for the three-item subscale "Compassion", demonstrated at least acceptable internal consistency (all α values $\geq .70$, mean inter-item correlations $> .30$).

Table 4. Internal consistencies of SLB-LF-97, SLB-SF-65, and subscales across gender

	Whole Sample (N = 214)		Males (N = 60)		Females (N = 154)	
	α	Mean Inter-item correlations	α	Mean Inter-item correlations	α	Mean Inter-item correlations
Long-Form Service Leadership Behavior Scale (SLB-LF-97)	0.97	0.26	0.97	0.27	0.97	0.25
Short-Form Service Leadership Behavior Scale (SLB-SF-65)	0.96	0.28	0.96	0.29	0.96	0.27
Subscale 1: *Problem-Solving*	0.90	0.59	0.91	0.64	0.89	0.56
Subscale 2: *Self-leadership and Life-long Learning*	0.90	0.51	0.90	0.50	0.90	0.51
Subscale 3: *Non-cognitive Intrapersonal Competences*	0.88	0.42	0.90	0.47	0.86	0.39
Subscale 4: *Distributed Leadership*	0.79	0.44	0.78	0.43	0.79	0.44
Subscale 5: *Integrity*	0.84	0.46	0.85	0.49	0.83	0.45
Subscale 6: *Caring Behavior*	0.74	0.34	0.76	0.35	0.72	0.34
Subscale 7: *Compassion*	0.61	0.35	0.61	0.37	0.59	0.34
Subscale 8: *Self-reflection*	0.88	0.65	0.91	0.73	0.87	0.62
Subscale 9: *Service Provision*	0.73	0.40	0.70	0.36	0.73	0.41
Subscale 10: *Positive Social Relationship*	0.85	0.65	0.88	0.70	0.83	0.61
Subscale 11: *Communication Skills*	0.81	0.52	0.86	0.61	0.78	0.47
Subscale 12: *Fairness*	0.86	0.61	0.88	0.64	0.85	0.59

Note. α = Cronbach's alpha value.

Despite the seemingly unacceptable alpha values (i.e., 0.59 to 0.61), inspection of the range of mean inter-item correlations of subscale "Compassion" (i.e., 0.34 to 0.37) revealed that they all fell within the range (i.e., 0.20 to 0.40) of "optimal level of homogeneity" (p. 114) defined by Briggs and Cheek (41). In short, the present findings provided support for the high reliability of the different forms of the behavior scale and its subscales.

Validity assessment: Correlation with external criterion measures

Confirming Hypotheses 1 to 4, correlational findings (see Table 5) revealed a significant ($p <. 05$, two-tailed), positive correlation between the SLB-SF-65 (and almost all the subscales) and the *Revised Servant Leadership Profile*, *Interpersonal Reactivity Index* (including the composite score and the two subscales), *Moral Self-Concept*, and *Leadership Efficacy*, respectively. Hypothesis 5 was also supported as the *Systemic Thinking Scale* (ST) was significantly and positively associated with the SLB-SF-65 alongside its subscales (see Table 5). Echoing Hypothesis 7, despite the statistical significance ($p <.05$, two-tailed), the SLB-SF-65 was only mildly correlated (r = 0.25) to the *Paternalistic Leadership Scale* (PTL). Similar findings (see Table 5) emerged when the subscales were correlated with PTL (rs ranging from 0.04 to 0.25), further supporting Hypothesis 7.

Meanwhile, contrary to Hypothesis 6, both SLB-SF-65 and the subscales were positively correlated to the *Hierarchical Thinking Scale* (see Table 5). This may be attributable to the non-mutual exclusiveness of *Hierarchical* (HT) and *Systemic Thinking* (ST) whereby people can be both hierarchical and systemic thinkers (17). Hence, it is possible that the present positive link between HT and SLB-SF-65 ($r = 0.30$) was due to the moderate correlation between ST and SLB-SF-65 ($r = 0.51$) and that of HT and ST ($r = 0.44$). Indeed, once ST was controlled for, the HT-SLB-SF-65 correlation was no longer significant ($p = .17$, two-tailed). In contrast, the ST-SLB-SF-65 link ($r = 0.44$) remained to be moderate even after controlling for HT. In short, while these results seemingly contradicted Hypothesis 6, further scrutiny revealed a pattern of findings that resonated with Wielkiewicz's (17) conceptualization of HT and ST.

Furthermore, utilizing the statistical package *cocor* (42) which allows the comparison of strengths between two pairs of correlation coefficients using Steiger's (43) z-test, the results (see Table 6) highlighted that out of all significant associations, the SLB-SF-65 was most strongly correlated to the *Revised Servant Leadership Profile* ($r = 0.78$) while considerably more weakly associated with the *Paternalistic Leadership Scale* ($r = 0.25$) as well as the *Hierarchical Thinking Scale* ($r = 0.30$). Taken together, these findings are generally supportive of the convergent validity of the SLB-SF-65—which was shown to consistently correlate with various constructs theorized to underscore the behavioral qualities characteristic of an elite Service Leader.

Table 5. Correlations with external criterion scales (and subscales)

	RSLP	PTL	IRI	IRI-EC	IRI-PT	MSC	HT	ST	LEF
Long-Form Service Leadership Behavior Scale (SLB-LF-97)	0.81	0.26	0.51	0.28	0.56	0.75	0.28	0.51	0.56
Short-Form Service Leadership Behavior Scale (SLB-SF-65)	0.78	0.25	0.46	0.25	0.52	0.72	0.30	0.51	0.55
Subscale 1: *Problem-Solving*	0.33	0.04$^{n.s.}$	0.11$^{n.s}$	-0.04$^{n.s.}$	0.22	0.27	0.20	0.28	0.43
Subscale 2: *Self-leadership and Life-long Learning*	0.58	0.24	0.26	0.09$^{n.s.}$	0.34	0.55	0.28	0.47	0.42
Subscale 3: *Non-cognitive Intrapersonal Competences*	0.52	0.10$^{n.s.}$	0.30	0.16	0.34	0.44	0.18	0.29	0.44
Subscale 4: *Distributed Leadership*	0.66	0.21	0.39	0.16	0.49	0.57	0.21	0.49	0.34
Subscale 5: *Integrity*	0.67	0.20	0.40	0.21	0.46	0.66	0.25	0.37	0.45
Subscale 6: *Caring Behavior*	0.71	0.24	0.39	0.22	0.42	0.65	0.22	0.44	0.33
Subscale 7: *Compassion*	0.49	0.15	0.43	0.42	0.29	0.49	0.04$^{n.s.}$	0.30	0.13$^{n.s.}$
Subscale 8: *Self-reflection*	0.35	0.17	0.30	0.20	0.30	0.36	0.27	0.38	0.29
Subscale 9: *Service Provision*	0.58	0.22	0.44	0.26	0.47	0.55	0.15	0.35	0.29
Subscale 10: *Positive Social Relationship*	0.54	0.14	0.37	0.24	0.38	0.54	0.10$^{n.s.}$	0.20	0.49
Subscale 11: *Communication Skills*	0.53	0.18	0.35	0.23	0.34	0.48	0.19	0.30	0.51
Subscale 12: *Fairness*	0.67	0.25	0.39	0.18	0.48	0.56	0.30	0.37	0.41

Note. N= 214. RSLP: RSLP: Revised Servant Leadership Profile; PTL: Paternal Leadership; IRI: Interpersonal Reactivity Index; IRI-EC: Subscale "Empathic Concern"; IRI: PT: Subscale "Perspective Taking"; MSC: Moral Self-Concept; HT: Hierarchical Thinking about leadership; ST: Systematic Thinking about leadership; LEF: Leadership Efficacy. Unless otherwise specified by the superscript "n.s." which denotes statistical non-significance ($p >. 05$, two-tailed), all correlation coefficients are significant at $p <.05$ (two-tailed).

Table 6. Comparison of the strength of correlations between SLB-SF-65 with the criterion scales

Correlations with the external criterion measures (and subscales)			Z-scores of difference between *r*s with SLB-SF-65:							
	Cronbach's alpha (Mean inter-item correlations)	*r*	PTL	IRI	IRI-EC	IRI-PT	MSC	HT	ST	LEF
1. RSLP	0.93 (0.42)	0.782***	8.91	6.92	8.89	6.14	2.51	8.47	6.04	4.96
2. PTL	0.79 (0.43)	0.249***	—	-2.71	$0.04^{n.s.}$	-3.65	-7.30	$-0.69^{n.s.}$	-3.55	-4.09
3. IRI	0.73 (0.17)	0.462***	—	—	5.94	$-1.64^{n.s.}$	-5.57	1.97	$-0.77^{n.s.}$	$-1.44^{n.s.}$
4. IRI-EC	0.67 (0.23)	0.245***	—	—	—	-3.96	-8.18	$-0.54^{n.s.}$	-3.50	-4.13
5. IRI-PT	0.66 (0.24)	0.523***	—	—	—	—	-4.12	2.95	$0.20^{n.s.}$	$-0.49^{n.s.}$
6. MSC	0.88 (0.49)	0.716***	—	—	—	—	—	6.62	4.09	3.22
7. HT	0.83 (0.26)	0.297***	—	—	—	—	—	—	-2.96**	-3.65
8. ST	0.84 (0.28)	0.511***	—	—	—	—	—	—	—	$-0.64^{n.s.}$
9. LEF	0.84 (0.41)	0.553***	—	—	—	—	—	—	—	—

Note. N= 214. ***p <.001 (two-tailed). RSLP: Revised Servant Leadership Profile; PTL: Paternal Leadership; IRI: Interpersonal Reactivity Index; IRI-EC: Subscale "Empathic Concern"; IRI: PT: Subscale "Perspective Taking"; MSC: Moral Self-Concept; HT: Hierarchical Thinking; ST: Systematic Thinking; LEF: Leadership Efficacy. Unless otherwise specified by the superscript "n.s." which denotes statistical non-significance, all other Z-scores of difference were significant at p <.05 (two-tailed) (i.e., |Z-score| > 1.96).

DISCUSSION

Utilizing a sample of 231 PolyU students, the present study attempted to examine the internal consistency, factorial validity, and convergent validity of the 97-item long-form of the Service Leadership Behavior Scale (SLB-LF-97). Moreover, findings of the EFA suggested the retention of 65 items which formed the short-form of the behavior scale (SLB-SF-65). Besides recording meritorious internal consistency, the SLB-SF-65 and the subscales were shown to correlate significantly and positively with all the external criterion measures. Specifically, by confirming six out of seven hypotheses (i.e., Hypotheses 1 to 5 and 7), the present correlational findings underscored the convergent validity of the SLB-SF-65. In short, the present results not only vouch for the psychometric property of the 65-item SLB-SF-65, but also its utility in serving as a sound measurement tool to help evaluate whether an individual has exhibited adequate behavioral qualities representative of a genuine Service Leader.

There are several key contributions of this work. First, amidst the scanty evidence base of assessment inventory about leadership especially in the Chinese context (8, 12), the SLB-SF-65 constitutes a timely addition to the literature. As remarked by Ho and Nesbit (44), the interdependent construal of interpersonal relationships unique to a collectivist society such as China could constitute a fundamentally different interpretation of leadership. Hence, it is imperative that objective measurement tool be tailor-made for the Chinese population, especially considering that China accounts for about 20% of the global population. Second, the present paper informs the literature of Service Leadership education. Considering the paucity in robust evaluation methodologies as regards leadership training programs (13), the SLB-SF-65 would be useful for implementers attempting to gauge the effectiveness of a Service Leadership training program. A successful training should, in principle, enhance trainees' propensity to display behavioral qualities representative of a true Service Leader which can be operationalized by a post-program improvement in one's SLB-SF-65 score. Third, as a precursor to a validation study involving 4,486 Hong Kong undergraduates (i.e., the main event of "The Project"), the present findings justify the inclusion of the 65-item SLB-SF-65 by underscoring its excellent internal consistency and strong convergent validity. Moreover, the preliminary item-screening and eventual trimming of the scale did not only add to the ease of administration, but also facilitate the elicitation of quality responses which are crucial to the ensuing large-scale validation study.

Nonetheless, there are certain issues worthy of our attention. One glaring concern would be the legitimacy of the present EFA attributable to the sample size of the present study (N= 214). As the present subjects-to-variables (i.e., STV) ratio only amounts to 2.23, which is below the commonly adopted "rule-of-thumb" STV ratio of 5 (see (45) for a list of "rule-of-thumb" STV ratios), there is inevitably a concern of under-sampling. However, previous research (e.g., 46, 47) had staunchly challenged the validity and utility of those "rules of thumbs", as these researchers maintained that sampling adequacy should also depend on other factors such as communalities and size of loadings. Particularly, MacCallum and colleagues (45) specified that good recovery of population factors can be achieved "with communalities in the range of 0.5" (p. 96) and "a somewhat larger sample in the range of 100 to 200" (p. 96). Given that both these criteria were met in the present analysis (i.e., N= 214; average communality = 0.53), there is no reason to outright dismiss the meaningfulness of the present EFA findings just because of the low STV ratio. Of course, there is a need to further assess the stability of the factors extracted because it is easy for multivariate statistics to capitalize on chance.

Additionally, owing to the exploratory nature of the present dimensionality assessment, there is a need to conduct a confirmatory factor analysis (CFA) to further examine the absolute and relative model fit of the current twelve-factor solution to participants' responses (20). Nevertheless, due to the sample size concern as outlined above, conducting a CFA by further splitting the present sample into two halves is just not workable. Therefore, to better ascertain the stability and fit indices of the current twelve-factor solution, both EFA and CFA need to be administered in the ensuing large-scale validation study (N= 4,486) as mentioned above.

Furthermore, contrary to Hypothesis 6, the SLB-SF-65 was positively correlated to the *Hierarchical Thinking Scale* measuring people's orientation toward leadership as a "leader-centric" concept whereby leaders ought to take the lion's share of blames or credits for the organizational outcomes (17, 48). As abovementioned, the non-mutual exclusiveness of Hierarchical (HT) and Systemic Thinking (ST) (17), coupled with the present positive, moderate correlation between the two and that between ST and SLB-SF-

65, may account for the present positive association between HT and SLB-SF-65. Indeed, Wielkiewicz and colleagues (48) contended that an elite leader should in theory "embrace these two forms of leadership (beliefs)" (p. 4) owing to their more sophisticated understanding on and experience with leadership. Taken together, it is conceivable that the positive link between HT and SLB-SF-65 was attributable to those "elite leaders" in the present sample who scored high on both HT and ST. Findings from the partial correlation analyses implied just that. As ST was controlled for, the positive HT-SLB-SF-65 association became non-existent, while the ST-SLB-SF-65 link remained highly significant and moderate even after controlling for HT. Nevertheless, the question why is Service Leadership behavior insignificantly, instead of negatively, linked to Hierarchical Thinking remains an interesting research topic to be examined in future.

Notwithstanding the above concerns, the present paper constitutes a pioneer assessment on the convergent and factorial validity of the Service Leadership Behavior Scale. Not only did the current findings strongly corroborate the psychometric soundness of the SLB-LF-97, they also provided a glimpse into an interpretable factorial structure of SLB-LF-97 which warrants further empirical scrutiny. More importantly, as the precursor to the main event of "The Project", the current study serves a preliminary screening purpose which informs the list of scale items worthy of inclusion in the upcoming large-scale validation study. Last but not least, the current paper helps to bridge a well-documented literature gap in the systematic evaluation of Service Leadership education (8, 13) by introducing a valid and reliable tool to measure people's behavioral qualities as a good Service Leader.

Acknowledgments

The validation project is financially supported by the Victor and William Fung Foundation. The preparation for this paper is supported by the Foundation and the Endowed Professorship in Service Leadership Education at The Hong Kong Polytechnic University. This chapter is an updated version of a publication in the special issue "Development and validation of assessment tools on service leadership knowledge, attitude and behavior" edited by Daniel TL Shek, Xiaoqin Zhu and Joav Merrick published in the International Journal of Child and Adolescent Health, 2018;11(4).

References

[1] Antonelli C, Fassio C. The economics of the light economy: Globalization, skill biased technological change and slow growth. Technol Forecast Soc Change 2014;87:89-107.

[2] Castells M. The service economy and postindustrial society: A sociological critique. Int J Health Serv 1976;6:595-607.
[3] Chung PPY. Service reborn: The knowledge, skills, and attitudes of service companies. 1st ed. New York: Lexingford, 2012.
[4] Fung VK. Development of the service economy in Hong Kong: Challenges and opportunities. In: Shek DTL, Chung PPY, eds. Promoting Service Leadership qualities in university students. Singapore: Springer, 2015:xi-xiii.
[5] Chung PPY. Where there is no vision, the people will perish. In: Shek DTL, Chung PPY, eds. Promoting Service Leadership qualities in university students: The case of Hong Kong. Singapore: Springer, 2015:xv-xviii.
[6] Shek DTL, Chung PPY, Lin L, Leung H, Ng ECW. Service Leadership under the Service Economy. In: Chin JL, Trimble JE, Garcia JE, eds. Global and culturally diverse leaders and leadership: New dimensions and challenges for business, education and society, 1st ed. Bingley, UK: Emerald, 2018:143-61.
[7] Shek DTL, Chung PPY, Yu L, Merrick J, eds. Service Leadership curriculum and higher education reform in Hong Kong. Int J Disabil Hum Dev 2015;14:297-406.
[8] Shek DTL, Chung PPY. Service Leadership education for university students: Seven unfinished tasks. In: Shek DTL, Chung PPY, eds. Promoting Service Leadership qualities in university students. Singapore: Springer, 2015:225-32.
[9] Chung PPY, Bell AH. 25 Principles of service leadership, 1st ed. New York: Lexingford Publishing, 2015.
[10] Chung PPY, Elfassy R. The 12 dimensions of a service leader, 1st ed. New York: Lexingford Publishing, 2016.
[11] Shek DTL, Lin L. Core Beliefs in the Service Leadership model proposed by the Hong Kong Institute of Service Leadership and Management. Int J Disabil Hum Dev 2015;14:233-42.
[12] Shek DTL, Lin L. Validation of the Service Leadership Knowledge Scale: Criterion-Related validity. In: Shek DTL, Chung PPY, Lin L, Merrick J, eds. Service Leadership education for university students. New York: Nova Science, 2017:189-204.
[13] Shek DTL, Lin L. Evaluating Service Leadership programs with multiple strategies. In: Shek DTL, Chung PPY, eds. Promoting Service Leadership qualities in university students: The case of Hong Kong. Singapore: Springer, 2015:197-211.
[14] Shek DTL, Lin L, Leung H, Yu L, Ma CMS, Li X. Development and validation of the Service Leadership Knowledge Scale in a Chinese context. In: Shek DTL, Chung PPY, Lin L, Merrick J, eds. Service Leadership education for university students. New York: Nova Science, 2017:163-88.
[15] Hwang JY, Plante T, Lackey K. The development of the Santa Clara Brief Compassion Scale: An abbreviation of Sprecher and Fehr's Compassionate Love Scale. Pastoral Psychol 2008;56:421-8.
[16] King DB, DeCicco TL. A viable model and self-report measure of spiritual intelligence. Int J Transpersonal Stud 2009;28:68-85.
[17] Wielkiewicz RM. The Leadership Attitudes and Beliefs Scale: An instrument for evaluating college students' thinking about leadership and organizations. J Coll Stud Dev 2000;41:335-47.
[18] Yukl G. Effective leadership behavior: What we know and what questions need more attention. Acad Manag Perspect 2012;26:66-85.
[19] Field AP. Discovering statistics using IBM SPSS statistics, 4th ed. London: Sage, 2013.
[20] Cohen RJ, Swerdlik ME. Psychological testing and assessment: An introduction to tests and measurement, 6th ed. New York: McGraw-Hill, 2005.
[21] Page D, Wong PTP. A conceptual framework for measuring Servant Leadership. In: Adjibolooso SBSK, ed. The human factor in shaping the course of history and development. Lanham, MD: University Press of America, 2000:69-109.
[22] Wong PTP, Page D. Servant Leadership: An opponent-process model and the Revised Servant Leadership Profile. Virginia Beach, VA: Regent University, 2003.
[23] Aycan Z, Kanungo RN, Mendonca M, Yu KC, Deller J, Stahl G, et al. Impact of culture on human resource management practices: A 10-country comparison. Appl Psychol 2000;49:192-221.

[24] Farh J-L, Cheng B-S. A cultural analysis of paternalistic leadership in Chinese organizations. In: Li JT, Tsui AS, Welden E, eds. Management and organizations in the Chinese context. London: Palgrave, 2000:84-127.

[25] Pellegrini EK, Scandura TA. Paternalistic leadership: A review and agenda for future research. J Manage 2008;34:566-93.

[26] Aketa Y. On a framework for and measures of empathy: An organizational model of empathy by Davis, and a preliminary study of a multidimensional empathy scale (IRI-J). Psychol Rep Sophia Univ 1999;23:19-31. [Japanese]

[27] Gilet A-L, Mella N, Studer J, Grühn D, Labouvie-Vief G. Assessing dispositional empathy in adults: A French validation of the Interpersonal Reactivity Index (IRI). Can J Behav Sci 2013;45:42-8.

[28] Siu AMH, Shek DTL. Validation of the Interpersonal Reactivity Index in a Chinese context. Res Soc Work Pract 2005;15:118-26.

[29] Davis MH. Measuring individual differences in empathy: Evidence for a multidimensional approach. J Pers Soc Psychol 1983;44:113-26.

[30] Cheng CHK. The Chinese Adolescent Self-Esteem Scales (CASES): A user manual. Hong Kong: City University of Hong Kong Press, 2005.

[31] Murphy SE. The contribution of leadership experience and self-efficacy to group performance under evaluation apprehension. Dissertation. Seattle: WA: University of Washington, 1992.

[32] Hannah ST, Avolio BJ, Luthans F, Harms PD. Leadership efficacy: Review and future directions. Leadersh Q 2008;19:669-92.

[33] Tabachnick BG, Fidell LS. Using multivariate statistics, 5th ed. Boston, MA: Pearson Education, 2007.

[34] Velicer WF. Determining the number of components from the matrix of partial correlations. Psychometrika 1976;41:321-7.

[35] Courtney MGR. Determining the number of factors to retain in EFA: Using the SPSS R-Menu V 2.0 to make more judicious estimations. Pract Assess Res Eval 2013;18:1-14.

[36] Warne RT, Larsen R. Evaluating a proposed modification of the Guttman rule for determining the number of factors in an exploratory factor analysis. Psychol Test Assess Model 2014;56:104-23.

[37] Mullin EM. Scale development: Heterosexist attitudes in women's collegiate athletics. Meas Phys Educ Exerc Sci 2013;17:1-21.

[38] Shek DTL, Chung PPY, Leung H. Manufacturing economy vs. service economy: Implications for Service Leadership. Int J Disabil Hum Dev 2015;14:205-15.

[39] Shek DTL, Yu L, Ma CMS, Sun RCF, Liu TT. Development of a credit-bearing Service Leadership subject for university students in Hong Kong. Int J Adolesc Med Health 2013;25:353-61.

[40] O'Connor BP. SPSS and SAS programs for determining the number of components using parallel analysis and Velicer's MAP test. Behav Res Methods Instrum Comput 2000;32:396-402.

[41] Briggs SR, Cheek JM. The role of factor analysis in the development and evaluation of personality scales. J Pers 1986;54:106-48.

[42] Diedenhofen B, Musch J. cocor: A comprehensive solution for the statistical comparison of correlations. PLoS ONE 2015;10:e0121945. doi:10.1371/journal.pone.

[43] Steiger JH. Tests for comparing elements of a correlation matrix. Psychol Bull 1980;87:245-51.

[44] Ho J, Nesbit PL. A refinement and extension of the self-leadership scale for the Chinese context. J Manag Psychol 2009;24:450-76.

[45] MacCallum RC, Widaman KF, Zhang S, Hong S. Sample size in factor analysis. Psychol Methods 1999;4:84-99.

[46] Preacher KJ, MacCallum RC. Exploratory factor analysis in behavior genetics research: Factor recovery with small sample sizes. Behav Genet 2002;32:153-61.

[47] MacCallum RC, Widaman KF, Preacher KJ, Hong S. Sample size in factor analysis: The role of model error. Multivariate Behav Res 2001;36:611-37.

[48] Wielkiewicz RM, Fischer DV, Stelzner SP, Overland M, Sinner AM. Leadership attitudes and beliefs of incoming first-year college students: A multi-institutional study of gender. J Leadersh Educ 2012;11:1-25.

SECTION TWO: VALIDATION

In: Service Leadership ISBN: 978-1-53614-852-7
Editors: Daniel TL Shek, Xiaoqin Zhu, Li Lin et al.

Chapter 7

CONTENT VALIDATION OF A SERVICE LEADERSHIP BEHAVIOR SCALE IN HONG KONG

Daniel TL Shek[1-6,*], PhD, FHKPS, BBS, SBS, JP, Jing Wu[1], PhD, Li Lin[1], PhD and Xiang Li[1], PhD

[1]Department of Applied Social Sciences, The Hong Kong Polytechnic University, Hong Kong, PR China,
[2]Centre for Innovative Programmes for Adolescents and Families, The Hong Kong Polytechnic University, Hong Kong, PR China,
[3]Department of Social Work, East China Normal University, Shanghai, PR China,
[4]Kiang Wu Nursing College of Macau, Macau, PR China,
[5]Hong Kong Institute of Service Leadership and Management, Hong Kong, PR China
[6]Division of Adolescent Medicine, Department of Pediatrics, Kentucky Children's Hospital, University of Kentucky School of Medicine, Lexington, Kentucky, US

ABSTRACT

In this chapter we report the development of the 97-item Service Leadership Behavior Scale (i.e., SLB-LF-97) based on the Service Leadership framework proposed by Po Chung. To understand the content validity of the scale, the content validity of the developed items was examined. A panel of experts (n = 3) was formed to assess the content validity of the scale items in different domains (service provision, competence, character, caring, commitment to continuous improvement, and distributed leadership) in terms of relevance,

[*] Correspondence: Daniel TL Shek, PhD, FHKPS, BBS, SBS, JP, Associate Vice President (Undergraduate Programme), Chair Professor of Applied Social Sciences and Li and Fung Professor in Service Leadership Education, Department of Applied Social Sciences, The Hong Kong Polytechnic University, Hung Hom, Hong Kong, PR China. E-mail: daniel.shek@polyu.edu.hk.

clarity, and representativeness on each item. Results indicated that the SLB-LF-97 has an excellent content validity indexed by relevance, clarity, and representativeness for the whole scale and the different categories. The findings suggest the scale and subscales of the Service Leadership Behavior Scale possess excellent content validity.

INTRODUCTION

Desirable leadership characteristics vary with the characteristics of different economic systems. The leadership qualities required by service economy are different from those required by manufacturing economy. Generally speaking, leadership in the manufacturing economy was regarded as inflexible, task-focused, and authority-based. In contrast, effective leadership in the service economy is characterized by people orientation, relationship orientation and service orientation (1). Hong Kong has a service-oriented economy where the service industries shared 92.2% of the Gross Domestic Product (GDP) in 2016 (2). With respect to the growth of service economy in the global context, Chung (3) proposed the notion of service leadership and developed the Service Leadership and Management Model (SLAM). As defined by Chung (3), service leadership "is about satisfying needs by consistently providing quality personal service to everyone one comes into contact with, including one's self, others, groups, communities, systems, and environments". It is also believed that effective service leadership is a function of leadership competencies, character, and caring disposition (4).

Although the notion of service leadership is newly proposed, its related components are not brand-new. Compared with other mainstream leadership theories and approaches, service leadership shares some similar features, such as the emphasis on integrity (5). Nevertheless, the service leadership model has its distinctive features that are seldom mentioned in other theories. To begin with, not a single leadership theory emphasizes the importance of the service orientation, including servant leadership theory (6), authentic leadership theory (7), and ethical leadership theory (8). Besides, these theories primarily conceptualize leadership at the individual level, dealing with the leadership behaviors of self and/or others. For example, while authentic leadership is mostly dependent on leaders' behaviors in self-reflection, self-management, and self-improvement (7), service leadership theory adopts a more systematic multi-level perspective towards the service for self, others, as well as the ecological system (4).

Besides, some leadership theories argue that excellent leadership primarily relies on the competencies or certain personal qualities of the leaders. For example, managerial competencies are the core elements for top-down leadership theory (9), while a set of born characteristics is proposed to determine the success of a leader according to the trait approach to leadership (10). In contrast, the service leadership framework asserts that competencies and character are not enough for an effective leader in the modern service economy (3). The SLAM framework suggests three components that determine effective leadership, including moral character, leadership competencies, and caring disposition (for short, $E = MC^2$). This framework not only highlights the importance of service leaders' personal qualities and competencies but also establishes a more comprehensive and systematic model to explain how these characteristics contribute to effective leadership (5).

Furthermore, although both service leadership and servant leadership focus on the development of followers through mentoring and teaching (11), servant leaders only focus on the followers rather than the leaders. Moreover, service leadership considers that everyone could be a leader and leadership requires life-long continuous improvement. Lastly, another new feature that service leadership goes beyond the other existing theories is that the SLAM framework incorporates Chinese cultural values and the philosophies of Buddhism, Confucianism, and Taoism (3). The incorporation helps to look at moral character from an integrated perspective. Overall speaking, service leadership theory is multidisciplinary in nature that it covers leadership in different domains (12).

As university students are the future leaders in society, service leadership education is essential for youths (13). With the collaborative partnership of the Victor and William Fung Foundation, the Hong Kong Institute of Service Leadership & Management Limited (HKI-SLAM), and the eight universities funded by the University Grants Committee in Hong Kong, the Fung Service Leadership Initiative (SLI) was initiated in 2012 to promote service leadership education. The Hong Kong Polytechnic University (PolyU), among the eight universities, has developed and provided credit-bearing courses and non-credit-bearing programs/workshops on service leadership within the SLAM curriculum framework (14). Both qualitative and quantitative evaluation strategies have supported the positive influences on the leadership capacities of students who have participated in the courses or programs (15-17). In general, the service leadership education has obtained great achievement and recognition among university students.

Although some initiatives on service leadership education have been launched, there is little empirical research that assesses the qualities of service leaders. A survey of the literature shows that leadership behavior scales based on different leadership theories have been used, such as the Multifactor Leadership Questionnaire (MLQ) (18) that allows individuals to measure their own transformational, transactional, and passive-avoidant leadership behaviors. However, the MLQ has been criticized by researchers for having problematic construct validity issues as it focuses primarily on transformational leadership, rather than the other two leadership styles (19). Other specific leadership behavior scales were largely developed with respect to its corresponding leadership theory, which has different conceptualizations from the Service Leadership theory. For example, the Transformational Leadership Inventory (20), the Authentic Leadership Inventory (ALI) (21), and the Servant Leadership Behavior Scale (22) were developed according to corresponding leadership theories. Therefore, there is an urgent need to develop a measurement specifically for the Service Leadership theory.

To fill this gap and to strengthen the assessment component of service leadership education, the Research Team at The Hong Kong Polytechnic University (PolyU) embarked on a research project entitled "Development and Validation of Measures Based on the Service Leadership Model". In this project, three scales on service leadership (knowledge, attitude, and behavior) were developed and validated. Previous studies have documented the processes of developing the Service Leadership Attitude Scale and Knowledge Scale (23, 24). Results of both studies showed that the items developed were perceived to be relevant, clear, and representative of the constructs of service leadership attitude and knowledge. In this paper, we reported the development of the 97-item Service Leadership Behavior Scale (SLB-LF-97) and its related content validation findings.

Generally speaking, three steps were involved in developing an assessment tool, including domain identification, item generation, and instrument formation (25). For the present study, the SLB-LF-97 was developed based on the groundwork of the HKI-SLAM curriculum framework (3), 7 core beliefs of service leadership (26), 12 dimensions of the personal quality of service leadership (5), 25 principles of service leaders (4), and the existing literature. Specifically, the developed scale attempted to cover the behavior of service leaders in the following key domains:

1. **Service provision** – According to the Service Leadership theory, it is essential for service leaders to satisfy the needs of self, others, and systems, which is elaborated in the Core Belief 1 of the SLAM framework (26). Also, as advocated by The Principle of Service Mindset (1), service leaders must have genuine care for others' needs. However, unlike servant leadership theory or spiritual leadership theory which overemphasizes followers' needs and neglects leaders' needs (5), service leadership theory adopts a more balanced approach in looking at the needs of the followers and leaders.
2. **Competence** – The traditional leadership approaches emphasize management skills or expertise (9), which is more applicable to the manufacturing economy. In contrast, leadership competency in the service economy has a broader coverage focusing on the importance of intrapersonal and interpersonal competencies (3). Four types of intrapersonal competencies are concerned the most in the service leadership education (27). First, intelligence quotient (IQ) is closely related to job performance as well as leadership performance (28). The IQ of an effective service leader is manifested in good problem-solving, critical thinking, logical reasoning, and analytical abilities (27). The second intrapersonal competence is emotional quotient (EQ), which is one of the most recognized non-intellectual factors that contribute to our work and daily life (29). The ability to understand, recognize, and manage emotions of oneself and others will undoubtedly enhance the performance and leadership at work (30). The other two essential intrapersonal competencies for service leaders are adversity quotient (AQ) and spiritual quotient (SQ). AQ addresses the ability to accept and successfully bounce back from failure, misfortune, or

other adversity situations (31), while SQ is regarded as the ability to use meaning, faith, and other spiritual resources to solve problems (32). A competent service leader possesses and utilizes intrapersonal competencies to serve oneself, others, and systems.

In addition, interpersonal competencies are also among the core personal attributes that service leaders should promote (33). Five task domains of interpersonal competence were identified by Buhrmester, Furman, Wittenberg, and Reis (34), which included initiating relationships, self-disclosure, emotional support, conflict managing, and asserting personal thoughts and feelings. Besides, the SLB-LF-97 incorporates Chinese philosophy to enrich the model. As such, six components of interpersonal competencies are considered in the SLB-LF-97: passionate about people; positive social relationships; assertiveness; collaboration and cooperation with people; conflict resolution; and communication skills. Specifically, service leaders are supposed to be people-oriented (*"yi ren wei ben"*) and develop positive and healthy relationships with others. Meanwhile, an effective service leader shows great verbal and non-verbal communication skills, through which one could develop and maintain collaborative relationships with teammates and other people, as well as assert one's own rights when having conflicts. In short, service leaders with good interpersonal competencies can appreciate different opinions (*"he er bu tong"*) and create constructive ways to resolve interpersonal conflicts.

3. **Character** – Complying with the Principle of Competence, Character, and Care (4), and the Principle of Personal Ethics (4), leaders in the service economy are required to exhibit positive characters that are morally valued, which make followers more willing to work with them (35). In Western cultures, Park, Peterson, and Seligman (36) developed the VIA Classification and listed 24 virtues in action, such as integrity, gratitude, forgiveness, and bravery. However, Eastern cultural philosophies, particularly, Confucianism also uphold some traditional character strengths, such as benevolence ("*ren*"), affection ("*ai*"), and forgiveness (*"shu"*) (37). The SLB-LF-97 synthesizes the Eastern and Western cultures and highlights the service leadership virtues by integrity, fairness, humility, and acting as an ethical role model.
4. **Caring** – This category covers the quality of caring disposition of the service leaders. The Principle of Trust, Fairness, Respect, and Care implies that successful service experiences cannot exist without caring service leaders (4). A competent and moral service leader should also show concern for others and oneself (38). Two aspects of caring disposition are measured in the SLB-LF-97. On the one hand, good service leadership involves the qualities of concern, such as empathy and compassion. On the other hand, caring leaders provide care for others by loving, supporting, and developing others.

5. **Commitment to continuous improvement** – The need for continuous improvement is one of the key characteristics of the service leadership model (5). The HK-SLAM model emphasizes self-leadership and growth mindset, rather than the notion of "inborn" or "elite" leadership (26). Besides, only through continuous professional and personal improvement could one be well prepared to serve oneself as well as others. Therefore, effective service leaders should make efforts to promote self-leadership, self-reflection, and life-long learning.
6. **Distributed leadership** – In response to the core belief of service leadership that "every day, every human occupies a position of leadership and possesses the potential to improve his leadership quality and effectiveness" (Core Belief 2) (26), distributed leadership style in the service economy encourages and empowers every teammate to voice out and contribute their insights to the team decision-making. Meanwhile, distributed leaders would show trust and respect to followers by acknowledging and respecting their views and abilities.

A well-developed Service Leadership Behavior Scale is indispensable for educators and researchers to empirically investigate students' changes after taking service leadership education. Such a scale serves as an instrument for assessing one's qualities of service leadership, which enables researchers to further validate the theory and hypotheses proposed by the service leadership model, such as the principle $E = MC^2$. Based on the Service Leadership model, the PolyU Research Team drafted a total of 97 items for the Service Leadership Behavior Scale. However, before formally utilizing the scale and interpreting scores with confidence, the validation process is a highly critical step in the test development (39). To obtain judgmental evidence on whether the scale and items could adequately represent the content of service leadership behavior, content validation procedure was conducted in the present study.

Content validation was defined as "the degree to which elements of an assessment instrument are relevant to and representative of the targeted construct for a particular assessment purpose" (40, p.238), or "whether or not the items sampled for inclusion on the tool adequately represent the domain of content addressed by the instrument" (41, p.155). One of the most frequently utilized approaches for content validation in previous research is the engagement of "content experts" (42), in which several knowledgeable people in a specialized area discuss and have consensus on the quality and representativeness of the instrument items. To minimize errors arising from subjective assessment and artificial consensus (43), content validity index (CVI) (44) was employed in the current study, which provides quantitative judgment evidence for the content validity of the test, including relevance, clarity, and representativeness (44). In the present study, a panel of experts was invited to evaluate the items of the SLB-LF-97. Based on the quantitative and qualitative content validation findings, revisions were made to improve the scale.

OUR STUDY

The present study documented the development of the SLB-LF-97 and evaluated its content validation. Based on a thorough examination of the tenets of the Service Leadership Model (3) and leadership literature (e.g., spiritual quotient, 32), an item pool on the behaviors and qualities of service leaders was established. The following six categories are included in the SLB-LF-97:

C1. Service provision (4 items). Items in this category assess respondents' tendency of having a sensitivity to individuals' needs and providing good service to others.

C2. Competence (38 items). This category addresses behaviors and qualities representing intrapersonal and interpersonal competencies within the framework of HKI-SLAM (27, 33). For the intrapersonal competencies, items measure individuals' IQ, EQ, AQ, and SQ. For the interpersonal competencies, items assess "passionate about people", "positive social relationship", "assertiveness", "collaboration and cooperation with people", "conflict resolution", and "communication skills". Basically, intrapersonal and interpersonal competencies are covered under this domain.

C3. Character (14 items). Items in this category measure a well-developed personal code of ethics as characterized by integrity, fairness, humanity, and whether a person is acting as an ethical role model.

C4. Caring (15 items). This category underlines caring disposition defined by the Service Leadership Model (3), including notions that deeply embedded in Chinese virtues, such as items assessing "guan xin" (concern) and "zhao gu" (providing care).

C5. Commitment to continuous improvement (13 items). This category involves the notion that effective service leaders put self-development efforts aiming at ethically improving their competencies, abilities, willingness, and resources to satisfy the needs of others. Based on the 25 principles of service leadership (4), items evaluating individuals' self-leadership, self-reflection, and life-long learning were constructed.

C6. Distributed leadership (13 items). Items in this category assess the three core characteristics of distributed service leadership, including shared decision-making, empowerment of teammates, and trust and respect.

Three experts familiar with the Service Leadership literature were invited to assess the extent to which the SLB-LF-97 measured what it was intended to measure. All experts had a doctoral degree and were involved in the curriculum development and/or the teaching of the subject "Service Leadership" and they have professional knowledge in Service Leadership, especially the framework of the HKI-SLAM.

Instrument

A self-administered questionnaire was distributed to the three experts. They evaluated the content validity for each item in the following aspects:

1) **Relevance**, the extent to which the item falls within the body of knowledge of the SLAM framework. Experts were asked to judge on a 4-point rating scale: 1 = *Irrelevant*, 2 = *Unable to assess the relevance without item revision* or *item is in need of revision or otherwise would no longer be relevant*, 3 = *Relevant but needs minor amendment*, 4 = *Relevant.*
2) **Clarity**, the extent to which the item is concise, accurate, and direct. Experts were asked to judge on a 4-point rating scale: 1 = *Very unclear,* 2 = *Unclear,* 3 = *Clear,* 4 = *Very clear.*
3) **Representativeness**, the extent to which the item adequately represents and encompasses the corresponding concept. Experts were asked to judge on a 4-point rating scale: 1 = *Very unrepresentative*, 2 = *Unrepresentative*, 3 = *Representative*, 4 = *Very representative.*

Meanwhile, the experts were requested to give justifications or suggested modifications if they had negative ratings (option 1 or 2) on the items. After rating the individual items, the experts were also invited to judge the overall quality of the scale via the following questions:

1) Does this batch of items cover all the essential behaviors of qualities within the service leadership framework?
2) Is there any additional behavior(s) or qualities that you regard essential to service leader? If yes, please list the additional point(s) below.
3) Does this batch of items adequately represent the behavior(s) or qualities in service leadership?
4) Any other comments (open-ended question).

Experts' ratings were used to analyze the content validity of the scale, while their written feedbacks and suggestions would direct further revisions of the developed items.

FINDINGS

With reference to the previous studies, the I-CVI index for each item was computed as the number of experts giving a rating of 3 or 4, divided by the number of experts (i.e., 3) — that is, the proportion in agreement about relevance, clarity, or representativeness. Then, the S-CVI/ave for each category was an average score of the I-CVIs for all the items. As shown in Table 1, most of the items indicated good I-CVIs. Items that with an I-CVI value lower than 1.00 were modified according to the experts' comments. For example, the original item 24 "I have passion for people" was revised to "I show passion for other people's welfare" because one rater considered that the original expression was too subjective and abstract. For the whole scale, the S-CVI/ave manifested excellent content validity (see Table 1). For each category, the S-CVI/aves for all subscales were also very good (see Table 2).

Table 1. The frequency of I-CVI and the S-CVI/ave for the whole scale

	Number of items (percentage)		
I-CVI	**Relevance**	**Clarity**	**Representativeness**
0.33	0 (0%)	1 (1.0%)	0 (0%)
0.67	5 (5.2%)	10 (10.3%)	3 (3.1%)
1.00	92 (94.8%)	86 (88.7%)	94 (96.9%)
S-CVI/ave	.98	.96	.99

Table 2. The S-CVI/ave for the subscales

			S-CVI/ave		
No.	**Domains**	**No. of items**	**Relevance**	**Clarity**	**Representativeness**
	Service provision	4	1.00	1.00	1.00
	Competence	38	.98	.91	.99
	Character	14	.93	.98	.95
	Caring	15	1.00	.98	1.00
	Commitment to continuous improvement	13	1.00	1.00	1.00
	Distributed leadership	13	1.00	1.00	1.00

DISCUSSION

The primary purpose of the present study was to develop the SLB-LF-97 as well as to ensure the measure is relevant to the framework, appropriate and clear, and could represent the concept of service leadership. The construction and validation of a Service Leadership Behavior Scale could help educators and researchers to assess the behaviors and related qualities in an effective service leader as outlined by the HK-SLAM framework (3) in a valid manner. The content validity index (CVI) method based on expert ratings has been widely used to quantify content validity (44). In the Hong Kong context, researchers also have used this approach to develop and validate scales (e.g., 45, 46). Both item-level content validity index (I-CVI) and average scale-level content validity index (S-CVI/ave) were calculated in the present study.

Results showed favorable results based on the views of three experts. First, all experts agreed that almost all items were relevant to the HK-SLAM framework and only 5 items needed minor revisions. Second, one item was rated as unclear, ten items were regarded as in need of revision, and the rest 86 items were rated as clear by all three experts. Third, all but 3 items were judged as representative of the framework by all the three raters. Based on the judges' suggestions, scale developers have carried out revisions of the wording. Therefore, according to the three experts' judgments, the developed items for the SLB-LF-97 could successfully measure what it was intended to measure. Some sample items for each category are presented in the Appendix.

Theoretically, the development of Service Leadership Behavior Scale is valuable for the leadership literature. A sound understanding of leader behavior and leadership effectiveness can hardly be achieved without research findings based on rigorous assessments. Thus, well-established instruments would help further validate the theoretical propositions and hypotheses of the service leadership model. Although past research has yielded a number of measurements on leader behavior, such as Servant Leadership Behavior Scale (22) and Leader Behavior Description Questionnaire (LBDQ) (47), there is a need to develop new Service Leadership measures because it is a new type of leadership theory. The present study helped with an initial check on the content validity of Service Leadership Behavior Scale and also highlighted the criteria of effective service leadership behaviors.

Practically, a validated measurement is indispensable for effective service leadership education. Although the eight universities in Hong Kong were involved in the Fung Service leadership initiative, no systematic effort has been made to develop appropriate assessment tools to assess service leadership behavior. With the development of the Service Leadership Behavior Scale, the effectiveness of leadership education could then be examined. A simple evaluation strategy would be to collect both pretest and posttest data before and after the training program.

It is noteworthy that there are several limitations of the present study. First, although the involvement of three raters fulfills the minimum requirement of numbers of experts proposed by Lynn (48), future studies could invite more parties to help increase its generalizability, such as scholars from other universities, management professionals who have been trained with service leadership qualities, or students who excellently finished the study of service leadership courses (40). Second, there is still a need for the continued refinement and validation of the scale. For example, psychometric properties of the scale including reliability and validity should be verified (49). Furthermore, theoretical and empirical relationships among service leadership behavior, attitude, and knowledge should also be explored. This process could also provide support for the construct validity of the measures. Despite the abovementioned limitations, the present study contributes to our understanding of the service leadership qualities. It also provides another valid measurement to evaluate service leadership education programs (23, 24).

ACKNOWLEDGMENTS

The validation project is financially supported by the Victor and William Fung Foundation. The preparation for this paper is supported by the Foundation and the Endowed Professorship in Service Leadership Education at The Hong Kong Polytechnic University. This chapter is an updated version of a publication in the special issue "Development and validation of assessment tools on service leadership knowledge, attitude and behavior" edited by Daniel TL Shek, Xiaoqin Zhu and Joav Merrick published in the International Journal of Child and Adolescent Health, 2018;11(4).

APPENDIX: SAMPLE ITEMS (WITH ADAPTATION) OF THE SERVICE LEADERSHIP BEHAVIOR SCALE (SLB-LF-97)

Categories	Sample items
C1. Service provision	I provide service to others according to their specific needs. Readiness to serve: A good leader serves others with a genuine heart.
C2. Competence	*IQ:* When there is any issue that is out of my expectation, I can quickly come up with a workable solution on the spot.
	EQ: I can manage my negative emotions well so that it will not negatively affect my work.
	SQ: I have faith to deal with challenges in my life.
	AQ: Adversity such as failure and setback usually makes me stronger rather than weaker.
	Passionate about people: I value the well-being of other people.
	Positive social relationships: I am able to create a positive rapport with other people.
	Assertiveness: I uphold my own principles and stand firm to reject tasks that I think inappropriate.
	Collaboration and cooperation with people: I am good at collaborating with other people.
	Conflict resolution: I negotiate with others when we have conflict.
	Communication skills: I am able to effectively convey my thoughts and ideas to others.
C3. Character	*Integrity:* I am honest with people.
	Fairness: I treat people around me equally without favoritism.
	Humility: I recognize my limitations.
	Role model: People regard me as a person with ethical behavior.
C4. Caring	*Concern:* I am able to feel what other people are experiencing.
	Provide care: I do good things for other people without expecting them to return the favor.
C5. Commitment to continuous improvement	*Self-leadership:* I constantly seek to improve my character.
	Self-reflection: I give time to closely examine my own thoughts and behavior.
	Life-long learning: I keep learning new skills.
C6. Distributed leadership	*Shared decision-making:* When making decisions, I welcome critiques from my teammates.
	Empowerment of teammates: I delegate my power and authority to my teammates to facilitate their work.
	Trust and respect: I trust my teammates to make good decisions.

REFERENCES

[1] Shek DTL, Chung PPY, Leung H. Manufacturing economy vs. service economy: Implications for service leadership. Int J Disabil Hum Dev 2015;14(3):205-15.

[2] The World Bank. Services, value added (% of GDP) 2016. URL: https://data.worldbank.org/indicator/NV.SRV.TOTL.ZS.

[3] Chung PPY. Hong Kong Institute of Service Leadership and Management Curriculum Framework. Hong Kong: Hong Kong Institute of Service Leadership and Management, 2011.

[4] Chung PPY, Bell AH. The 25 Principles of Service Leadership. New York: Lexingford Publishing, 2015.

[5] Shek DTL, Chung PPY, Leung H. How unique is the service leadership model? A comparison with contemporary leadership approaches. Int J Disabil Hum Dev 2015;14(3):217-31.

[6] Van Dierendonck D. Servant leadership: A review and synthesis. J Manage 2011;37(4):1228-61.

[7] Cooper CD, Scandura TA, Schriesheim CA. Looking forward but learning from our past: Potential challenges to developing authentic leadership theory and authentic leaders. Leadersh Q 2005;16(3):475-93.

[8] Brown ME, Treviño LK, Harrison DA. Ethical leadership: A social learning perspective for construct development and testing. Organ Behav Hum Decis Process 2005;97(2):117-34.

[9] Kezar A. Bottom-up/top-down leadership: Contradiction or hidden phenomenon. J Higher Educ 2012;83(5):725-60.

[10] Fleenor JW. Trait approach to leadership. In: Rogelberg SG, ed. Encyclopedia of Industrial Organizational Psychology. Thousand Oaks, CA: Sage, 2011:830-2.

[11] Shek DTL, Lin L. Leadership and mentorship: Service leaders as mentors of the followers. Int J Disabil Hum Dev 2015;14(4):351-9.

[12] Shek DTL, Sun RCF, Liu TT. Evolution and realms of service leadership and leadership models. Int J Disabil Hum Dev 2015;14(3),243-54.

[13] Shek DTL, Chung PPY, Lin L, Merrick J. Service leadership education for University students. In Shek DTL, Chung PPY, Merrick J, eds. Service leadership education for University students. New York: Nova Science, 2017:3-8.

[14] Shek DTL, Sun RCF, Lin L, Leung H, Siu AMH, Ma CMS, Yu L, Law MYM. Service leadership education at the Hong Kong Polytechnic University. Int J Adolesc Med Health. In Shek DTL, Chung PPY, Lin L, Merrick J, eds. Service leadership education for University students. New York: Nova Science, 2017:83-92.

[15] Shek DTL, Lin, L. Evaluating service leadership programs with multiple strategies. In: Shek DTL, Chung PPY, eds. Promoting service leadership qualities in university students: The case of Hong Kong. Quality of life in Asia, vol. 6. Singapore: Springer, 2015:197-211.

[16] Shek DTL, Zhu XQ, Lin L. Evaluation of an Intensive Service Leadership Course in Mainland China. Int J Child Adolesc Health 2017;10(2):223-31.

[17] Shek DTL, Yu L, Ma CMS, Sun RCF, Liu TT. Development of a credit-bearing service leadership subject for university students in Hong Kong. Int J Adolesc Med Health 2013;25(4):353-61.

[18] Bass BM, Avolio BJ. Multifactor Leadership Questionnaire. Palo Alto, CA: Consulting Psychologists Press, 1990.

[19] Schriesheim CA, Cogliser CC. Construct validation in leadership research: Explication and illustration. Leadersh Q 2010;20(5):725-36.

[20] Castro SL, Schriesheim CA. Transformational leadership: A summary of the behavioral dimensions of the construct and an assessment of the validity of new scales measuring each dimension. Paper presented at the Academy of Management Meetings, Chicago, IL, 1998.

[21] Neider LL, Schriesheim CA. The Authentic Leadership Inventory (ALI): Development and empirical tests. Leadersh Q 2011;22(6):1146-64.

[22] Sendjaya S. Development and Validation of the Servant Leadership Behavior Scale. Melbourne, Australia: Monash University, 2005.

[23] Shek DTL, Lin L, Leung H, Yu L, Ma CMS, Li X. Development and validation of the service leadership knowledge scale in a Chinese context. In Shek DTL, Chung PPY, Lin L, Merrick J, eds. Service leadership education for University students. New York: Nova Science, 2017:163-88.
[24] Shek DTL, Lin L, Leung H, Yu L, Ma CMS, Li X. Content validation of the service leadership attitudes scale. In Shek DTL, Chung PPY, Lin L, Merrick J, eds. Service leadership education for University students. New York: Nova Science, 2017:205-26.
[25] Carmines EG, Zeller RA. Reliability and validity assessment. Beverly Hills, CA: Sage, 1979.
[26] Shek DTL, Lin L. Core beliefs in the service leadership model proposed by the Hong Kong Institute of Service Leadership and Management. Int J Disabil Hum Dev 2015;14(3):233-42.
[27] Shek DTL, Lin L. Intrapersonal competence and service leadership. Int J Disabil Hum Dev 2015;14(3):255-63.
[28] Shek DTL, Sun RCF. Promoting leadership and intrapersonal competence in university students: what can we learn from Hong Kong? Int J Disabil Hum Dev 2012;11(3):221-8.
[29] Schutte NS, Malouff JM, Hall LE, Haggerty DJ, Cooper JT, Golden CJ, Dornheim L. Development and validation of a measure of emotional intelligence. Pers Individ Diff 1998;25(2):167-77.
[30] Wong CS, Law KS. The effects of leader and follower emotional intelligence on performance and attitude: An exploratory study. Leadersh Q 2002;13(3):243-74.
[31] Stoltz PG. Adversity quotient: turning obstacles into opportunities. New York: John Wiley, 1997.
[32] King DB, DeCicco TL. A Viable Model and Self-Report Measure of Spiritual Intelligence. Int J Transpers Stud 2009;28(1):68-85.
[33] Shek DTL, Yu L, Siu AMH. Interpersonal competence and service leadership. Int J Disabil Hum Dev 2015;14(3):265-74.
[34] Buhrmester D, Furman W, Wittenberg MT, Reis HT. Five domains of interpersonal competence in peer relationships. J Pers Soc Psychol 1988;55(6):991-1008.
[35] Shek DTL, Yu L. Character strengths and service leadership. Int J Disabil Hum Dev 2015;14(4):299-307.
[36] Park N, Peterson C, Seligman ME. Strengths of character and well-being. J Soc Clin Psychol 2004;23(5):603-19.
[37] Shek DTL, Sun RCF, Liu TT. Character strengths in Chinese philosophies: Relevance to service leadership. Int J Disabil Hum Dev 2015;14(4):309-18.
[38] Shek DTL, Li X. The role of caring disposition in service leadership. Int J Disabil Hum Dev 2015;14(4):319-32.
[39] Beck CT, Gable RK. Ensuring content validity: An illustration of the process. J Nurs Meas 2001;9(2):201-15.
[40] Haynes SN, Richard DCS, Kubany ES. Content validity in psychological assessment: a functional approach to concepts and methods. Psychol Assess 1995;7(3):238-47.
[41] Waltz CF, Strickland OL, Lenz ER. Measurement in nursing and health research, 3rd ed. NewYork: Springer, 2005.
[42] Grant JS, Davis LL. Selection and use of content experts for instrument development. Res Nurs Health 1997;20(3):269-74.
[43] Delgado-Rico E, Carrctero-Dios H, Ruch W. Content validity evidences in test development: An applied perspective. Int J Clin Health Psychol 2012;12(3):449-60.
[44] Polit DF, Beck CT, Owen SV. Is the CVI an acceptable indicator of content validity? Appraisal and recommendations. Res Nurs Health 2007;30(4):459-67.
[45] Chung V, Wong E, Griffiths S. Content validity of the integrative medicine attitude questionnaire: perspectives of a Hong Kong Chinese expert panel. J Altern Complement Med 2007;13(5):563-70.
[46] Leung JTY, Shek DTL. "All I can do for my child"–development of the Chinese Parental Sacrifice for Child's Education Scale. Int J Disabil Hum Dev 2011;10(3):201-8.
[47] Hemphill JL. Leader behavior associated with the administrative reputations of college departments. J Educ Psychol 1955;46(7):385-401.
[48] Lynn MR. Determination and quantification of content validity. Nurs Res 1986;35:382-5.
[49] Mazzetti G, Schaufeli WB, Guglielmi D, Depolo M. Overwork climate scale: Psychometric properties and relationships with working hard. J Manage Psychol 2016;31(4):880-96.

In: Service Leadership
Editors: Daniel TL Shek, Xiaoqin Zhu, Li Lin et al.
ISBN: 978-1-53614-852-7

Chapter 8

VALIDATION OF THE SERVICE LEADERSHIP KNOWLEDGE SCALE: FACTORIAL AND CONVERGENT VALIDITY

Daniel TL Shek[1-6,*], PhD, FHKPS, BBS, SBS, JP, Lawrence K Ma[1], PhD, Lu Yu[1], PhD and Loretta MK Leung[7], MEd

[1]Department of Applied Social Sciences, The Hong Kong Polytechnic University, Hong Kong, PR China,
[2]Centre for Innovative Programmes for Adolescents and Families, The Hong Kong Polytechnic University, Hong Kong, PR China,
[3]Department of Social Work, East China Normal University, Shanghai, PR China,
[4]Kiang Wu Nursing College of Macau, Macau, PR China,
[5]Hong Kong Institute of Service Leadership and Management Limited, Hong Kong, PR China,
[6]Division of Adolescent Medicine, Department of Pediatrics, Kentucky Children's Hospital, University of Kentucky School of Medicine, Lexington, Kentucky, US
[7]Student Affairs Office, The Education University of Hong Kong, Hong Kong, PR China

* Correspondence: Daniel TL Shek, PhD, FHKPS, BBS, SBS, JP, Associate Vice President (Undergraduate Programme), Chair Professor of Applied Social Sciences and Li and Fung Professor in Service Leadership Education, Department of Applied Social Sciences, The Hong Kong Polytechnic University, Hung Hom, Hong Kong, PR China. E-mail: daniel.shek@polyu.edu.hk.

ABSTRACT

Building on the previous work regarding the assessment tools developed based on the Service Leadership Education model, this chapter reports a large-scale validation study on the Service Leadership Knowledge Scale. A total of 4,486 Hong Kong undergraduates recruited from eight universities funded by the government were administered the Service Leadership Knowledge Scale (Short-Form) with 50 items (SLK-SF-50). After the initial internal consistency assessment, 40 items were retained to form the trimmed version (SLK-SF-40). Confirmatory factor analysis provided support for the hypothesized one-factor structure of the SLK-SF-40 and correlation analyses showed that the scale score was significantly related to different theoretically relevant constructs. The findings demonstrated that the trimmed Service Leadership Knowledge Scale (SLK-SF-40) is an objective measure in gauging individuals' knowledge about Service Leadership.

INTRODUCTION

As a result of the structural shifts in the global economic makeup over the past few decades, Hong Kong has transitioned from a manufacturing-based economy to a service-oriented economy (1). Not only is such a transition characterized by the *production* aspects such as variability of the production process and GDP compositions and share of employment (1), the *people* aspects such as leaders' and organizations' perceptions of human nature and knowledge or competencies needed to excel also constitute the defining attributes of this transformation (2). Owing to the evolution from an *Industrial* to a *Service* Age mentality (3), Chung (4, 5) argued passionately for the need of undergraduates in Hong Kong to learn effective leadership in a service economy, which is key to their survival and personal development in today's ultra-competitive business environment.

Against such a backdrop, a large-scale project entitled the "Fung Service Leadership Education Initiative", financially supported by the Victor and William Fung Foundation and with the collaborative effort of the Hong Kong Institute of Service Leadership and Management Limited (HKI-SLAM) and the University Grants Committee (UGC), was implemented in eight UGC-funded universities in Hong Kong. Po Chung, Chairman of HKI-SLAM, instigated the concept of Service Leadership education targeting Hong Kong's undergraduates (i.e., SLAM framework). Specifically, the SLAM framework maintains that effective Service Leadership is embodied by "a leader or service provider possessing relevant situational task *competencies* plus being judged by superiors, peers, and subordinates as possessing *character* and exhibiting *care*" (6, p. 354). Accordingly, the principle "**E**ffective leadership = **M**oral character * **C**ompetencies * **C**aring disposition", summarized by the equation $E = MC^2$, is highly emphasized within the SLAM framework (6).

As each university would devise her curriculum on the nurturance of effective leadership attributes (i.e., MC^2) (7), it is imperative that systematic evaluation research is conducted to gauge the effectiveness of these independently developed curricula (8).

Particularly, Shek and Lin (9) argued that it is important to assess students' knowledge, attitudes, and behavior to assess an educational program's effectiveness. To facilitate the evaluation of Service Leadership education across universities, the research team at The Hong Kong Polytechnic University (PolyU) developed the long-form Service Leadership Knowledge Scale (SLK-LF-200; 200 items) to measure students' mastery of the fundamental knowledge points on the SLAM framework (10). The assessment tool includes 200 multiple-choice scale items in seven domains based on the SLAM framework and the relevant literature (10). These seven domains include the i) general descriptions of Service Leadership, ii) three realms of Service Leadership, iii) the belief that "Everyone can be a leader", iv) the principle "$E = MC^2$", v) manufacturing versus service economy, vi) distinction of Service Leadership and other leadership theories, and vii) other knowledge points in SLAM framework.

Utilizing a posttest-only control design, Shek and Lin (9) attempted to examine the criterion-related validity of the SLK-LF-200 with an undergraduate sample. The experimental group consisted of 67 students who took a three-credit "Service Leadership" course at the PolyU, whereas the control group was composed of 94 conveniently recruited PolyU students who had never taken the course. Inspection of each item revealed that the former significantly outscored the latter on 63 items. A follow-up inspection of these 63 criterion-valid items, led by the first author of this chapter, resulted in a further removal of 13 items due to duplication or face validity concerns. Ultimately, 50 items were retained to form the short-form of the Service Leadership Knowledge Scale (SLK-SF-50).

While Shek and colleagues (9, 10) pioneered the criterion and content validation of the initial knowledge scale (i.e., SLK-LF-200), the dimensionality and convergent validity of the short form (i.e., SLK-SF-50) remain to be ascertained. Against such a background, utilizing the responses of 4,486 undergraduates in Hong Kong, this chapter is primarily concerned with the psychometric properties of the 50-item SLK-SF-50 based on a large sample of students. Despite the fact that seven dimensions were theorized to be subsumed under the original scale (SLK-LF-200), the removal of three-quarters of items suggests that a re-examination of the trimmed scale's (i.e., SLK-SF-50) dimensionality is necessary. Considering that the knowledge scale operationalizes respondents' understanding of Service Leadership as "knowledge points" they acquired, and that a composite score which denotes overall proficiency is computed (9, 10), there is an implicit assumption that the knowledge scale is indeed unidimensional as the items cohere around one latent "knowledge" dimension (11, 12). Hence, the proposed factor structure of the scale is a one-factor structure of the SLK-SF-50.

Convergent validity, which can be derived from "correlations with measures purporting to measure related constructs" (13), is also crucial in scale development as it informs whether the instrument can adequately probe into the target construct (14). Utilizing several validated measures of relevant constructs outlined in the SLAM framework (see 15), including i) *Servant Leadership*, ii) *moral self-concept*, iii) *leadership efficacy*, and iv) *empathy*, this study sought to establish the convergent validity of the SLK-SF-50 via examining its correlations with these external measures.

OUR STUDY

Altogether 4,486 undergraduates (mean age: 20.47 years; SD: 1.67) from eight UGC-funded institutions completed the Short-Form Service Leadership Scale (SLS) validation study via an online platform. There were 1,517 (33.8%) male and 2,969 (66.2%) female respondents. The majority were aged 20 to 24 years (68.4%), had neither taken any credit-bearing Service Leadership (SL) subjects (74.3%) nor participated in any non-credit-bearing SL events a priori (82.0%), had previous work experience (91.4%), and had formerly served in leadership positions (61.4%). Additionally, 77.1% sat the Hong Kong Diploma of Secondary Education Examination (HKDSE). Table 1 highlights the demographic information for the present sample.

Procedures

All participants were administered the SLS online survey via the mySurvey@PolyU electronic survey system in March 2017. Students were asked to complete the survey in a self-administered fashion. Each participating university had her version of the online survey because the additional information asked is not the same. While the scale items were identical throughout, there were items probing into the respondents' demographics (e.g., faculty or school) and contact information of the person-in-charge that were unique to each university. The research objectives and guidelines on how to complete the questionnaire were detailed in the invitation emails and on the survey webpage. It was reiterated to students that it would take 45 to 60 minutes to conscientiously complete the whole survey. Each participant was given a supermarket voucher by the end of the study valued at HK$100 or US$12.80. Students indicated their consent or refusal to participate at the opening page.

Table 1. Basic demographic information for the current working sample (N = 4,486)

Demographic variables		N= 4,486
Valid responses from eligible participants from:	The Hong Kong Polytechnic University (PolyU)	1,000 (22.3%)
	The Chinese University of Hong Kong (CUHK)	505 (11.3%)
	The Education University of Hong Kong (EdUHK)	500 (11.1%)
	Hong Kong Baptist University (HKBU)	517 (11.5%)
	City University of Hong Kong (CityU)	464 (10.3%)
	Lingnan University (LU)	500 (11.1%)
	The University of Hong Kong (HKU)	500 (11.1%)
	Hong Kong University of Science and Technology (HKUST)	500 (11.1%)

Demographic variables		N= 4,486
Gender	Male	1,517 (33.8%)
	Female	2,969 (66.2%)
Age Group	15 to 19 years	1,344 (30.0%)
	20 to 24 years	3,070 (68.4%)
	25 to 29 years	69 (1.5%)
	30 years or above	3 (0.1%)
Year commencing on one's undergraduate study	2016	1,533 (34.2%)
	2015	1,164 (25.9%)
	2014	897 (20.0%)
	2013	742 (16.5%)
	2012 or before	150 (3.3%)
Number of credit-bearing Service Leadership (SL) courses taken*	0	2,962 (74.3%)
	1	951 (23.9%)
	2	71 (1.8%)
	3	2 (0.1%)
Number of non-credit-bearing SL events participated	0	3,680 (82.0%)
	1	506 (11.3%)
	2	230 (5.1%)
	3	62 (1.4%)
	4 or more	8 (0.2%)
Other leadership training taken	Yes	1,955 (43.6%)
	No	2,531 (56.4%)
Previous work experience	With work experience	4,102 (91.4%)
	Without work experience	384 (8.6%)
Self-proclaimed knowledge of Service Leadership	No knowledge	916 (20.4%)
	Little knowledge	1,590 (35.4%)
	Some knowledge	1,774 (39.5%)
	A lot of knowledge	195 (4.3%)
	All the knowledge	11 (0.2%)
Leadership position ever taken	Yes	2,753 (61.4%)
	No	1,753 (38.6%)
Entrance Exam	Hong Kong Diploma of Secondary Education Examination (HKDSE)	3,484 (77.1%)
	Hong Kong Advanced Level Examination (HKALE)	71 (1.6%)
	National College Entrance Examination (NCEE) in mainland China	221 (4.9%)
	Associate Degree/Higher Diploma in Hong Kong	495 (11.0%)
	Others (e.g., GCE A-Levels, IB, etc.)	215 (4.8%)
Grade Point Average	Mean converted Grade Point Average out of 4.00 (SD)	2.89 (0.45)
Time of completion	Average time (in minutes) taken to complete the survey (SD)	69.98 (383.13)

Note. *EdUHK does not provide any credit-bearing SL modules for her students.

Table 2. Number of cases retained in the main analyses

Participating universities	"Completed" cases as per record in mySurvey	Declined	Multiple participations	Deleted due to ineligibility of participants	Cases retained for the main analyses
EdUHK	506	0	6	0	500
CityU	477	0	3	10	464
HKUST	514	1	12	1	500
CUHK	511	2	0	4	505
LU	509	0	6	3	500
HKU	508	1	2	5	500
HKBU	522	2	0	3	517
PolyU	1008	0	4	4	1000
Total	4555	6	33	30	4486

Participants' completed electronic responses were downloaded as an EXCEL file for a preliminary data cleaning process before being converted to an SPSS file and a DAT file for statistical analyses. Several procedures were involved regarding the 4,555 completed responses as recorded. First, six cases of which students refused to participate were removed. Thirty more cases were excluded due to ineligibility of participants. These included a) participants completing the wrong survey (i.e., University A's students completed the survey designed for University B's students), and b) participants revealing themselves to be non-undergraduates (e.g., postgraduates) in those open-ended questions. Furthermore, thirty-three cases of multiple participations—as per inspection of participants' student ID—were excluded from the main analyses. Accordingly, 4,486 cases were retained for further analyses. Table 2 features a breakdown of the number of cases retained for the present sample.

Table 3. Three sample items of the SLK-SF-50

Items	Options	Model Answer
8. A manager under the service economy wants to hire someone. Based on the Service Leadership model, which of the following advice would you give him/her?	A. Hire for qualifications, train for character B. Hire for character, train for skills C. Hire for attitude, train for character D. Hire for efficiency, train for mindset	B
22. In the four options below, which one belongs to an attribute of intelligence quotient (IQ)?	A. Raw power B. Attractiveness C. Sexual orientation D. Problem-solving skills	D
37. Which of the following statements is inconsistent with the concept of "respect"?	A. Showing off one's strength B. Accepting and appreciating differences C. Accepting and appreciating oneself D. Serving as a key element in nurturing authentic relationship	A

Note. All sample items were slightly re-phrased due to copyright concern.

Instruments

The current questionnaire comprised items of the short-forms of the Service Leadership scales, including that of i) the Service Leadership Attitude Scale (SLA-SF-73; 73 items), ii) the Service Leadership Behavior Scale (SLB-SF-65; 65 items), and iii) the Service Leadership Knowledge Scale (SLK-SF-50; 50 items). The present chapter is primarily concerned about the validation of the 50-item SLK-SF-50.

Developed based on the HKI-SLAM framework, twenty-five principles of Service Leadership (16), twelve dimensions of a Service Leader (3) and the relevant literature (e.g., 15), a 200-item Service Leadership Knowledge Scale (i.e., SLK-LF-200) was designed to "capture the essential knowledge points of Service Leadership model in the format of multiple-choice questions" (10). Fifty items were ultimately retained to form the SLK-SF-50, following Shek and Lin's (9) criterion-validation study and a follow-up item screening. Table 3 features three sample items and the model answers. Participants' responses were coded based on accuracies. Each *correct* answer would earn the participants one point, whereas an *incorrect* answer entitles them to zero point. The scale items are in English.

Several well-validated inventories from the leadership and personality literature were also utilized, with the objective to establish the convergent validity of the SLA-SF-73, the SLB-SF-65, and the SLK-SF-50. These external criterion scales included the Revised Servant Leadership Profile (RSLP; 20 items), Leadership Efficacy Scale (LEF; 8 items), the Moral Self-Concept (MSC; 8 items), and the Interpersonal Reactivity Index (IRI; 14 items). A few forced-choice and open-ended items assessing students' background demographics were also included.

1. **Revised Servant Leadership Profile (RSLP):** Developed by Wong and Page (17), the RSLP measures *Servant Leadership* as a multidimensional construct. Twenty items from five factors relevant to the SLAM framework—namely, i) *Empowering and developing others* (five items), ii) *Serving others* (seven items), iii) *Open, participatory leadership* (two items), iv) *Inspiring leadership* (two items), and v) *Integrity and authenticity* (four items)—were adopted at present. Items were rated on a seven-point Likert scale, with a higher score indicating a greater alignment with a Servant Leader's mentality. Reliability analyses showed an excellent internal consistency of RSLP (α = 0.94; mean inter-item correlations = 0.46).
2. **Leadership Efficacy Scale (LEF):** LEF was developed by Murphy (18) as a measure of one's perceived "generalized capability in the leadership role" (19, p. 270). The LEF, which was utilized in the present study, entails eight items which are rated on a five-point Likert scale. Higher scores indicate one's perceived capability that he/she could lead effectively. Reliability analyses highlighted the acceptable internal consistency of LEF on the present sample (α = 0.72; mean inter-item correlations = 0.25).
3. **Moral Self-Concept (MSC):** As a subscale under the Chinese Adolescent Self-Esteem Scales developed and validated by Cheng (20), the eight-item MSC measures participants' self-evaluation on facets of i) *Conduct and virtues*, ii) *Self-control and discipline*, and iii) *Altruism*. A slightly modified, English-translated version of the MSC—which operates on a seven-point Likert scale—was adopted in the present study. A higher score reflects a greater perceived importance of *morality* to oneself, which is a fundamental attribute of effective Service Leadership according to the SLAM framework (21). Reliability analyses revealed a high internal consistency among the items (α = 0.83; mean inter-item correlations = 0.44).
4. **Interpersonal Reactivity Index (IRI):** Developed by Davis (22), the IRI constitutes the most widely adopted assessment tool of empathy. Not only was the IRI validated cross-culturally (e.g., 23, 24), some suggested that it was the sole "published measure that allows a multi-dimensional assessment of empathy" (25, p. 620). Two subscales

of IRI, namely i) *Perspective Taking* (PT; seven items) and ii) *Empathic Concern* (EC; seven items), were adopted for the current study. Items were rated on a five-point Likert scale, with a higher score indicating a "higher level of empathy which is an essential quality of ethical leadership" (26, p. 44). Component scores for subscales PT and EC were computed alongside a composite IRI score. Cronbach's alpha coefficients of the subscales PT, EC, and the composite IRI score were 0.58, 0.62, and 0.74, respectively.

Data analysis plan

SPSS Statistics version 24.0 (IBM) was used for the descriptive statistical analyses (i.e., demographics) and examination of internal consistency and construct validity. Owing to the dichotomous nature (i.e., *correct* versus *incorrect*) of the coded responses, assessment of the factorial structure of the SLK-SF-50 (i.e., Confirmatory factor analysis [CFA]) was conducted using Mplus version 6.12 (27).

We first inspected the reliability indices of the 50-item SLK-SF-50. A Kuder-Richardson 20 coefficient of 0.93 was observed, suggesting excellent reliability. Ten items with item-total correlations below 0.30 were excluded from the ensuing CFA. We then re-examined the reliability indices of the 40-item, trimmed SLK-SF-50 (i.e., SLK-SF-40 hereafter). Regarding CFA, the proposed one-factor structure was tested using the robust weighted least squares (WLSMV) estimator, which is appropriate for categorical items (28).

We examined the model fit using several indices including, a) Bentler-Bonett Nonnormed Fit Index (NNFI), b) comparative fit index (CFI), c) root mean square error of approximation (RMSEA; including also the 90% confidence interval [90% CI]), and d) weighted root-mean-square residual (WRMR). Based on the recommendations in the literature (29-31), a model with a NNFI exceeding 0.95, a CFI greater than 0.95, a RMSEA lower than 0.05 (with an upper CI value below 0.08), and a WRMR smaller than 0.90 would be considered an 'excellent' fit. Models with a 'good' fit should produce indices close to the above standards (28). We also reported the STDY metric for each item, which denotes the change in standard deviation units of outcomes (as per unit change in predictor). The STDY metric represents each item's standardized factor loading (32).

Lastly, the total scale score was correlated with the different criterion measures. Considering that the knowledge preached in the Service Leadership curriculum covers domains on *Servant Leadership*, *leadership efficacy*, *morality*, and *empathy*, we would predict a positive correlation between the SLK-SF-40 with each of these external criterion scales (and subscales). Correlational analyses with other Service Leadership scales (and subscales) under validation were also administered. Data of the entire sample (N = 4,486) were utilized throughout every step of the present validation study. Specifically, we hypothesized that the SLK-SF-40 would be positively and significantly correlated with i)

RSLP, ii) LEF, iii) MSC, and iv) IRI (subscales EC and PT). We expected the SLK-SF-40 to also correlate positively with the validated versions of the SLA-SF-73 and SLB-SF-65 (and the subscales), considering that all these scales were constructed to assess the same underlying topic with different focuses (i.e., knowledge, attitude, and behavior).

FINDINGS

After removing ten items with low item-total correlations, reliability analyses revealed the excellent internal consistency of the 40 items retained (α = 0.94, mean inter-item correlations = 0.28). All items had a corrected item-total correlation above 0.31.

Confirmatory factor analysis

Table 4 presents the model-fit indices of the proposed single-factor structure of SLK-SF-40, alongside the criteria for goodness-of-fit evaluation as abovementioned. Overall, the NNFI, CFI, and RMSEA all suggested that the present proposed one-factor structure fit excellently with the current data (29-31), while the WRMR exceeded the proposed cut-off of 0.90, suggesting a model misspecification (33). Nevertheless, Newsom (34) cautioned against the sole reliance on WRMR as the only indicator of fit as it "does not always give sensible results (p. 3)", and there is evidence (e.g., 35) that the three other metrics adopted at present (i.e., NNFI, CFI, and RMSEA) could perform well with categorical model estimations. Taken together, the examination of the goodness-of-fit indices offers preliminary support to the one-factor solution of SLK-SF-40.

We also scrutinized the individual parameter estimates of the present proposed one-factor solution. Table 5 presents every item's i) standardized factor loading (i.e., STDY estimates), ii) R-squared, iii) accuracy rate, iv) residual variance, and v) item-total correlations. As addressed in the table, the factor loadings and R-squared of all the SLK-SF-40 items were positive and significant at p <.001. The STDY estimates ranged from moderate to strong (0.32 to 0.90). No spurious findings were observed regarding the standard errors. These findings, in conjunction with the goodness-of-fit indices (see Table 4), again gave support to the proposed one-factor structure of the knowledge scale. Accordingly, this single-factor model was accepted as the final factorial solution, and each respondent's SLK-SF-40 score was computed via a simple summation of their *correct* responses to the 40 items.

Table 4. Model fit indices for the one-factor structure of SLK-SF-40

Model Tested	χ^2	Df	WRMR	NNFI	CFI	RMSEA (pclose)	RMSEA (90% C.I.)
One-factor	3,492.44	740	1.725	0.985	0.984	0.029 (1.00)	0.028/0.030
Criterion for goodness-of-fit	-	-	≤ 0.90	≥ 0.95	≥ 0.95	≤ 0.05	≤ 0.08

Note. WRMR= weighted root-mean-square residual; NNFI= Bentler-Bonett Nonnormed Fit Index; CFI= comparative fit index; RMSEA= root mean square error of approximation; pclose= probability of RMSEA $\leq$ 0.05; 90% CI= 90% Confidence Intervals (lower value/ upper value).

Table 5. Individual parameter estimates of the one-factor SLK-SF-40 (N= 4,486)

Items	Mean* (Standard Deviation)	Accuracy Rate**	Standardized factor loadings	R-squared	Residual variance	Corrected Item-total Correlations
SLK-01	0.391 (0.488)	39.12%	0.528	0.279	0.721	0.396
SLK-02	0.751 (0.433)	75.06%	0.545	0.297	0.703	0.396
SLK-03	0.830 (0.376)	83.01%	0.646	0.417	0.583	0.433
SLK-05	0.742 (0.438)	74.19%	0.537	0.289	0.711	0.391
SLK-06	0.439 (0.496)	43.87%	0.419	0.175	0.825	0.316
SLK-08	0.612 (0.487)	61.21%	0.570	0.325	0.675	0.444
SLK-10	0.447 (0.497)	44.72%	0.597	0.356	0.644	0.461
SLK-11	0.523 (0.500)	52.25%	0.522	0.272	0.728	0.399
SLK-12	0.607 (0.489)	60.65%	0.535	0.287	0.713	0.415
SLK-13	0.740 (0.439)	73.99%	0.831	0.690	0.310	0.621
SLK-14	0.592 (0.492)	59.16%	0.718	0.515	0.485	0.565
SLK-15	0.396 (0.489)	39.59%	0.676	0.456	0.544	0.509
SLK-16	0.604 (0.489)	60.43%	0.878	0.770	0.230	0.699
SLK-17	0.673 (0.469)	67.32%	0.869	0.755	0.245	0.682
SLK-18	0.597 (0.490)	59.74%	0.901	0.813	0.187	0.726
SLK-19	0.673 (0.469)	67.32%	0.558	0.311	0.689	0.422
SLK-20	0.624 (0.484)	62.44%	0.838	0.703	0.297	0.667
SLK-21	0.675 (0.468)	67.50%	0.570	0.324	0.676	0.433
SLK-22	0.685 (0.465)	68.46%	0.760	0.578	0.422	0.577
SLK-23	0.619 (0.486)	61.93%	0.819	0.672	0.328	0.652
SLK-24	0.542 (0.498)	54.19%	0.603	0.363	0.637	0.469
SLK-25	0.568 (0.495)	56.82%	0.755	0.570	0.430	0.598
SLK-26	0.594 (0.491)	59.38%	0.748	0.559	0.441	0.583
SLK-28	0.664 (0.472)	66.41%	0.316	0.100	0.900	0.653
SLK-30	0.672 (0.469)	67.23%	0.833	0.693	0.307	0.568
SLK-31	0.536 (0.499)	53.63%	0.731	0.534	0.466	0.573
SLK-32	0.552 (0.497)	55.19%	0.739	0.546	0.454	0.522
SLK-33	0.399 (0.490)	39.88%	0.662	0.438	0.562	0.494
SLK-34	0.536 (0.499)	53.59%	0.651	0.424	0.576	0.665
SLK-36	0.375 (0.484)	37.47%	0.820	0.673	0.327	0.462
SLK-38	0.429 (0.495)	42.93%	0.617	0.381	0.619	0.478
SLK-39	0.358 (0.480)	35.84%	0.618	0.382	0.618	0.318

Items	Mean* (Standard Deviation)	Accuracy Rate**	Standardized factor loadings	R-squared	Residual variance	Corrected Item-total Correlations
SLK-41	0.608 (0.488)	60.81%	0.430	0.185	0.815	0.616
SLK-42	0.514 (0.500)	51.38%	0.772	0.596	0.404	0.580
SLK-44	0.343 (0.475)	34.26%	0.731	0.534	0.466	0.366
SLK-45	0.526 (0.499)	52.56%	0.497	0.247	0.753	0.591
SLK-46	0.649 (0.477)	64.87%	0.757	0.572	0.428	0.437
SLK-47	0.539 (0.499)	53.92%	0.563	0.317	0.683	0.343
SLK-48	0.363 (0.481)	36.31%	0.442	0.196	0.804	0.314
SLK-50	0.566 (0.496)	56.58%	0.421	0.177	0.823	0.575

Note. * Each correct (incorrect) response was coded "1" ("0"). ** Accuracy Rate = (Number of correct responses)/ (Total responses, i.e., 4,486) *100%. All standardized factor loadings and R^2 metrics were statistically significant at p <.001 (two-tailed).

Validity analyses: Correlation with external criterion scales (and subscales)

Confirming our hypotheses, findings of the correlational analyses (see Table 6) indicated that the SLK-SF-40 scores correlated significantly (all *p*s <.001) and positively with all external criterion scales (and subscales). Utilizing the *cocor* statistical package (36) which allows comparisons of strengths of association across two pairs of correlation coefficients (e.g., Steiger's (37) computation of z-score using average correlations), the findings (see Table 6) indicated that amongst the significant associations, the SLK-SF-40 correlated most strongly with the *Interpersonal Reactivity Index* (r = 0.438, N = 4,486) and least with the *Leadership Efficacy* (r = 0.125, N = 4,486). These findings should give substance to the convergent validity of the SLK-SF-40 as it was demonstrated to relate positively and significantly to a myriad of well-validated measures (e.g., IRI and MSC) on constructs that were highly emphasized in the SLAM framework (e.g., empathy and morality).

Table 6. Correlations between SLK-SF-40 and the presently adopted external criterion scales

Correlations with the external criterion scales (and subscales)			Z-scores of difference between *r*s with SLK-SF-40 (36,37):				
	α (MITC)	*r*	MSC	LEF	IRI	IRI-EC	IRI-PT
1. RSLP	0.94 (0.46)	0.200***	-16.17***	4.83***	-16.92***	-14.15***	-10.09***
2. MSC	0.83 (0.44)	0.361***	—	15.11***	-6.25***	-4.31***	1.12
3. LEF	0.72 (0.25)	0.125***	—	—	-18.83***	-16.76***	-13.09***
4. IRI	0.74 (0.17)	0.438***	—	—	—	2.97**	12.91***
4a. IRI- EC	0.62 (0.19)	0.419***	—	—	—	—	5.64***
4b. IRI- PT	0.58 (0.19)	0.346***	—	—	—	—	—

Note. **p <.01 (two-tailed). ***p <.001 (two-tailed). MITC: Mean inter-item correlations. RSLP: Revised Servant Leadership Profile; MSC: Moral Self-Concept; LEF: Leadership Efficacy; IRI: Interpersonal Reactivity Index; IRI-EC: Subscale "Empathic Concern"; IRI: PT: Subscale "Perspective Taking".

Table 7. Correlations between SLK-SF-40 and other Service Leadership scales (and subscales) under validation

Correlations with other Service Leadership Scales under validation			Z-scores of difference between *r*s with SLK-SF-40 (36,37)[a]														
	α (MITC)	*r*	SLB-SF-38-F2	SLB-SF-38-F3	SLB-SF-38-F4	SLB-SF-38-F5	SLB-SF-38-F6	SLB-SF-38-Total	SLA-SF-46-F1	SLA-SF-46-F2	SLA-SF-46-F3	SLA-SF-46-F4	SLA-SF-46-F5	SLA-SF-46-F6	SLA-SF-46-F7	SLA-SF-46-F8	SLA-SF-46-Total
1.SLB-SF-38-F1	0.91 (0.53)	0.203***	-5.93	12.03	-0.20$^{n.s.}$	6.39	21.47	3.32	-7.57	-8.78	3.06	8.76	-11.35	-2.05	8.91	-10.53	-12.44
2.SLB-SF-38-F2	0.87 (0.42)	0.269***	—	16.39	5.56	10.44	26.85	11.54	-3.36	-5.08	8.01	13.51	-7.81	2.31	13.37	-7.42	-8.87
3.SLB-SF-38-F3	0.87 (0.50)	0.047**	—	—	-12.57	-5.26	9.64	-14.88	-16.03	-17.07	-6.42	-0.48$^{n.s.}$	-18.95	-10.93	0.53$^{n.s.}$	-17.40	-20.59
4.SLB-SF-38-F4	0.86 (0.55)	0.205***	—	—	—	6.06	20.81	2.92	-7.19	-8.71	3.18	8.77	-11.25	-1.82$^{n.s.}$	9.17	-10.59	-12.14
5.SLB-SF-38-F5	0.87 (0.56)	0.117***	—	—	—	—	13.36	-5.80	-12.20	-13.09	-2.22	3.35	-15.34	-7.05	4.06	-14.54	-16.32
6.SLB-SF-38-F6	0.85 (0.65)	-0.097***	—	—	—	—	—	-25.32	-23.05	-24.12	-15.34	-9.03	-25.78	-18.11	-7.35	-23.05	-28.03
7.SLB-SF-38-Total	0.96 (0.37)	0.178***	—	—	—	—	—	—	-9.59	-10.91	1.61$^{n.s.}$	7.67	-13.46	-3.74	7.92	-11.54	-15.12
8.SLA-SF-46-F1	0.90 (0.46)	0.315***	—	—	—	—	—	—	—	-2.35	12.83	18.20	-5.98	6.73	15.51	-4.97	-8.93
9.SLA-SF-46-F2	0.87 (0.47)	0.337***	—	—	—	—	—	—	—	—	14.30	18.90	-3.52	7.80	17.93	-3.96	-5.44
10.SLA-SF-46-F3	0.86 (0.47)	0.155***	—	—	—	—	—	—	—	—	—	8.28	-17.20	-5.85	7.01	-12.12	-24.59
11.SLA-SF-46-F4	0.85 (0.53)	0.055***	—	—	—	—	—	—	—	—	—	—	-21.46	-11.92	1.05$^{n.s.}$	-16.15	-27.97
12.SLA-SF-46-F5	0.83 (0.56)	0.373***	—	—	—	—	—	—	—	—	—	—	—	11.05	19.00	-2.09	-0.54$^{n.s.}$
13.SLA-SF-46-F6	0.82 (0.49)	0.235***	—	—	—	—	—	—	—	—	—	—	—	—	10.41	-8.53	-13.48
14.SLA-SF-46-F7	0.70 (0.54)	0.037***	—	—	—	—	—	—	—	—	—	—	—	—	—	-18.97	-22.18
15.SLA-SF-46-F8	0.79 (0.42)	0.411***	—	—	—	—	—	—	—	—	—	—	—	—	—	—	1.92$^{n.s.}$
16.SLA-SF-46-Total	0.93 (0.28)	0.377***	—	—	—	—	—	—	—	—	—	—	—	—	—	—	—

Note. [a]Unless otherwise specified by the superscript "n.s." which denotes statistical non-significance, all other Z-scores of difference were significant at $p < .05$ (two-tailed) (i.e., |Z-score| > 1.96). ** $p < .01$ (two-tailed). *** $p < .001$ (two-tailed). MITC: Mean inter-item correlations. SLB-SF-38-Total: Scale score of the six-factor, 38-item Service Leadership Behavior (SLB) Scale; SLA-SF-46-Total: Scale score of the eight-factor, 46-item Service Leadership Attitude (SLA) Scale; SLB-SF-38-F1: SLB Factor 1 "Self-improvement and self-reflection"; SLB-SF-38-F2: SLB Factor 2 "People and principles orientation"; SLB-SF-38-F3: SLB Factor 3 "Resilience"; SLB-SF-38-F4: SLB Factor 4 "Social competence"; SLB-SF-38-F5: SLB Factor 5 "Problem-solving"; SLB-SF-38-F6: SLB Factor 6 "Mentorship"; SLA-SF-46-F1: SLA Factor 1 "Vision and competence"; SLA-SF-46-F2: SLA Factor 2 "People orientation"; SLA-SF-46-F3: SLA Factor 3 "Caring disposition"; SLA-SF-46-F4: SLA Factor 4 "Ethical role model"; SLA-SF-46-F5: SLA Factor 5 "Social competence"; SLA-SF-46-F6: SLA Factor 6 "Self-understanding and reflection"; SLA-SF-46-F7: SLA Factor 7 "Positive view about human beings"; SLA-SF-46-F8: SLA Factor 8 "Unchangeable and dark human nature".

Validity analyses: Correlation with other Service Leadership scales under validation

As detailed in Table 7, the SLK-SF-40 correlated significantly (all *ps* <.001) and positively with both composite scores of the six-factor, 38-item Service Leadership Behavior (i.e., SLB-SF-38) scale ($r = 0.178$, N = 4,486) and the eight-factor, 46-item Service Leadership Attitude (i.e., SLA-SF-46) scale ($r = 0.337$, N = 4,486). Discussions regarding the validations of both SLB-SF-38 and SLA-SF-46 are featured in two other papers within the current issue. The SLK-SF-40 also correlated positively with almost all the subscales of SLB-SF-38 and SLA-SF-46. These findings are consistent with our hypotheses that the three concurrently administered Service Leadership scales are positively and significantly associated with one another.

Furthermore, comparison via the *cocor* package highlighted that the strengths of correlations between SLK-SF-40 and SLA-SF-46 (and the subscales) were overall significantly greater (*ps* <.05) than those of SLK-SF-40 and SLB-SF-38 (and its subscales). These findings suggested that while individuals knowing more about Service Leadership may be more prone to *think* or *feel* (i.e., attitude) and to *act* (i.e., behavior) as an effective Service Leader, there seems to be a weaker tie between "knowing" and "practicing what one was preached".

DISCUSSION

The primary purpose of this study was to examine the factorial validity and convergent validity of the Service Leadership Knowledge Scale in a sample of Hong Kong undergraduates. Reliability analyses highlighted the excellent internal consistency amongst the 40 items which formed the SLK-SF-40. Consistent with our predictions, results of the CFA corroborated the unidimensionality of the SLK-SF-40, as both the goodness-of-fit indices and individual parameter estimates indicated that the proposed one-factor solution fits excellently with the data. Furthermore, the SLK-SF-40 correlated significantly and positively with all the external criterion scales. The SLK-SF-40 also correlated positively with the two other Service Leadership scales. Both these correlational findings offer convergent evidence for the SLK-SF-40, as instruments measuring i) the same underlying construct (i.e., SLB-SF-38 and SLA-SF-46) and ii) theoretically relevant constructs (i.e., IRI, MSC) all related consistently and positively to the SLK-SF-40. In summary, the present findings underscore the adequacy of SLK-SF-40 in measuring students' knowledge in Service Leadership.

While the findings overall support the validity and reliability of the SLK-SF-40, there are observations worthy of attention. First, the effect sizes of the *Knowledge-Servant*

Leadership correlation ($r = 0.20$) and the *Knowledge-Efficacy association* ($r = 0.13$) are noticeably smaller compared to that of the *Knowledge-Empathy* ($r = 0.44$) and the *Knowledge-Moral Self-concept* ($r = 0.36$) associations. These findings may reflect the differential coverage of the constructs within the SLAM framework. As discussed above, *Moral character* constitutes the cornerstone of the SLAM framework (i.e., the "$E = MC^2$" principle). Likewise, empathy is extensively covered as a fundamental attribute of *Caring Disposition* (38). *Servant Leadership* and *Leadership Efficacy*, by contrast, are not as central to the SLAM framework despite being two highly relevant constructs. In particular, the disregard of self-interest, which is a hallmark attribute in the *Servant Leadership* theory (39), is even at odds with a Core Belief of the SLAM framework (21).

Second, comparison of the correlational strengths underlined a discrepancy between the *Knowledge-Attitude* ($r = 0.34$) tie vis-à-vis the *Knowledge-Behavior* association ($r = 0.18$), implying that Service Leadership may be easier-said-than-done. However, as theorized in the Theory of Planned Behavior (TPB) (39), while *attitude* and perceived behavioral control (which involves *knowledge*) constitute two key contributors of behavioral intention (BI), BI is also determined by a perception of whether a particular behavior would lead to others' approval (i.e., normative beliefs [NB]). In other words, although both *attitude* and *knowledge* are essential to the formation of intent to behave like a Service Leader, there is an additional element in NB (perception of whether acting as a Service Leader would be well-received by relevant others) to be taken into consideration. Hence, the current observed differential correlation strengths amongst knowledge, attitude, and behavior are actually in line with the TPB (39). This would be an interesting direction for future research.

As a continuation of the PolyU research team's effort, the current study marks the concluding step of the creation (plus validation) of the assessment tool aimed to measure people's understanding of Service Leadership. Specifically, the present paper came up with a much-shortened version of the knowledge scale (i.e., SLK-SF-40) which was demonstrated to be valid and reliable. Not only is a shorter survey easier to administer, crucially, meta-analytic review findings had also consistently pointed to how shorter questionnaires are linked to higher response rates and avoidance of low-quality data due to response burden (40, 41). In response to Shek et al.'s (10) appeal to develop an assessment instrument which facilitates cross-institutional comparisons on students' understanding of the SLAM framework, alongside adding to the literature on systematic evaluation of Service Leadership education, the present study produced a refined, "participant-friendly", and most importantly, a psychometrically sound measurement tool in the SLK-SF-40.

All in all, in conjunction with the previous studies, there is a strong evidence base for the different versions of the Service Leadership Knowledge Scale. In future, more work could be done to further examine the criterion-related validity of the different versions of the scale. Besides, the relationship between Service Leadership knowledge and actual Service Leadership behavior deserves investigation using longitudinal research designs.

ACKNOWLEDGMENTS

The validation project is financially supported by the Victor and William Fung Foundation. The preparation for this chapter is supported by the Foundation and the Endowed Professorship in Service Leadership Education at The Hong Kong Polytechnic University. This chapter is an updated version of a publication in the special issue "Development and validation of assessment tools on service leadership knowledge, attitude and behavior" edited by Daniel TL Shek, Xiaoqin Zhu and Joav Merrick published in the International Journal of Child and Adolescent Health, 2018;11(4).

REFERENCES

[1] Shek DTL, Chung PPY, Leung H. Manufacturing economy vs. service economy: Implications for Service Leadership. Int J Disabil Hum Dev 2015;14:205-15.

[2] Shek DTL, Leung H. Service Leadership qualities in university students through the lens of student well-being. In: Shek DTL, Chung PPY, eds. Promoting Service Leadership qualities in university students: The case of Hong Kong. Singapore: Springer, 2015:1-16.

[3] Chung PPY, Elfassy R. The 12 dimensions of a service leader, 1st ed. New York: Lexingford, 2016.

[4] Chung PPY. Service reborn: The knowledge, skills, and attitudes of service companies, 1st ed. New York: Lexingford, 2012.

[5] Chung PPY. Where there is no vision, the people will perish. In: Shek DTL, Chung PPY, eds. Promoting Service Leadership qualities in university students: The case of Hong Kong. Singapore: Springer, 2015:xv-xviii.

[6] Shek DTL, Yu L, Ma CMS, Sun RCF, Liu TT. Development of a credit-bearing Service Leadership subject for university students in Hong Kong. Int J Adolesc Med Health 2013;25:353-61.

[7] Shek DTL, Chung PPY, eds. Promoting Service Leadership qualities in university students: The case of Hong Kong. Singapore: Springer, 2015.

[8] Shek DTL, Lin L. Evaluating Service Leadership programs with multiple strategies. In: Shek DTL, Chung PPY, eds. Promoting Service Leadership qualities in university students: The case of Hong Kong. Singapore: Springer, 2015:197-211.

[9] Shek DTL, Lin L. Validation of the Service Leadership Knowledge Scale: Criterion-related validity. In: Shek DTL, Chung PPY, Lin L, Merrick J, eds. Service Leadership education for university students. New York: Nova Science, 2017:189-204.

[10] Shek DTL, Lin L, Leung H, Yu L, Ma CMS, Li X. Development and validation of the Service Leadership Knowledge Scale in a Chinese context. In: Shek DTL, Chung PPY, Lin L, Merrick J, eds. Service Leadership education for university students. New York: Nova Science, 2017:163-87.

[11] DeMars CE. Item response theory: Understanding statistics measurement. New York: Oxford University Press, 2010.

[12] Piedmont RL. Factorial validity. In: Michalos AC, ed. Encyclopedia of Quality of Life and Well-being research. Netherlands: Springer, 2014:2148-9.

[13] Cohen RJ, Swerdlik ME. Psychological testing and assessment: An introduction to tests and measurement, 6th ed. New York: McGraw-Hill, 2005.

[14] Goodwin CJ. Research in psychology: Methods and design, 6th ed. New York: Wiley, 2009.

[15] Shek DTL, Chung PPY, Yu L, Merrick J, eds. Service Leadership education for university students: Experience of Hong Kong [Special issue]. Int J Disabil Hum Dev 2015;14:203-93.

[16] Chung PPY, Bell AH. 25 principles of service leadership, 1st ed. New York: Lexingford, 2015.

[17] Wong PTP, Page D. Servant Leadership: An opponent-process model and the Revised Servant Leadership Profile. Virginia Beach, VA: Regent University, 2003.
[18] Murphy SE. The contribution of leadership experience and self-efficacy to group performance under evaluation apprehension. Dissertation. Seattle: WA: University of Washington, 1992.
[19] Chemers MM, Watson CB, May ST. Dispositional affect and leadership effectiveness: A comparison of self-esteem, optimism, and efficacy. Pers Soc Psychol Bull 2000;26:267-77.
[20] Cheng CHK. The Chinese Adolescent Self-Esteem Scales (CASES): A user manual. Hong Kong: City University of Hong Kong Press, 2005.
[21] Shek DTL, Lin L. Core Beliefs in the Service Leadership model proposed by the Hong Kong Institute of Service Leadership and Management. Int J Disabil Hum Dev 2015;14:233-42.
[22] Davis MH. Measuring individual differences in empathy: Evidence for a multidimensional approach. J Pers Soc Psychol 1983;44:113-26.
[23] Albiero P, Ingoglia S, Lo Coco A. Contributo all'adattamento Italiano dell'Interpersonal Reactivity Index [A contribution to the Italian validation of the Interpersonal Reactivity Index]. Test Psicom Methodol 2006;13:107-25. [Italian]
[24] Siu AMH, Shek DTL. Validation of the Interpersonal Reactivity Index in a Chinese Context. Res Soc Work 2005;15:118-26.
[25] Shamay-Tsoory SG, Aharon-Peretz J, Perry D. Two systems for empathy: A double dissociation between emotional and cognitive empathy in inferior frontal gyrus versus ventromedial prefrontal lesions. Brain 2009;132:617-27.
[26] Shek DTL, Yu L. General University Requirements and holistic development in university students in Hong Kong. Int J Adolesc Med Health 2017;29:41-8.
[27] Muthén LK, Muthén BO. Mplus user's guide, 6th ed. Los Angeles, CA: Muthén Muthén, 2011.
[28] Rodebaugh TL, Holaway RM, Heimberg RG. The factor structure and dimensional scoring of the Generalized Anxiety Disorder Questionnaire for DSM-IV. Assessment 2008;15:343-50.
[29] Hu LT, Bentler PM. Evaluating model fit. In: Hoyle RH, ed. Structural equation modeling: Concepts, issues and applications. Thousand Oaks, CA: Sage, 1995:76-99.
[30] Hu LT, Bentler PM. Cutoff criteria for fit indexes in covariance structure analysis: Conventional criteria versus new alternatives. Struct Equ Modeling 1999;6:1-55.
[31] Kenny DA. Measuring model fit. 2015. URL: http://davidakenny.net/cm/fit.htm.
[32] Templin J. Confirmatory factor analysis: Introduction to structural equation modeling. 2012. URL: https://jonathantemplin.com/files/sem/sem12ersh8750/sem12ersh8750_lecture05.pdf.
[33] Yu C-Y. Evaluation of model fit indices for latent variable models with categorical and continuous outcomes. Dissertation. Los Angeles, CA: University of California, 2002.
[34] Newsom JT. Practical approaches to dealing with non-normal and categorical variables. 2015. URL: https://pdfs.semanticscholar.org/d6f1/7c3bf7253376ac2e3098544ba18ba3c55dbd.pdf?_ga=2.137211449.804333835.1526630013-801728712.1526630013.
[35] Beauducel A, Herzberg PY. On the performance of maximum likelihood versus means and variance adjusted weighted least squares estimation in CFA. Struct Equ Modeling 2006;13:186-203.
[36] Diedenhofen B, Musch J. cocor: A comprehensive solution for the statistical comparison of correlations. PLoS One 2015;10:e0121945. doi:10.1371/journal.pone.0121945.
[37] Steiger JH. Tests for comparing elements of a correlation matrix. Psychol Bull 1980;87:245-51.
[38] Shek DTL, Li X. The role of a caring disposition in Service Leadership. Int J Disabil Hum Dev 2015;14:319-32.
[39] Ajzen I. The theory of planned behavior. Organ Behav Hum Decis Process 1991;50:179-211.
[40] Edwards P, Roberts I, Clarke M, DiGuiseppi C, Pratap S, Wentz R, et al. Increasing response rates to postal questionnaires: Systematic review. BMJ 2002;324:1183-91.
[41] Rolstad S, Adler JA, Rydén A. Response burden and questionnaire length: Is shorter better? A review and meta-analysis. Value Health 2011;14:1101-8.

In: Service Leadership
Editors: Daniel TL Shek, Xiaoqin Zhu, Li Lin et al.
ISBN: 978-1-53614-852-7

Chapter 9

VALIDATION OF THE SERVICE LEADERSHIP ATTITUDE SCALE IN HONG KONG

Daniel TL Shek[1-6,*], PhD, FHKPS, BBS, SBS, JP, Alex YF Zhu[1], PhD, Lawrence K Ma[1], PhD and Li Lin[1], PhD

[1]Department of Applied Social Sciences, The Hong Kong Polytechnic University, Hong Kong, PR China
[2]Centre for Innovative Programmes for Adolescents and Families, The Hong Kong Polytechnic University, Hong Kong, PR China
[3]Department of Social Work, East China Normal University, Shanghai, PR China
[4]Kiang Wu Nursing College of Macau, Macau, PR China
[5]Hong Kong Institute of Service Leadership and Management Limited, Hong Kong, PR China
[6]Division of Adolescent Medicine, Department of Pediatrics, Kentucky Children's Hospital, University of Kentucky School of Medicine, Lexington, Kentucky, US

ABSTRACT

To cultivate leadership of university students under the service economy, there is a need to help them develop positive attitude towards service leadership. Unfortunately, validated service leadership attitude measures do not exist. In this chapter, validation of the Service Leadership Attitude Scale was reported. Based on the responses of 4,486 students, internal consistency, convergent validity and construct validity of the 73-item Service Leadership Attitude Scale (SLA-SF-73) were examined. Exploratory factor analyses further showed

* Correspondence: Daniel TL Shek, PhD, FHKPS, BBS, SBS, JP, Associate Vice President (Undergraduate Programme), Chair Professor of Applied Social Sciences and Li and Fung Professor in Service Leadership Education, Department of Applied Social Sciences, The Hong Kong Polytechnic University, Hung Hom, Hong Kong, PR China. E-mail: daniel.shek@polyu.edu.hk.

that seven stable factors (Vision and Competence, Social Competence, Caring Disposition, People Orientation, Self-Reflection and Self-Understanding, Positive Views about Human Beings, and Ethical Role Models) were abstracted from the final 46-item scale (SLA-SF-46E), providing support for the factorial validity of the scale.

INTRODUCTION

Hong Kong has shifted from a manufacture-oriented economy to a service economy since the 80s of the last century (1). Till the end of 2016, four service-oriented pillars including banking and investment services, tourism services, logistics transportation and business support services have become the key engines driving the Hong Kong economy (2). The number of working adults in the service-oriented sectors has increased from 3.14 million in 2011 to 3.31 million in 2016, accounting for 84.57% of all working adults (2), indicating the importance of service industries to the Hong Kong economy. Previous studies have devoted increasing attention to human capital and organizational climate in service sectors (3, 4), which are two primary mechanisms to obtain organizational success by influencing employees (5, 6). Although traditional research emphasizes the positive influence of the bundles of Human Resource Management (HRM) Practice on human capital and organizational climate, Jiang and his colleagues (7) found other than HRM, both human capital and organizational climate are also positively shaped by a new ideology of leadership, service leadership, in service-economies.

Jiang and his colleagues (7) adopted the definition of service leadership in the study of Schneider and his colleagues (8), which claimed service leadership is essentially a behavioral focus on improving the service quality of an organization. Chung (9) extended the scope (i.e., not service manufacturing) and claimed that service leadership is essentially a behavioral focus on consistently offering quality personal service to meet the demand at individual, organizational, and social levels. Based on the framework of the Hong Kong Institute of Service Leadership and Management Limited (HKI-SLAM) (10), service leadership is featured by seven core beliefs which increase the competiveness of the service-oriented economy in Hong Kong. First, service leaders believe service leadership is the service satisfying the needs of stakeholders at different levels, including individuals, groups, communities, systems and environments (10), which well responds to the service-dominant logic in the service-oriented economy that all social units compete with service, and compete through service (11). Second, service leaders believe everyone can be a leader to improve service effectiveness and quality anytime (10), which spurs service innovation as the core competency of a service organization (12). Third, service leadership supports the notion that leadership effectiveness and service satisfaction are jointly determined by task competencies, unique character and exhibiting care (10), which promotes the effectiveness of relationship marketing and emphasizes on keeping loyal customers by setting their satisfaction as priorities instead of emphasizing on the number of transactions completed. Researchers (1, 13) asserted that this is the most common strategy to retain customers in the service organizations. Fourth, service leaders believe that service leadership aims to ethically promote the competiveness, abilities, and willingness of offering service to others (10), which is a particular prerequisite of improving service quality in Hong Kong, where the economic return of service does not wholly depend on service quality. Fifth, service leadership is focused on consistently creating personal service to change the life of others, responding to the transformation of profit model from indiscriminate commodities in the manufacture-oriented economy to customized service in the service-oriented economy (14). Sixth, service leadership is seen as the longest and most competitive business model (10), which can be adopted as a main business model for Hong Kong, considering a majority of its domestic production is supported by service-related industries. Last, other than specific skills and knowledge, leadership competencies, appropriate character strengths and caring social dispositions are also key requirements for high status positions in the service-oriented economy (10), which highlight that the soft skills are valuable assets in leading people-oriented projects in the service organizations (11).

In order to maintain the competitiveness of the service-oriented economy of Hong Kong in the global market, strengthening the service leadership in the service organizations is a necessity. With the requirement of cognitive and social-emotional competence, service leadership should be introduced before joining the labor market. Hence, the best time to conduct the related education is during tertiary education. To achieve this goal, HKI-SLAM and the Victor and William Fung Foundation cooperated and founded the Fung Service Leadership Education Initiative in 2012, and William Fung Foundation resolved to allocate HK$40 million to design and conduct education programs of service leadership among college students in eight publically funded tertiary institutions in Hong Kong. The initiative aimed at promoting service leadership among local college students. Although the eight universities designed and implemented the courses and projects based on their own needs, there is a call for valid scales measuring service leadership attitude, knowledge and behavior to evaluate the effectiveness of these courses and projects as well as comparing the evaluation outcomes cross eight universities.

In the framework of cognitive and behavioral development, attitude plays an important mediation role connecting knowledge and behavior (15-17). Knowledge can positively shape attitude, which in turn leads to the formation of a behavioral intention (15). Ajzen (15) argued the more favorable the attitude, the stronger should be the person's intention to perform the specific behavior under consideration. Unfortunately, although attitude to service leadership is important, there has been no valid scales measuring service leadership attitude in Hong Kong-based college students. To fill the gap, a 132-item scale (SLA-LF-132) was initially developed to measure service leadership attitude among local college students by our team based on the SLAM framework, 25 principles of service leadership (18), 12 dimensions of a service leader (19) and relevant literature authored by Shek and his colleagues (20, 21). The 132-item scale showed good content validity (22). Based on the preliminary criterion-related validation results which are unpublished, 73 items were retained as the short version (SLA-SF-73). In this chapter we aim to explore the internal consistency, convergent validity and factorial validity of these 73 items.

OUR STUDY

The participants were sampled from undergraduate students of eight publically funded universities in Hong Kong. Students from each university were invited to fill out a customized online survey. The purpose of the research and how the data would be used were presented to students at the title page of the survey. Students were informed they have the rights to stop the online survey anytime. The title page also revealed that all information would be kept confidential and the individual identity of students would not be disclosed at any point. Students were informed that a supermarket voucher worth HK$100 (roughly equivalent to US$13) would be given to them upon successful completion of the whole survey with 252 items which would be completed within 45-60 minutes. The survey would not be activated unless students gave formal consent to be the participants of this study.

The online survey covered the measures of service leadership attitude, knowledge, behavior, external criterion measures and demographic attributes. It was administered in English. The link to online survey was offered to students with the assistance of administrators in eight universities. The data were collected between late March and early June, 2017.

Measures

1) **Service Leadership Attitude Scale (SLA-SF-73).** Students were invited to respond to 73 items on a 6-point Likert scale ranging from "1" (strongly disagree) to "6" (strongly agree).
2) **Service Leadership Knowledge Scale (SLK-SF-40)**. The original 200-item scale (SLK-LF-200) was also developed based on the literature related to the SLAM framework, service leadership and service leader (18-21). The 200-item scale showed good content validity (23). The initial criterion validation study shortened the 200 items to 63 items (24). After considering the face validity and duplication of the items, 63 items were further shortened into 50 items (SLK-SF-50). After evaluating the internal consistency, 50 items were shortened into 40 items (SLK-SF-40). Factor analyses reported in a book chapter in this book showed that the scale possessed excellent factorial validity. These 40 items were used in this study and presented in the form of multiple choice questions. Value "1" was assigned to

all correct answers and Value "0" was assigned to all incorrect answers. The Cronbach's alpha cross all items was 0.93 (mean inter-item correlations = 0.21). The score of service leadership knowledge was calculated as the sum of all 40 items. A higher total score indicates a higher level of knowledge.

3) **Service Leadership Behavior Scale (SLB-SF-38).** Based on the aforementioned literature on service leadership and other published work on leadership (25, 26), a 97-item scale (SLB-LF-97) was developed to measure the extent to which the respondents demonstrated the behaviors that are representative of a service leader. On the basis of a Principal Axis Analysis (PAA) conducted, 97 items were shortened into 65 items (SLB-SF-65). After one round of Principal Component Analysis (PCA, see book chapter in this book) and one round of Confirmatory Factor Analysis (CFA) conducted, 65 items were further shortened into 38 items (SLB-SF-38), which demonstrated good convergent validity. Six stable factors were identified in the 38 items. They were Self-Improvement and Self-Reflection, People and Principle Orientation, Resilience, Social Competence, Problem-Solving, and Mentorship. The 38 items were adopted in this study. The items were formulated as statements, and responses were given on 6-point Likert items (1: very dissimilar to me; 6: very similar to me). The Cronbach's alpha cross all 38 items was 0.96. The Cronbach's alpha of the items of six subscales ranged from 0.85 to 0.91(mean inter-item correlations ranged from 0.42 to 0.65). The score of service leadership behavior was calculated as the mean of all 38 items.
4) **Revised Servant Leadership Profile (RSLP).** RSLP is a 20-item instrument measuring attitudes toward servant leadership, commitment to developingothers in the service, skills concerning servant leadership and capacity of leading a team in the service (27). For each item, the respondent was invited to respond on a 7-point Likert scale with options ranging from "1" (strongly disagree) to "7" (strongly agree). The Cronbach's alpha cross all items is 0.94 (mean inter-item correlations = 0.46). The total score of Servant Leadership was calculated as the mean of all 20 items.
5) **Moral Self-Concept (MSC).** The Chinese Adolescent Self-Esteem Scales (CASES) consists of 60 items measuring overall self-esteem and six specific self-esteem including Cognitive, Family, Social, Moral, Body Image, and Physical Performance (28). MSC is one of them consisting of 8 items (29), which was used to assess the moral self-concept of university students in this study. Students were invited to respond to a 7-point Likert scale with response options ranging from "1" (strongly disagree) to "7" (strongly agree). The Cronbach's alpha cross all items was 0.83 (mean inter-item correlations = 0.44). The total score of MSC was calculated as the mean of all 8 items.
6) **Leadership Efficacy (LEF).** LEF was measured by the 8-item scale developed by Murphy (30) with the focus on assessing the generalized capability in the

leadership role (31). Participants were invited to respond to items with a 5-point Likert scale with responses ranging from "1" (strongly disagree) to "5" (strongly agree). Three items were reversely coded. The Cronbach's alpha cross all items was 0.72 (mean inter-item correlations = 0.25). The total score of LEF was calculated as the mean of all 8 items.

7) **Interpersonal Reactivity Index (IRI).** IRI is a 28-item self-reported scale in which 7-item subscales were extracted: Empathic Concern (EC), Perspective Taking (PT), Fantasy (FS) and Personal Distress (PD) (32). The present study only measured the first two aspects with a total of 14 items. Participants were invited to respond on a 5-point Likert scale ranging from "1" (Does not describe me well) to "5" (Describe me very well). The Cronbach's alpha cross all items was 0.74 (mean inter-item correlations = 0.17), while the Cronbach's alpha cross EC and PT were 0.62 and 0.59 respectively (mean inter-item correlations were 0.19 for both measures). The score of interpersonal reactivity, empathic concern, and perspective thinking were calculated as the mean of relevant items.

Data analysis

The item-total correlation of each of 73 items was examined using SPSS 23 (IBM, New York), and those with item-total correlation less than 0.25 were dropped. Then we randomly and evenly split the data into two sets: A and B. Set A was adopted for main analysis and Set B was only used to test the factorial structural stability. We performed the Principal Components Analysis (PCA) with varimax rotation to investigate the factor structure. Coefficients of congruence (33) were computed to test the factorial stability by quantifying the similarity of the factor structure across two subsamples. Only items with the factor loading equaled to or above 0.50 were retained. Regarding reliability, the Cronbach's alpha value was adopted to examine the internal consistency. For convergent validity, correlation analysis was used to evaluate the association between the scores of SLA (and its subscales) and the scores of SLK-SF-40, SLB-SF-38 (and its subscales), RSLP, MSC, LEF, IRI, EC and PT respectively.

Considering the attitude of service-oriented organizational citizenship is positively related with the related knowledge (34), we hypothesized SLA would be positively correlated with SLK-SF-40 (Hypothesis 1). As how one believes about leadership to some extent directs one's behavior when performing the duties as a leader (15, 17), it was hypothesized that SLA would be positively associated with SLB-SF-38 and its subscales (Hypothesis 2a to 2f). Given that the basic propositions are consistent with those of service leadership, it was hypothesized that SLA would be positively correlated with RSLP (Hypothesis 3). Considering service leaders normally believe that good leaders must be of high moral quality (22), this study hypothesized that SLA would be positively associated with MSC (Hypothesis 4). Considering service leaders should have a positive attitude toward a commitment to continuous improvement in service leadership (22) and that positive attitude is positively correlated with self-efficacy (15), it was hypothesized that SLA would be positively associated with LEF (Hypothesis 5). As service leaders should have multiple intrapersonal and interpersonal competencies (22), so SLA would be expected to be positively correlated with IRI (Hypothesis 6). Besides, as s service leaders are expected to exhibit care to peers and subordinates, and empathic concern is an important prerequisite to exhibit care (35), SLA would be expected to be positively correlated with EC (Hypothesis 7). Considering service leadership model posits that service quality should be judged by service receivers and the service provided based on the needs of service receivers is more likely to lead to their satisfaction (36), SLA would also be expected to be positively correlated with PT (Hypothesis 8).

WHAT WE FOUND

A total of 4,555 completed questionnaires were received by the research team. After excluding those declining to participate (n = 6), multiple participation (n = 33), ineligible responses (n = 30), the final sample consisted of 4,486 undergraduate students. Around 500 students were affiliated to each university except for The Hong Kong Polytechnic University, whose sample was doubled to around 1,000. Among the 4,486 respondents (i.e., Mean age = 20.47; SD = 1.67), 1,517 (33.8%) were male and 2,969 (66.2%) were female. The full data set was randomly split into two sets: Set A contained 2,246 respondents, whereas Set B was composed of 2,240 respondents.

Factor structure

After checking the item-total correlation coefficients, 9 items with values less than 0.25 were deleted from the original 73-item scale. To avoid double loading and to derive a conceptually meaningful picture, a seven-factor solution was tested. The solution could explain for 53.67% of the whole variance. The factor loading of all items was over 0.30. Table 1 reports the factor loadings of all items. Seven factors identified were Vision and Competence (18 items), Social Competence (8 items), Caring Disposition (13 items), People Orientation (11 items), Self-Reflection and Self-Understanding (5 items), Positive Views about Human Beings (3 items), and Ethical Role Models (6 items). Based on this finalized factor structure, the coefficient of congruence across two subsamples was 0.97 and the coefficient of congruence of each subscale ranged from 0.96 to 0.98 (see Table 2), indicating that the seven-factor structure across two subsamples was almost the same (33). After removing 18 items with the factor loading less than 0.50 to keep a more robust factor solution, the finalized 7-factor scale contained 46 items (SLA-SF-46E). In another paper under preparation, CFA was further conducted to look at the factor structure of the scale.

Table 1. Factorial structural of Service Leadership Attitude Scale (SLA-SF-73) using varimax rotation (N = 2,246)

	Factor loading of component						
	1	2	3	4	5	6	7
Vision and Competence							
SL22	**0.64**	0.05	0.19	0.26	0.14	0.07	0.17
SL27	**0.61**	0.24	0.17	0.13	0.19	0.10	0.10
SL23	**0.60**	-0.01	0.16	0.14	0.10	0.06	0.25
SL21	**0.59**	0.16	0.17	0.32	0.17	0.11	0.15
SL26	**0.59**	0.21	0.16	0.22	0.22	0.02	0.13
SL15	**0.58**	0.02	0.16	0.37	0.11	-0.04	0.12
SL28	**0.58**	0.36	0.12	0.20	0.19	0.12	0.07
SL20	**0.58**	0.19	0.11	0.31	0.17	0.02	0.11
SL33	**0.55**	0.25	0.24	0.13	0.13	0.07	0.19
SL14	**0.52**	0.11	0.08	0.39	0.20	0.00	0.06
SL24	**0.51**	0.21	0.18	0.34	0.12	0.07	0.14
SL30	**0.49**	0.16	0.23	0.15	0.08	0.10	0.30
SL36	**0.48**	0.41	0.14	0.18	0.15	0.04	0.13
SL16	**0.48**	0.17	0.18	0.39	0.19	-0.08	0.06
SL19	**0.47**	0.20	0.17	0.34	0.13	-0.04	0.18
SL34	**0.47**	0.40	0.23	0.22	0.18	0.08	0.12
SL25	**0.45**	0.31	0.12	0.29	0.23	0.11	0.07
SL31	**0.44**	0.44	0.13	0.33	0.16	0.09	0.07
Social Competence							
SL37	0.38	**0.57**	0.17	0.31	0.16	0.10	0.08
SL35	0.39	**0.54**	0.17	0.29	0.22	0.06	0.08
SL38	0.39	**0.52**	0.16	0.27	0.15	0.06	0.12
SL41	0.37	**0.50**	0.21	0.29	0.26	0.05	0.11
SL40	0.30	**0.43**	0.23	0.21	0.21	0.11	0.22
SL49	0.14	**0.42**	0.35	0.36	0.15	-0.10	0.31
SL42	0.15	**0.41**	0.32	0.16	0.10	0.14	0.34
SL29	0.26	**0.37**	0.17	0.16	-0.04	0.18	0.32
Caring Disposition							
SL56	0.12	0.13	**0.64**	0.16	0.11	0.18	0.30
SL57	0.26	0.11	**0.63**	0.17	0.19	0.10	0.14
SL58	0.31	0.06	**0.60**	0.16	0.21	0.05	0.08
SL59	0.37	-0.02	**0.59**	0.10	0.23	0.04	0.14
SL55	0.12	0.15	**0.56**	0.04	0.08	0.20	0.25
SL53	0.12	0.25	**0.56**	0.19	0.05	0.10	0.38
SL54	0.07	0.18	**0.55**	0.17	0.06	0.23	0.36
SL60	0.34	0.09	**0.51**	0.21	0.29	0.03	0.10
SL52	0.18	0.28	**0.51**	0.23	0.12	0.08	0.31

	Factor loading of component						
	1	2	3	4	5	6	7
SL51	0.16	0.36	**0.48**	0.36	0.14	0.03	0.29
SL50	0.15	0.34	**0.47**	0.31	0.13	-0.09	0.32
SL48	0.13	0.31	**0.38**	0.30	0.19	0.02	0.32
SL32	0.21	0.10	**0.35**	-0.01	-0.14	0.34	0.27
People Orientation							
SL11	0.30	0.28	0.12	**0.62**	0.19	0.14	0.05
SL08	0.35	0.17	0.09	**0.60**	0.25	0.15	0.06
SL09	0.36	0.10	0.17	**0.59**	0.20	0.15	0.08
SL10	0.35	0.10	0.10	**0.58**	0.21	0.18	0.09
SL12	0.24	0.18	0.25	**0.58**	0.00	0.03	0.14
SL07	0.27	0.18	0.12	**0.56**	0.19	0.17	0.10
SL02	0.18	0.06	0.11	**0.54**	0.09	0.27	0.22
SL17	0.25	0.21	0.34	**0.54**	-0.02	-0.06	0.16
SL01	0.20	0.20	0.08	**0.53**	0.08	0.25	0.19
SL13	0.39	0.16	0.15	**0.53**	0.13	0.06	0.04
SL18	0.32	0.14	0.34	**0.49**	0.00	-0.11	0.25
Self-Reflection and Self-Understanding							
SL68	0.30	0.23	0.08	0.26	**0.61**	-0.01	0.13
SL66	0.27	0.27	0.17	0.19	**0.68**	0.03	0.11
SL65	0.21	0.16	0.14	0.14	**0.68**	0.05	0.21
SL67	0.26	0.19	0.21	0.18	**0.64**	-0.01	0.15
SL64	0.20	-0.05	0.19	0.06	**0.53**	0.02	0.14
Positive Views About Human Being							
SL04	0.02	0.06	0.09	0.14	0.03	**0.73**	0.13
SL03	0.04	0.05	0.16	0.21	-0.04	**0.71**	0.13
SL73	0.14	0.08	0.30	0.10	0.19	**0.33**	0.03
Ethical Role Model							
SL44	0.18	0.11	0.22	0.13	0.16	0.05	**0.74**
SL46	0.13	0.05	0.23	0.10	0.08	0.15	**0.70**
SL47	0.08	0.05	0.28	0.11	0.15	0.16	**0.67**
SL45	0.24	0.10	0.18	0.13	0.18	0.02	**0.66**
SL43	0.28	0.14	0.16	0.14	0.15	0.04	**0.62**
SL39	0.02	0.33	0.30	0.07	0.05	0.30	**0.40**

Table 2. Coefficients of congruence across two subsamples (N = 4,486)

	Between two random sub-samples
Service Leadership Attitude Scale (SLA-SF-73)	0.97
SLA-SF-73 - Vision and Competence	0.98
SLA-SF-73 - Social Competence	0.97
SLA-SF-73 - Caring Disposition	0.98
SLA-SF-73 - People Orientation	0.97
SLA-SF-73 - Self-Reflection and Self-Understanding	0.97
SLA-SF-73 - Positive Views About Human Being	0.96
SLA-SF-73 - Ethical Role Model	0.97

Internal consistency and convergent validity

Full SLA-SF-46E and its seven subscales demonstrated high internal consistency. The Cronbach's value of full SLA-SF-46E scale was 0.96 and those of subscales were between 0.70 and 0.91 (see Table 3), showing good internal consistency. As expected, the scores of SLA-SF-46E and seven subscales were all positively correlated with those of SLK-SF-40, SLB-SF-38, RSLP, MSC, LEF, IRI, EC, and PT (see Table 4). Consistently, the scores of SLA-SF-46E and seven subscales were found positively associated with the scores of each subscale of SLB-SF-38 (see Table 5). The findings supported all hypotheses, establishing the convergent validity of SLA-SF-46E and seven subscales among Hong Kong undergraduate students.

Table 3. Internal consistency of Service Leadership Attitude Scale (SLA-SF-46E) and external criterions scales (N = 2,246)

	α	Mean Inter-item correlations
Service Leadership Attitude Scale (SLA-SF-46E)	0.96	0.36
SLA-SF-46E - Vision and Competence	0.91	0.46
SLA-SF-46E - Social Competence	0.84	0.56
SLA-SF-46E - Caring Disposition	0.89	0.47
SLA-SF-46E - People Orientation	0.89	0.46
SLA-SF-46E - Self-Reflection and Self-Understanding	0.82	0.49
SLA-SF-46E - Positive Views About Human Being	0.70	0.54
SLA-SF-46E - Ethical Role Model	0.85	0.53
Service Leadership Knowledge Scale (SLK-SF-40)	0.93	0.21
Service Leadership Behavioral Scale (SLB-SF-38)	0.96	0.38
SLB-SF-38 - Self-Improvement and Self-Reflection	0.91	0.53
SLB-SF-38 - People and Principles Orientation	0.87	0.42
SLB-SF-38 - Resilience	0.87	0.50
SLB-SF-38 - Social Competence	0.86	0.55
SLB-SF-38 - Problem-Solving	0.87	0.56
SLB-SF-38 - Mentorship	0.85	0.65
Revised Servant Leadership Scale (RSLP)	0.94	0.46
Moral Self-Concept Scale (MSC)	0.83	0.44
Leadership Efficacy Scale (LEF)	0.72	0.25
Interpersonal Reactivity Index (IRI)	0.74	0.17
IRI - Empathic Concern	0.62	0.19
IRI – Perspective Taking	0.59	0.19

Table 4. Correlation coefficients with external criterion scales and other Service Leadership scales (N = 2,246)

	SLK-SF-40	SLB-SF-38	RSLP	MSC	LEF	IRI	EC	PT
SLA-SF-46E	0.29	0.58	0.59	0.55	0.24	0.40	0.33	0.37
SLA-SF-46E-F1	0.37	0.46	0.46	0.50	0.18	0.38	0.33	0.34
SLA-SF-46E-F2	0.17	0.50	0.53	0.45	0.20	0.33	0.28	0.30
SLA-SF-46E-F3	0.17	0.50	0.53	0.45	0.20	0.33	0.28	0.30
SLA-SF-46E-F4	0.33	0.47	0.50	0.49	0.20	0.37	0.32	0.34
SLA-SF-46E-F5	0.24	0.47	0.44	0.44	0.19	0.29	0.22	0.29
SLA-SF-46E-F6	0.04	0.26	0.29	0.21	0.13	0.13	0.11	0.11
SLA-SF-46E-F7	0.04	0.42	0.45	0.36	0.16	0.25	0.20	0.23

Note. SLK-SF-40: One-factor Service Leadership Knowledge Scale (40 items); SLB-SF-38: Six-factor Service Leadership Behavior Scale (38 items); RSLP: Revised Servant Leadership Profile; MSC: Moral Self-Concept; LEF: Leadership Efficacy; IRI: Interpersonal Reactivity Index; EC: IRI- Empathic Concern; PT: IRI-Perspective Taking. SLA-SF-46E-F1: Vision and Competence; SLA-SF-46E-F2: Social Competence; SLA-SF-46E-F3: Caring Disposition; SLA-SF-46E-F4: People Orientation; SLA-SF-46E-F5: Self-Understanding and Reflection; SLA-SF-46E-F6: Positive View About Human Beings; SLA-SF-46E-F7: Ethical Role Model. All correlations are significant at the level of 0.01(two-tailed).

Table 5. Correlation coefficients with subscales of SLB-SF-38

	SLB-SF-38-F1	SLB-SF-38-F2	SLB-SF-38-F3	SLB-SF-38-F4	SLB-SF-38-F5	SLB-SF-38-F6
SLA-SF-46E	0.52	0.62	0.38	0.50	0.36	0.35
SLA-SF-46E-F1	0.48	0.55	0.33	0.45	0.36	0.25
SLA-SF-46E-F2	0.43	0.53	0.27	0.44	0.29	0.19
SLA-SF-46E-F3	0.43	0.53	0.34	0.42	0.28	0.39
SLA-SF-46E-F4	0.43	0.54	0.29	0.44	0.28	0.23
SLA-SF-46E-F5	0.44	0.47	0.30	0.40	0.33	0.24
SLA-SF-46E-F6	0.36	0.42	0.31	0.31	0.22	0.38
SLA-SF-46E-F7	0.21	0.26	0.21	0.22	0.13	0.24

Note. SLB-SF-38-F1: Self-Improvement and Self-Reflection; SLB-SF-38-F2: People and Principles Orientation; SLB-SF-38-F3: Resilience; SLB-SF-38-F4: Social Competence; SLB-SF-38-F5: Problem-Solving; SLB-SF-38-F6: Mentorship. SLA-SF-46E-F1: Vision and Competence; SLA-SF-46E-F2: Social Competence; SLA-SF-46E-F3: Caring Disposition; SLA-SF-46E-F4: People Orientation; SLA-SF-46E-F5: Self-Understanding and Reflection; SLA-SF-46E-F6: Positive View About Human Beings; SLA-SF-46E-F7: Ethical Role Model. All correlations are significant at the level of 0.01(two-tailed).

DISCUSSION

This study reported the shortening of the SLA-LF-73 from 73 items to 46 items after factor analyses based on 4,468 college students in Hong Kong, and tested the reliability, convergent validity and factorial validity of the 46-item scale. Exploratory factors analyses showed that seven factor emerged from the scale and this seven-factor structure was stable across two sub-samples of Hong Kong college students. Based on the cut-offs of inter-item correlation and factor loading, 73 items were further shortened into 46 items. The findings suggested that both the full scale and seven sub-scales demonstrated excellent reliability status. In addition, both the 46-item scale and all seven sub-scales demonstrated convergent validity, which is proven by their significant correlations with SLK-SF-40, SLB-SF-38 (and sub-scales), RSLP, MSC, LEF, IRI, EC, and PT.

As expected, there were positive correlations between SLA-SF-46E and SLK-SF-40, echoing to a series of previous findings that knowledge and information establish the understanding of importance of a subject, shaping positive attitudes toward it at the next stage (33, 37). SLA-SF-46E was found positively correlated with SLB-SF-38 and its subscales, which is consistent with the theory of planned behavior that positive attitude is able to shape positive behavior through behavioral intentions (15). There were positive correlations detected between SLA-SF-46E and RSLP, echoing the common philosophy and practices of both service leadership and servant leadership that enrich the lives of individuals and create a caring environment (27). Besides, SLA-SF-46E was positively correlated with MSC, which is consistent with the core philosophy of service leadership that service leaders should possess moral character and practice following the principles of integrity, fairness, and humanity (22). For service leaders, the strong motivation of being ethical role models make them take efforts to shape their moral character and improve their moral self-concept, causing the strong positive correlations between SLA-SF-46E and MSC. As expected, SLA-SF-46E was positively correlated with LEF as confidence is normally generated from the behavior and experience and positive attitude always drives positive behaviors (38). SLA-SF-46E was found positively correlated with IRI, echoing the core belief of service leadership that service leaders should demonstrate interpersonal and intrapersonal competencies in terms of the willingness of collaborating with peers, the capacity of addressing conflicts within a team, and capabilities in constructing communication channels to promote information exchange (22). More specific, the positive correlations between SLA-SF-46E and EC are consistent with the literature that empathic concern increases the likelihood of exhibiting care, which is believed to be one of the core practices of service leaders (35). The positive correlations between SLA-SF-46E and PT echo the literature that thinking from the perspective of service receivers is positively associated with their satisfaction on the service received (36).

This study helps to develop a briefer and focused measure of service leadership attitude for Hong Kong undergraduate students. The SLA-SF-46E is important to local universities in view of the need to objectively evaluate service leadership programs, which has long-term impacts on the healthy operation of the Hong Kong's service economy.

Although current study makes a sound contribution, some limitations should be noted. First, the study examined service leadership attitude and behavior by directly asking students only without checking the accuracy of their answers by comparing with the assessment from the perspective of teachers and peers. Similar to other self-report measures, it is noteworthy that social desirability may cloud the findings. Comparatively, their attitudes and behavior may be more accurately recognized by teachers and peers, suggesting future studies should invite teachers and peers to rate the same items. Second, the data in this study are from eight publically funded universities only. It is noteworthy that there are a number of undergraduate students studying in the self-funded tertiary institutions. Future studies might consider extending the sample of this study to cover students in self-funded tertiary institutions. Third, as the sample adopted in this study is essentially a convenient sample, there is a problem of generalizability of the findings, which should be addressed in future studies.

ACKNOWLEDGMENTS

The validation project is financially supported by the Victor and William Fung Foundation. The preparation for this paper is supported by the Foundation and the Endowed Professorship in Service Leadership Education at The Hong Kong Polytechnic University. This chapter is an updated version of a publication in the special issue "Development and validation of assessment tools on service leadership knowledge, attitude and behavior" edited by Daniel TL Shek, Xiaoqin Zhu and Joav Merrick published in the International Journal of Child and Adolescent Health, 2018;11(4).

REFERENCES

[1] Sin LYM, Tse ACB, Yau OHM, Lee JSY, Chow R. The effect of relationship marketing orientation on business performance in a service-oriented economy. J Serv Mark 2002;16(7):656-76.

[2] Census and Statistics Department. Hong Kong Annual Digest of Statistics. Hong Kong: Census and Statistics Department, 2017.

[3] Ployhart RE, Van Iddekinge, CH, MacKenzie Jr, WI. Acquiring and developing human capital in service contexts: The interconnectedness of human capital resources. Acad Manage J 2011;54(2):353-68.

[4] Ployhart RE, Weekley JA, Ramsey J. The consequences of human resource stocks and flows: A longitudinal examination of unit service orientation and unit effectiveness. Acad Manage J 2009;52(5):996-1015.

[5] Nyberg AJ, Moliterno TP, Hale Jr D, Lepak DP. Resource-based perspectives on unit-level human capital: A review and integration. J Manage 2014;40(1):316-46.

[6] Schneider B, Ehrhart MG, Macey WH. Organizational climate and culture. Annu Rev Psychol 2013;64:361-88.

[7] Jiang K, Chuang CH, Chiao YC. Developing collective customer knowledge and service climate: The interaction between service-oriented high-performance work systems and service leadership. J Appl Psychol 2015;100(4):1089-106.

[8] Schneider B, Ehrhart MG, Mayer DM, Saltz JL, Niles-Jolly K. Understanding organization-customer links in service settings. Acad Manage J 2005;48(6):1017-32.

[9] Chung PPY. Hong Kong Institute of Service Leadership and Management curriculum framework. Hong Kong: Hong Kong Institute of Service Leadership and Management, 2011.

[10] Shek, DTL, Lin L. Core beliefs in the service leadership model proposed by the Hong Kong Institute of Service Leadership and Management. Int J Disabil Hum Dev 2015;14(3):233-42.

[11] Lusch RF, Vargo SL, O'Brien M. Competing through service: Insights from service-dominant logic. J Retailing 2007;83(1):5-18.

[12] Kandampully J. Innovation as the core competency of a service organisation: the role of technology, knowledge and networks. Eur J Innovat Manage 2002;5(1):18-26.

[13] Harker MJ. Relationship marketing defined? An examination of current relationship marketing definitions. Market Intell Plann 1999;17(1):13-20.

[14] Fornell C, Johnson MD, Anderson EW, Cha J, Bryant BE. The American customer satisfaction index: Nature, purpose, and findings. J Mark 1996;60(4):7-18.

[15] Ajzen I. The theory of planned behavior. Organ Behav Hum Decis Process 1991;50(2):179-211.

[16] Arcury TA. Environmental attitude and environmental knowledge. Hum Organ 1990;49(4):300-4.

[17] Bass BM, Steidlmeier P. Ethics, character, and authentic transformational leadership behavior. Leadersh Q 1999;10(2):181-217.

[18] Chung PPY, Bell AH. 25 principles of service leadership, 1st ed. New York: Lexingford Publishing, 2015.

[19] Chung PPY, Elfassy R. The 12 dimensions of a service leader: Manage your personal brand for the service age, 1st ed. New York: Lexingford Publishing, 2016.

[20] Shek DTL, Chung PPY, Yu L, Merrick J., eds. Service leadership curriculum and higher education reform in Hong Kong [Special issue]. Int J Disabil Hum Dev 2015;14(4):297-406.

[21] Shek, DTL., Chung PPY, Yu L, Merrick J, eds. Service leadership education for university students: Experience of Hong Kong [Special issue]. Int J Disabil Hum Dev 2015;14(3):203-4.

[22] Shek DTL, Lin L, Leung H, Yu L, Ma CMS, Li X, eds. Content validation of the service leadership attitudes scale. In: Shek DTL, Chung PPY, Lin L, Merrick J, eds. Service leadership education for university students. New York: Nova Science, 2017:205-26.

[23] Shek DTL, Lin L, Leung H, Yu L., Ma, CMS, Li X. Development and validation of the service leadership knowledge scale in a Chinese context. In: Shek DTL, Chung PPY, Lin L, Merrick J Eds. Service leadership education for university students. New York: Nova Science, 2017:163-88.

[24] Shek DTL, Lin L. Validation of the service leadership knowledge scale: Criterion-related validity. In: Shek DTL, Chung PPY, Lin L, Merrick J, eds. Service leadership education for university students. New York: Nova Science, 2017:189-204.

[25] Hwang JY, Plante T, Lackey, K. The development of the Santa Clara Brief Compassion Scale: An abbreviation of Sprecher and Fehr's Compassionate Love Scale. Pastoral Psychol 2008;56(4):421-8.

[26] Wielkiewicz RM. The leadership attitudes and beliefs scale: An instrument for evaluating college students' thinking about leadership and organizations. J Coll Stud Dev 2000;41(3):335-47.

[27] Wong PTP, Page D. Servant Leadership: An opponent-process model and the Revised Servant Leadership Profile.Canada: Trinity Western University, 2003.

[28] Cheng CHK, Watkins D. Age and gender invariance of self-concept factor structure: An investigation of a newly developed Chinese self-concept instrument. Int J Psychol 2000;35(5):186-93.

[29] Cheng CHK. The Chinese Adolescent Self-Esteem Scales (CASES): A user manual. Hong Kong: City University of Hong Kong Press, 2005.

[30] Murphy SE. The contribution of leadership experience and self-efficacy to group performance under evaluation apprehension. Dissertation. Seattle: WA: University of Washington, 1992.

[31] Chemers MM, Watson CB, May ST. Dispositional affect and leadership effectiveness: A comparison of self-esteem, optimism, and efficacy. Pers Soc Psychol Bull 2000;26(3):267-77.

[32] Davis MH. Measuring individual differences in empathy: Evidence for a multidimensional approach. J Pers Soc Psychol 1983;44(1):113-26.

[33] Lorenzo-Seva U, Ten Berge JM. Tucker's congruence coefficient as a meaningful index of factor similarity. Methodology (Gott) 2006:2(2):57-64.
[34] Bettencourt LA, Gwinner KP, Meuter ML. A comparison of attitude, personality, and knowledge predictors of service-oriented organizational citizenship behaviors. J Appl Psychol 2001;86(1):29-41.
[35] Mercer SW, Maxwell M, Heaney D, Watt GC. The consultation and relational empathy (CARE) measure: Development and preliminary validation and reliability of an empathy-based consultation process measure. Fam Pract 2004;21(6):699-705.
[36] Zeithaml VA. Consumer perceptions of price, quality, and value: A means-end model and synthesis of evidence. J Mark 1988;52(3):2-22.
[37] Zhu X, Xie X. Effects of knowledge on attitude formation and change toward genetically modified foods. Risk Anal 2015;35(5):790-810.
[38] Daugherty T, Logan K., Chu, SC, Huang SC. Understanding consumer perceptions of advertising: A theoretical framework of attitude and confidence. Lubbock, TX: American Academy of Advertising, 2008.

In: Service Leadership
Editors: Daniel TL Shek, Xiaoqin Zhu, Li Lin et al.
ISBN: 978-1-53614-852-7

Chapter 10

CONVERGENT AND FACTORIAL VALIDATION OF THE SERVICE LEADERSHIP BEHAVIOR SCALE

Daniel TL Shek[1-6,*], PhD, FHKPS, BBS, SBS, JP, Lawrence K Ma[1], PhD, Cecilia MS Ma[1], PhD and A Reza Hoshmand[7], PhD

[1]Department of Applied Social Sciences, The Hong Kong Polytechnic University, Hong Kong, PR China
[2]Centre for Innovative Programmes for Adolescents and Families, The Hong Kong Polytechnic University, Hong Kong, PR China
[3]Department of Social Work, East China Normal University, Shanghai, PR China
[4]Kiang Wu Nursing College of Macau, Macau, PR China
[5]Hong Kong Institute of Service Leadership and Management Limited, Hong Kong, PR China
[6]Division of Adolescent Medicine, Department of Pediatrics, Kentucky Children's Hospital, University of Kentucky School of Medicine, Lexington, Kentucky, US
[7]General Education Office, Hong Kong Baptist University, Hong Kong, PR China

* Correspondence: Daniel TL Shek, PhD, FHKPS, BBS, SBS, JP, Associate Vice President (Undergraduate Programme), Chair Professor of Applied Social Sciences and Li and Fung Professor in Service Leadership Education, Department of Applied Social Sciences, The Hong Kong Polytechnic University, Hung Hom, Hong Kong, PR China. E-mail: daniel.shek@polyu.edu.hk.

ABSTRACT

Utilizing a sample of 4,486 Hong Kong undergraduates recruited from eight government-funded universities, this chapter reports the findings of a cross-institution validation study on the Service Leadership Behavior Scale (Short-Form) with 65 items (SLB-SF-65). Specifically, we examined the internal consistency, convergent validity, as well as the dimensionality of the SLB-SF-65. Results of the exploratory factor analysis indicated that six factors could be extracted with 48 items retained in the trimmed version of the scale (SLB-SF-48) with a stable factor structure. Besides, the overall scale showed excellent internal consistency and was positively correlated to a myriad of theoretically relevant constructs. In short, the present findings underscored the adequacy of the trimmed Service Leadership Behavior Scale (SLB-SF-48) as an objective assessment to gauge whether one possesses the behavioral qualities of a Service Leader.

INTRODUCTION

As an emergent leadership paradigm in advanced economies (1, 2), the Service Leadership paradigm, contrary to the traditional elitist leadership models, contends that leadership success should extend beyond discipline-oriented knowledge or task-specific competencies (i.e., the "hard (or *product*) skills") to cover "soft (or *process*) skills" including interpersonal communication and intrapersonal qualities (3, 4). As Shek and colleagues (5) remarked, such a paradigm which "calls for leaders with qualities to serve others" (p. 164) and inspires a revamp in leadership initiative, informs education and research which are instrumental to Hong Kong where service takes up a whopping 92.2% of GDP (6). As such, Po Chung, Chairman of the Hong Kong Service Leadership and Management Limited (HKI-SLAM), initiated the notion of Service Leadership education targeting university students of Hong Kong (i.e., SLAM framework).

With the financial support of the Victor and William Fung Foundation and the collaborative effort of the HKI-SLAM and the government, a multi-year project entitled the "Fung Service Leadership Education Initiative" was implemented in eight government-funded universities. On the basis of the SLAM framework, each participating institution would design her own curriculum aimed to promote students' Service Leadership attributes (see 7). Specifically, Po Chung highlighted **C**ompetence (i.e., "Doing things right"), **M**oral character (i.e., "Doing the right things"), and **C**aring disposition (i.e., "Serving with unselfish intent") as the three defining attributes in building a leader's legitimacy and thereby contributing to leadership success (8, 9). Hence, the formula "E (Effective leadership) = M (Moral character) C^2 (Competence * Caring)" laid the conceptual foundation for the model of Service Leadership education (10).

To objectively assess qualities of effective Service Leaders (11), the research team at The Hong Kong Polytechnic University (PolyU) initiated a project entitled "Development and validation of measures based on the Service Leadership Model" ("The Project" hereafter) (5). Via developing and validating three scales on attitude, behavior, and knowledge corresponding to the three dimensions argued to define the educational success of Service Leadership (12), Shek and colleagues (5) endeavored to develop reliable and valid assessment tools to judge whether an individual is a good Service Leader. In this chapter, findings of a large-scale validation study of the Short-Form of Service Leadership Behavior Scale (SLB-SF-65) are reported.

The long-form Service Leadership Behavior Scale (SLB-LF-97) was developed to measure the "behavioral qualities a Service leader should demonstrate" (5, p. 165). Operating on a six-point Likert Scale (1: very dissimilar; 6: very similar), the SLB-LF-97 includes 97 items developed based on the SLAM framework, 25 principles of Service Leadership (8), and the leadership literature (e.g., 13-15). These 97 items cover four main dimensions, including i) service provision, ii) principle "$E= MC^2$," iii) commitment to continuous improvement, and iv) distributed leadership.

As part of "The Project" (see 5), a validation study involving 231 PolyU undergraduates was conducted in November 2016 to examine the psychometric properties and factorial structures of the 97-item SLB-LF-97. The results highlighted the excellent reliability of the SLB-LF-97 ($\alpha = 0.97$) and its moderate to strong correlations (*r*s ranging from 0.51 to 0.81) with several theoretically relevant constructs including Servant Leadership (16), empathy (17), moral self-concept (18), and leadership efficacy (19, 20). Meanwhile, findings of the exploratory factor analysis (EFA) suggested the removal of 32 items due to the double-loading (21) and insufficient-loading issues (i.e., loadings less than 0.40) (see 22). Ultimately, 65 items were retained to form the Short-Form of the Service Leadership Behavior Scale (SLB-SF-65).

While the above unpublished study pioneered the convergent validation and the analysis of the dimensionality of the initial behavior scale (i.e., SLB-LF-97), there is a need to replicate the psychometric soundness and to re-examine the dimensionality of the trimmed scale using on a larger sample. As the main body of "The Project," the present study utilized a sample of 4,486 undergraduates to examine the item homogeneity, convergent and factorial validity of the 65-item SLB-SF-65. Specifically, this chapter is mainly focused on reporting the results of the EFA, in addition to analyses of the internal consistency and convergent validity of the SLB-SF-65.

OUR STUDY

Utilizing an e-platform, a total of 4,486 undergraduates (mean age: 20.47 years; SD: 1.67) from eight government-funded universities participated in the Service Leadership Scales validation study. Amongst the 4,486 respondents, 1,517 (33.8%) were males and 2,969 (66.2%) were females. An overwhelming proportion of the participants were aged 20 to 24 years (68.4%), had neither received any credit-bearing (74.3%) nor non-credit-bearing

(82.0%) training in Service Leadership, despite the fact that 64.4% had formerly served as a leader (such as being the chairperson of a student association). Furthermore, 77.1% sat the Hong Kong Diploma of Secondary Education Examination (HKDSE). Details regarding other demographic information of the present working sample are addressed in another chapter in this book.

Procedures

The data collection, which commenced in March 2017, was implemented via the mySurvey@PolyU electronic survey system. The research objectives, instructions on how to complete the present self-administered survey, participants' rights to voluntarily participate and withdraw, and the principle of data confidentiality were highlighted in the invitation documents and on the survey webpage. Participants were also informed that 45 to 60 minutes would be warranted to conscientiously complete the entire questionnaire. Students' informed consent was obtained at the start of the e-survey. Upon the completion of the study, each participant was entitled to a supermarket cash coupon valued at HK$100 (US$12.80).

Participants' completed responses were downloaded as an EXCEL file for a data-cleaning process before the conversion to an SPSS file for statistical analyses. Details on the various steps taken and criteria as regards the eligibility of the responses were reported in another chapter in this book. Ultimately, 4,486 cases were considered eligible for further analyses.

Instruments

The present e-survey was composed of items from the Short-Forms of the Service Leadership scales, including i) the Service Leadership Attitude Scale (SLA-SF-73; 73 items), ii) the Service Leadership Behavior Scale (SLB-SF-65; 65 items), and iii) the Service Leadership Knowledge Scale (SLK-SF-50; 50 items). The present chapter is primarily concerned with the validation of the 65-item Service Leadership Behavior Scale (SLB-SF-65).

Developed based on the SLAM framework, 25 principles of Service Leadership (8), and other published works on *leadership* (e.g., 15, 23), the 97-item Service Leadership Behavior Scale (i.e., SLB-LF-97) was constructed to examine the extent to which an individual demonstrates behaviors that are representative of a Service Leader. Sixty-five items were ultimately retained to form the SLB-SF-65, following an unpublished validation study involving 231 PolyU undergraduates as part of the project "Development and validation of measures based on the Service Leadership Model" (see 5). The SLB-SF-65, which is in English with a six-point Likert Scale (1: very dissimilar; 6: very similar), describes some leaders' behaviors whereby participants rate how each description resembles their behaviors if they are in a position to lead. Table 1 features four sample items of the SLB-SF-65.

Table 1. Four sample items of the SLB-SF-65

Items	Very Dissimilar to Me	Moderately Dissimilar to Me	Slightly Dissimilar to Me	Slightly Similar to Me	Moderately Similar to Me	Very Similar To Me
15. I trust myself in tackling difficulties in my life.	1	2	3	4	5	6
36. I have no problem letting others know my shortcomings.	1	2	3	4	5	6
49. I can motivate myself to achieve any goals I set.	1	2	3	4	5	6
64. I impose total control over duties assigned to other individuals. (Reverse-item)	1	2	3	4	5	6

Note. All sample items were slightly re-worded due to copyright issues.

Four other validated scales as listed below from the leadership and personality literature were also administered, with the aim of ascertaining the convergent validity of the SLA-SF-73, the SLB-SF-65, and the SLK-SF-50. These validated external inventories included the 20-item Revised Servant Leadership Profile (RSLP), the 8-item Leadership Efficacy Scale (LEF), the 8-item Moral Self-Concept Scale (MSC), plus 14 items selected from Interpersonal Reactivity Index (IRI). There were also forced-choice and open-ended items aimed to measure the respondents' demographics.

1. **Revised Servant Leadership Profile (RSLP):** The RSLP was developed by Wong and Page (24) to assess the multidimensional construct *Servant Leadership*. In this study, 20 items from five dimensions deemed relevant to the SLAM curriculum—including, i) *Empowering and developing others* (five items), ii) *Serving others* (seven items), iii) *Open, participatory leadership* (two items), iv) *Inspiring leadership* (two items), and v) *Integrity and authenticity* (four items)—were included. The RSLP operates on a seven-point Likert scale. A higher score indicates higher likelihood to behave like a *Servant Leader*. Reliability analyses underscored the high item homogeneity of RSLP ($\alpha = 0.94$; mean inter-item correlations = 0.45).
2. **Leadership Efficacy Scale (LEF):** Developed by Murphy (20), the LEF comprises eight items designed to tap into people's "confidence in their general leadership ability" (19, p. 270). Items were rated on a five-point Likert scale, with a higher score symbolizing one's perceived capability to take on a leadership role.

Reliability analyses demonstrated an acceptable internal consistency amongst the eight items ($\alpha = 0.73$; mean inter-item correlations = 0.27).

3. **Moral Self-Concept (MSC):** Developed and validated by Cheng (18) as a subscale under the Chinese Adolescent Self-Esteem Scales (CASES), the MSC, which consists of eight items, examines youngsters' self-appraisal on dimensions pertaining to i) *Conduct and virtues*, ii) *Self-control and discipline*, and iii) *Altruism*. Items were rated on a seven-point Likert scale, with a higher score indicative of one's value of *morality* to him/herself, which is a cornerstone of effective leadership based on the SLAM curriculum (25). In this study, we adopted the English-translated and slightly amended version of the MSC. Reliability assessment indicated a good internal consistency of the MSC on the current sample ($\alpha = 0.83$; mean inter-item correlations = 0.44).
4. **Interpersonal Reactivity Index (IRI):** Developed by Davis (17) and tested across nations and languages (see 26-28), the IRI is the most widely utilized inventory in assessing empathy as a multidimensional construct (29). The 14 items utilized in the present study were from subscales *Perspective Taking* (PT; seven items) and *Empathic Concern* (EC; seven items). All items were rated on a five-point Likert scale. A higher score, according to Shek and Yu (30), denotes a higher level of empathy which is crucial for effective leadership. Besides computing the component scores for both subscales, a composite IRI score was also calculated. Cronbach's alpha for subscales PT and EC and the composite IRI score were 0.59, 0.62, and 0.74, respectively.

We performed both exploratory (EFA) and confirmatory factor analyses (CFA) in the present validation study. SPSS statistics version 24.0 (IBM) was used to perform the EFA, descriptive analyses, and measurement of internal consistency and convergent validity. AMOS 24.0 (IBM) statistical package was utilized to perform the CFA. The present chapter is primarily concerned about reporting the findings of the PCA, the internal consistency and convergent validity of the 65-item SLB-SF-65. Details regarding the CFA and the final version of the behavior scale with 38 items will be addressed in another paper under preparation.

To explore the factorial structure of SLB-SF-65, we administered the EFA using the principal component analysis (PCA) with varimax rotation. The aggregate dataset (N= 4,486) was split into two random subsets, namely subset A (N= 2,246) and subset B (N= 2,240). The PCA was performed on subset A to explore the dimensionality of SLB-SF-65, whereby CFA was administered on subset B with the purpose of finalizing a factorial structure of the SLB-SF-65. Meanwhile, to establish the stability of the factorial structure, we performed the identical PCAs on subsets A and B. The Tucker's coefficients of congruence (r_c) were then computed to gauge the resemblance of factor structures across subsets A and B (31, 32).

Cronbach's alpha values and item-total correlations were computed to assess the internal consistency of the scale and the individual factor (i.e., subscale) derived. Regarding the assessment of convergent validity, the composite scores—computed via averaging respondents' ratings—of both the scale and the subscales were correlated with the four external criterion measures adopted at present. Since the SLAM curriculum which preaches the behavioral prerequisites of a Service Leader covers domains in *Servant Leadership*, *leadership efficacy*, *morality* and *empathy*, it is logical to hypothesize a positive and significant correlation between the behavior scale (and the subscales) and the i) RSLP, ii) LEF, iii) MSC, and iv) IRI (including subscales EC and PT). Correlational analyses with other Service Leadership scales under validation were also performed. Considering that all these scales were designed to tap into different dimensions (i.e., *knowledge*, *attitude*, and *behavior*) of Service Leadership, there is no reason not to expect significant positive correlations amongst the behavior scale (with the subscales) and the validated versions of the SLK-SF-50 and the SLA-SF-73 (and the subscales).

Findings

Table 2. Eigenvalues and total variance explained for the analyses on subset A and B

	Subset A (N= 2,246)		Subset B (N= 2,240)	
Factors	Eigenvalues	Total Variance Explained (%)	Eigenvalues	Total Variance Explained (%)
1	23.85	36.69	23.90	36.77
2	2.96	41.25	3.01	41.40
3	2.56	45.18	2.51	45.26
4	2.12	48.44	2.28	48.77
5	1.77	51.17	1.70	51.38
6	1.57	53.58	1.63	53.88
7	1.46	55.82	1.44	56.10
8	1.24	57.73	1.26	58.03
9	1.14	59.48	1.07	59.67
10	1.02	61.05	1.01	61.22
11	0.99	62.58	0.99	62.74

Note. Eigenvalues for the remaining factors are all below unity.

While ten factors were shown to have eigenvalues over unity across the two subsets (see Table 2), visual inspection of both scree plots and consideration of interpretability of the factor solution suggested that six factors which accounted for 53.58% of the total variance could be retained. Accordingly, the PCA was rerun on subset A specifying the extraction of six factors. The factor loadings of each item, eigenvalues, the percentage of variance explained by each factor, and the correlations amongst the factors and the entire scale are detailed in Table 3.

Table 3. Factor loadings of the SLB-SF-65 (N= 2,246)

	M	SD	Component								
			1	2	3	4	5	6	ITC	Retained for CFA?	Retained after CFA?
SLB-01	4.35	0.95	0.020	**0.501**	0.154	0.118	0.149	0.277	0.49	Yes	Yes
SLB-02	4.15	1.02	-0.036	0.388	0.206	0.091	0.113	0.403	0.44	No	No
SLB-03	4.46	0.88	0.146	0.434	0.131	0.233	0.228	0.232	0.56	No	No
SLB-04	4.39	0.99	0.233	0.168	0.207	0.134	**0.666**	0.110	0.57	Yes	Yes
SLB-05	4.21	1.01	0.204	0.066	0.253	0.139	**0.658**	0.225	0.56	Yes	Yes
SLB-06	4.55	0.98	0.237	0.170	0.231	0.110	**0.711**	0.055	0.58	Yes	Yes
SLB-07	4.52	0.98	0.235	0.181	0.200	0.090	**0.765**	0.051	0.58	Yes	Yes
SLB-08	4.50	0.99	0.194	0.165	0.148	0.139	**0.741**	0.083	0.55	Yes	Yes
SLB-09	4.39	0.97	0.184	0.135	0.166	0.216	**0.704**	0.155	0.57	Yes	No
SLB-10	4.58	0.99	0.241	0.290	0.340	0.228	0.226	-0.079	0.52	No	No
SLB-11	4.13	1.12	0.056	0.120	**0.691**	0.200	0.131	0.165	0.51	Yes	No
SLB-12	4.13	1.07	0.066	0.116	**0.702**	0.138	0.215	0.155	0.52	Yes	Yes
SLB-13	4.29	1.04	0.231	0.130	**0.563**	0.159	0.207	0.213	0.58	Yes	Yes
SLB-14	4.29	0.94	0.240	0.226	0.457	0.048	0.219	0.097	0.52	No	No
SLB-15	4.40	0.97	0.302	0.241	**0.529**	0.145	0.245	0.099	0.63	Yes	Yes
SLB-16	4.48	0.94	0.365	0.215	**0.525**	0.181	0.257	0.092	0.66	Yes	Yes
SLB-17	4.41	0.96	0.372	0.182	**0.532**	0.158	0.202	0.101	0.62	Yes	Yes
SLB-18	4.24	1.04	0.148	0.112	**0.652**	0.134	0.144	0.165	0.52	Yes	Yes
SLB-19	4.21	1.09	0.157	0.106	**0.670**	0.190	0.076	0.216	0.54	Yes	Yes
SLB-20	4.61	0.91	0.234	0.316	0.371	**0.564**	0.043	0.030	0.63	Yes	Yes
SLB-21	4.63	0.89	0.228	0.376	0.281	**0.611**	0.062	-0.017	0.64	Yes	Yes
SLB-22	4.66	0.90	0.230	0.391	0.212	**0.620**	0.052	-0.047	0.61	Yes	Yes
SLB-23	4.69	0.92	0.173	0.476	0.101	0.465	0.141	0.014	0.57	No	No
SLB-24	4.48	0.94	0.145	0.283	0.234	**0.642**	0.120	0.190	0.62	Yes	Yes
SLB-25	4.35	1.00	0.146	0.134	0.193	**0.661**	0.255	0.292	0.62	Yes	No
SLB-26	4.38	0.96	0.214	0.082	0.186	**0.545**	0.375	0.275	0.61	Yes	No
SLB-27	4.48	0.95	0.210	0.205	0.145	**0.557**	0.292	0.142	0.59	Yes	Yes
SLB-28	4.38	0.97	0.236	0.218	0.234	0.336	0.247	0.299	0.60	No	No
SLB-29	4.69	0.93	0.279	0.371	0.161	0.347	0.212	0.108	0.60	No	No

	M	SD	Component						ITC	Retained for CFA?	Retained after CFA?
			1	2	3	4	5	6			
SLB-30	4.69	0.94	0.222	0.461	0.159	0.273	0.113	0.124	0.57	No	No
SLB-31	4.70	0.91	0.331	0.379	0.142	0.400	0.189	0.126	0.64	No	No
SLB-32	4.53	0.94	0.225	**0.503**	0.157	0.232	0.118	0.205	0.60	Yes	Yes
SLB-33	4.23	0.98	0.111	0.419	0.355	0.070	0.057	0.406	0.56	No	No
SLB-34	4.49	0.90	0.222	0.437	0.295	0.109	0.217	0.288	0.63	No	No
SLB-35	4.25	1.03	0.085	0.385	0.302	0.074	0.068	0.450	0.53	No	No
SLB-36	4.13	1.13	0.062	0.312	0.181	0.086	-0.018	0.420	0.40	No	No
SLB-37	4.71	0.88	0.366	**0.553**	0.150	0.175	0.114	0.053	0.62	Yes	Yes
SLB-38	4.77	0.89	0.250	**0.623**	0.042	0.286	0.125	0.053	0.60	Yes	Yes
SLB-39	4.76	0.93	0.248	**0.620**	0.017	0.273	0.069	0.106	0.58	Yes	No
SLB-40	4.49	1.00	0.132	**0.533**	0.037	0.247	0.049	0.379	0.56	Yes	Yes
SLB-41	4.68	0.89	0.258	**0.569**	0.026	0.306	0.065	0.272	0.63	Yes	No
SLB-42	4.68	0.86	0.271	**0.534**	-0.029	0.310	0.080	0.340	0.62	Yes	Yes
SLB-43	4.36	0.98	0.279	0.240	0.102	0.248	0.209	**0.578**	0.63	Yes	Yes
SLB-44	4.20	1.05	0.201	0.250	0.113	0.153	0.121	**0.711**	0.57	Yes	Yes
SLB-45	4.17	1.04	0.223	0.224	0.125	0.130	0.127	**0.723**	0.57	Yes	Yes
SLB-46	4.32	1.10	0.455	0.002	0.262	0.221	0.070	0.369	0.53	No	No
SLB-47	4.54	0.99	**0.615**	0.058	0.186	0.254	0.112	0.295	0.61	Yes	No
SLB-48	4.61	0.94	**0.615**	0.302	0.153	0.150	0.122	0.165	0.65	Yes	Yes
SLB-49	4.48	0.98	**0.625**	0.040	0.225	0.245	0.136	0.323	0.64	Yes	Yes
SLB-50	4.39	1.03	**0.607**	0.057	0.236	0.210	0.146	0.324	0.63	Yes	Yes
SLB-51	4.67	0.89	**0.660**	0.296	0.115	0.171	0.223	0.081	0.67	Yes	Yes
SLB-52	4.65	0.95	**0.660**	0.303	0.089	0.103	0.167	0.035	0.60	Yes	Yes
SLB-53	4.60	0.92	**0.655**	0.277	0.091	0.113	0.232	0.094	0.63	Yes	No
SLB-54	4.56	0.96	**0.637**	0.250	0.104	0.103	0.172	0.116	0.60	Yes	Yes
SLB-55	4.68	0.92	**0.637**	0.315	0.150	0.122	0.216	0.041	0.65	Yes	Yes
SLB-56	4.72	0.89	**0.675**	0.306	0.162	0.139	0.175	0.087	0.67	Yes	Yes
SLB-57	4.61	0.92	**0.594**	0.340	0.178	0.161	0.150	0.113	0.66	Yes	No
SLB-58	4.58	0.95	**0.612**	0.312	0.193	0.097	0.160	0.125	0.65	Yes	Yes
SLB-59	4.46	0.92	0.445	0.342	0.199	0.146	0.148	0.297	0.65	No	No
SLB-60	4.72	0.89	0.393	**0.556**	0.185	0.113	0.147	0.067	0.64	Yes	Yes
SLB-61	4.56	0.92	0.315	**0.538**	0.258	0.037	0.171	0.132	0.62	Yes	No

Table 3. (Continued)

	M	SD	Component								
			1	2	3	4	5	6	ITC	Retained for CFA?	Retained after CFA?
SLB-62	4.62	0.87	0.278	**<u>0.584</u>**	0.221	0.048	0.110	0.067	0.58	Yes	Yes
SLB-63	4.43	0.93	0.226	0.462	0.226	0.002	0.149	0.262	0.54	No	No
SLB-64	3.23	1.27	-0.131	0.027	-0.153	0.066	-0.085	-0.543	-0.28	No	No
SLB-65	4.82	0.85	0.362	**<u>0.581</u>**	0.168	0.101	0.110	0.004	0.59	Yes	Yes
Eigenvalues			23.85	2.96	2.56	2.12	1.78	1.57			
Variance explained (%)			36.69	4.55	3.93	3.26	2.73	2.41			
Total variance (%)								53.58			
S1	4.59	0.71									
S2	4.64	0.63	0.72								
S3	4.29	0.76	0.61	0.56							
S4	4.51	0.72	0.63	0.68	0.63						
S5	4.43	0.80	0.59	0.50	0.60	0.55					
S6	4.24	0.90	0.56	0.60	0.51	0.52	0.44				
SLB-SF-65	4.46	0.57	0.87	0.87	0.80	0.82	0.72	0.69			
SLB-SF-48	4.50	0.60	0.88	0.86	0.80	0.82	0.74	0.69			

Note. N= 2,246. M: mean scores; SD: standard deviation. Bold and underlined values are the highest loadings by a variable among the factors which are over 0.50. ITC: item-total correlation. Forty-eight items were retained for the CFA in which 38 items were retained to form the finalized version of the scale. SLB-SF-65: 65-item Short-Form Service Leadership Behavior Scale; SLB-SF-48: the six-factor, 48-item solution to be subjected to CFA. S1: Subscale 1 (12 items, *Self-improvement and Self-reflection*); S2: Subscale 2 (12 items, *People and Principles Orientation*); S3: Subscale 3 (8 items, *Resilience*); S4: Subscale 4 (7 items, *Social Competence*); S5: Subscale 5 (6 items, *Problem-Solving*); S6: Subscale 6 (3 items, *Mentorship*). All correlation coefficients are statistically significant at $p < .001$ (two-tailed).

To assess the stability of this six-factor solution, we computed the coefficients of congruence (r_c) across subsets A (N= 2,246) and B (N= 2,240). As illustrated in Table 4, the value of r_c of SLB-SF-65 across subsets is 0.99, indicating that the six-factor structure was essentially identical across the two subsets (32). Additionally, the r_c of the six factors across these two random subsamples are all above 0.98 (see Table 4). In short, these findings corroborate the stability of the factors derived (33).

With the objective to simplify and thereby lead to a more stringent interpretability of the factorial structure, 17 items with loadings below 0.50 were removed (34, 35). The resultant 48-item, six-factor solution (SLB-SF-48) was then subjected to a confirmatory factor analysis (CFA), which will be discussed in detail in another paper under preparation. The six factors, each of which forms a subscale, were accordingly named "Self-improvement and Self-reflection" (items 47 to 58), "People and Principles Orientation" (items 1, 32, 37 to 42, 60 to 62, and 65), "Resilience" (items 11 to 13, 15 to 19), "Social Competence" (items 20 to 22, 24 to 27), "Problem-Solving" (items 4 to 9), and "Mentorship" (items 43 to 45).

Table 4. Coefficient of congruence across two subsamples

	Between two random subsamples (subset A: N= 2,246; subset B: N= 2,240)
Short-Form Service Leadership Behavior Scale (SLB-SF-65)	0.991
1: *Self-improvement and Self-reflection*	0.996
2: *People and Principles Orientation*	0.996
3: *Resilience*	0.989
4: *Social Competence*	0.982
5: *Problem-Solving*	0.993
6: *Mentorship*	0.988

Reliability of the measures

As detailed in Table 5a, the total scale (SLB-SF-65), trimmed scale (SLB-SF-48) and the subscales all demonstrated at least meritorious internal consistency (i.e., all α values >.80, mean inter-item correlations > .30) across subsets. Similar findings (i.e., all α values >.80, mean inter-item correlations > .30) emerged (see Table 5b) even when we further split the two subsamples based on the respondents' gender. All items, except for item 64 which was subsequently excluded from SLB-SF-48, had a corrected item-total correlation of at least 0.40 (see Table 4). Taken together, the present findings supported the high reliability of the SLB-SF-48 and its subscales.

Table 5a. Internal consistencies of SLB-SF-65, SLB-SF-48, and subscales across subsamples

	Entire Sample (N= 4,486)		Subset A (N= 2,246)		Subset B (N= 2,240)	
	α	Mean Inter-item correlations	α	Mean Inter-item correlations	α	Mean Inter-item correlations
SLB-SF-65	0.97	0.34	0.97	0.34	0.97	0.34
SLB-SF-48	0.97	0.38	0.97	0.37	0.97	0.38
1: *Self-improvement and Self-reflection*	0.93	0.53	0.93	0.53	0.93	0.53
2: *People and Principles Orientation*	0.90	0.44	0.90	0.44	0.91	0.45
3: *Resilience*	0.88	0.49	0.88	0.48	0.89	0.50
4: *Social Competence*	0.89	0.54	0.89	0.53	0.90	0.56
5: *Problem-Solving*	0.89	0.56	0.89	0.59	0.88	0.54
6: *Mentorship*	0.85	0.65	0.85	0.66	0.85	0.65

Note. α = Cronbach's alpha value. SLB-SF-65: 65-item Short-Form Service Leadership Behavior Scale; SLB-SF-48: the six-factor, 48-item solution to be subjected to CFA.

Table 5b. Internal consistencies of SLB-SF-65, SLB-SF-48, and subscales across gender

	Subset A (N= 2,246)				**Subset B (N= 2,240)**			
	Males (N= 775)		Females (N= 1,471)		Males (N= 742)		Females (N= 1,498)	
	α	Mean Inter-item correlations	α	Mean Inter-item correlations	α	Mean Inter-item correlations	α	Mean Inter-item correlations
SLB-SF-65	0.97	0.38	0.97	0.32	0.97	0.37	0.97	0.33
SLB-SF-48	0.97	0.42	0.96	0.35	0.97	0.40	0.96	0.36
Subscale 1	0.94	0.56	0.92	0.51	0.93	0.52	0.93	0.53
Subscale 2	0.91	0.45	0.90	0.43	0.92	0.48	0.89	0.41
Subscale 3	0.88	0.48	0.88	0.48	0.88	0.49	0.89	0.51
Subscale 4	0.90	0.55	0.88	0.52	0.90	0.56	0.89	0.55
Subscale 5	0.89	0.57	0.90	0.59	0.87	0.54	0.88	0.54
Subscale 6	0.83	0.62	0.87	0.68	0.84	0.63	0.85	0.66

Note. α = Cronbach's alpha value. SLB-SF-65: 65-item Short-Form Service Leadership Behavior Scale; SLB-SF-48: the six-factor, 48-item solution to be subjected to CFA. Subscale 1: *Self-improvement and Self-reflection*; Subscale 2: *People and Principles Orientation*; Subscale 3: *Resilience*; Subscale 4: *Social competence*; Subscale 5: *Problem-Solving*; Subscale 6: *Mentorship.*

Validity analyses: Correlation with external criterion scales (and subscales)

Consistent with our hypotheses, correlational findings (see Table 6a) revealed that the SLB-SF-48 scores (and the six subscales) correlated significantly (all *p*s <.001) and positively with all external criterion measures. Using the software package *cocor* (36) which permits comparisons of magnitude between two pairs of correlation coefficients (e.g., Steiger's (37) computation of z-score using average correlations), the findings (see Table 6b) revealed that amongst all significant correlations, the SLB-SF-48 correlated most robustly with the *Revised Servant Leadership Profile* (r = 0.790) and noticeably more modest with the *Interpersonal Reactivity Index* (r = 0.412). In summary, these findings shed light on the convergent validity of the SLB-SF-48, which was demonstrated to be positively linked with constructs (e.g., a Servant Leadership mindset and one's inner urge to uphold morality) theorized to delineate the behavioral prerequisites for a Service Leader (8, 9).

Table 6a. Correlations with external criterion scales (and subscales)

	External criterion scales					
	RSLP	MSC	LEF	IRI	IRI-EC	IRI-PT
SLB-SF-65	0.80	0.66	0.51	0.42	0.30	0.45
SLB-SF-48	0.79	0.65	0.53	0.41	0.29	0.43
1: *Self-improvement and Self-reflection*	0.69	0.59	0.42	0.35	0.24	0.39
2: *People and Principles Orientation*	0.78	0.69	0.37	0.54	0.44	0.51
3: *Resilience*	0.58	0.41	0.45	0.20	0.10	0.27
4: *Social Competence*	0.65	0.56	0.52	0.36	0.29	0.34
5: *Problem-Solving*	0.49	0.37	0.47	0.19	0.10	0.23
6: *Mentorship*	0.62	0.42	0.40	0.24	0.16	0.27

Note. N= 2,246. All correlation coefficients are statistically significant at p <.001 (two-tailed). SLB-SF-65: 65-item Short-Form Service Leadership Behavior Scale; SLB-SF-48: the six-factor, 48-item solution to be subjected to CFA. RSLP: Revised Servant Leadership Profile; MSC: Moral Self-Concept; LEF: Leadership Efficacy; IRI: Interpersonal Reactivity Index; IRI-EC: Subscale "Empathic Concern"; IRI: PT: Subscale "Perspective Taking."

Table 6b. Comparison of strength of correlations between SLB-SF-48 with the criterion scales

Correlations with the external criterion scales (and subscales)			Z-scores of difference between rs (36, 37) with SLB-SF-48:				
	α (MITC)	r	MSC	LEF	IRI	IRI-EC	IRI-PT
1. RSLP	0.94 (0.45)	0.790***	14.88***	18.45***	25.32***	29.16***	24.02***
2. MSC	0.83 (0.44)	0.648***	—	7.15***	15.28***	20.14***	13.28***
3. LEF	0.73 (0.27)	0.526***	—	—	5.41***	10.12***	4.44***
4. IRI	0.74 (0.17)	0.412***	—	—	—	12.67***	-2.15*
4a. IRI- EC	0.62 (0.19)	0.293***	—	—	—	—	-7.46***
4b. IRI- PT	0.59 (0.19)	0.433***	—	—	—	—	—

Note. N= 2,246. *p <.05 (two-tailed). ***p <.001 (two-tailed). α = Cronbach's alpha value. MITC: Mean inter-item correlations. RSLP: Revised Servant Leadership Profile; MSC: Moral Self-Concept; LEF: Leadership Efficacy; IRI: Interpersonal Reactivity Index; IRI-EC: Subscale "Empathic Concern"; IRI: PT: Subscale "Perspective Taking."

Validity analyses: Correlation with other Service Leadership scales under validation

As Table 7a shows, the SLB-SF-48 correlated significantly and positively with both the composite scores of the single-factor, 40-item Service Leadership Knowledge (i.e., SLK-SF-40) scale ($r = 0.170$), and the eight-factor, 46-item Service Leadership Attitude (i.e., SLA-SF-46) scale ($r = 0.565$). Details about the validation of SLK-SF-40 and SLA-SF-46 are addressed in two separate chapters in this book. The SLB-SF-48 also correlated positively with most of the subscales of SLA-SF-46. Regarding the six subscales of SLB-SF-48, they are mostly correlated positively and significantly with both the SLK-SF-40 and SLA-SF-46 (including the subscales), despite occasional non-significant or unexpected findings (see Table 7a).

Additionally, comparison of the strengths of correlation (see Table 7b) revealed that the strengths of associations between SLB-SF-48 and SLA-SF-46 (including the subscales) were, in general, significantly greater (*ps* <.05) than that of SLB-SF-48 and SLK-SF-40. These results indicated that the display of Service Leadership behaviors would be linked more to whether someone is prone to think or feel (i.e., attitude) like a Service Leader than him/her being more "book-smart" (i.e., knowledge) in the SLAM curriculum.

Table 7a. Correlations with other Service Leadership scales (and subscales) under validation

	SLK-SF-40	SLA-SF-46-F1	SLA-SF-46-F2	SLA-SF-46-F3	SLA-SF-46-F4	SLA-SF-46-F5	SLA-SF-46-F6	SLA-SF-46-F7	SLA-SF-46-F8	SLA-SF-46-Total
SLB-SF-65	0.17	0.52	0.48	0.51	0.43	0.47	0.48	0.27	-0.08	0.57
SLB-SF-48	0.17	0.52	0.47	0.50	0.42	0.47	0.47	0.26	-0.07	0.56
1: *Self-improvement and Self-reflection*	0.20	0.48	0.43	0.44	0.37	0.44	0.45	0.21	-0.03	0.52
2: *People and Principles orientation*	0.26	0.55	0.55	0.53	0.42	0.54	0.47	0.26	-0.01	0.62
3: *Resilience*	0.02$^{n.s.}$	0.31	0.27	0.33	0.30	0.26	0.29	0.21	-0.13	0.34
4: *Social Competence*	0.16	0.43	0.41	0.41	0.32	0.41	0.39	0.22	-0.03$^{n.s.}$	0.47
5: *Problem-Solving*	0.11	0.36	0.29	0.29	0.23	0.30	0.33	0.13	-0.05*	0.35
6: *Mentorship*	-0.12	0.24	0.22	0.38	0.38	0.19	0.24	0.24	-0.19	0.30

Note. N= 2,246. * p <.05 (two-tailed). "n.s." denotes statistical non-significance. Unless otherwise specified, all correlation coefficients are significant at p <.001 (two-tailed). SLB-SF-65: 65-item Short-Form Service Leadership Behavior Scale; SLB-SF-48: the six-factor, 48-item solution to be subjected to CFA. SLK-SF-40: Scale score of the single-factor, 40-item Service Leadership Knowledge Scale; SLA-SF-46-Total: Scale score of the eight-factor, 46-item Service Leadership Attitude (SLA) Scale; SLA-SF-46-F1: SLA Factor 1 "Vision and competence"; SLA-SF-46-F2: SLA Factor 2 "People orientation"; SLA-SF-46-F3: SLA Factor 3 "Caring disposition"; SLA-SF-46-F4: SLA Factor 4 "Ethical role model"; SLA-SF-46-F5: SLA Factor 5 "Social competence"; SLA-SF-46-F6: SLA Factor 6 "Self-understanding and reflection"; SLA-SF-46-F7: SLA Factor 7 "Positive view about human beings"; SLA-SF-46-F8: SLA Factor 8 "Unchangeable and dark human nature."

Table 7b. Comparison of strength of correlations between SLB-SF-48 and other Service Leadership scales under validation

Correlations with the external criterion scales (and subscales)			Z-scores of difference between *r*s (36, 37) with SLB-SF-48[a]								
	α (MITC)	*r*	SLA-SF-46-F1	SLA-SF-46-F2	SLA-SF-46-F3	SLA-SF-46-F4	SLA-SF-46-F5	SLA-SF-46-F6	SLA-SF-46-F7	SLA-SF-46-F8	SLA-SF-46-Total
1. SLK-SF-40	0.94 (0.28)	0.170***	-15.56	-13.63	-13.40	-9.21	-13.61	-12.58	-3.23	10.53	-18.99
2. SLA-SF-46-F1	0.90 (0.46)	0.515***	—	3.46	1.08$^{n.s.}$	5.47	3.86	3.02	11.07	20.88	-5.68
3. SLA-SF-46-F2	0.87 (0.47)	0.474***	—	—	-1.60$^{n.s.}$	2.93	0.50$^{n.s.}$	0.23$^{n.s.}$	9.60	19.57	-9.65
4. SLA-SF-46-F3	0.86 (0.46)	0.499***	—	—	—	5.39	2.04	1.74$^{n.s.}$	10.96	19.33	-5.98
5. SLA-SF-46-F4	0.85 (0.53)	0.419***	—	—	—	—	-2.57	-2.69	6.91	15.53	-10.23
6. SLA-SF-46-F5	0.84 (0.57)	0.467***	—	—	—	—	—	-0.17$^{n.s.}$	8.83	19.50	-9.50
7. SLA-SF-46-F6	0.82 (0.49)	0.470***	—	—	—	—	—	—	8.50	18.10	-7.13
8. SLA-SF-46-F7	0.70 (0.54)	0.261***	—	—	—	—	—	—	—	11.47	-15.37
9. SLA-SF-46-F8	0.78 (0.41)	-0.068**	—	—	—	—	—	—	—	—	-25.12
10. SLA-SF-46-Total	0.94 (0.28)	0.565***	—	—	—	—	—	—	—	—	—

Note. N= 2,246. ****p* <.001 (two-tailed). α = Cronbach's alpha value. MITC: Mean inter-item correlations. [a]Unless otherwise specified by the superscript "n.s." which denotes statistical non-significance, all other Z-scores of difference were significant at $p < .05$ (two-tailed) (i.e., |Z-score| > 1.96). SLK-SF-40: Scale score of the single-factor, 40-item Service Leadership Knowledge Scale; SLA-SF-46-Total: Scale score of the eight-factor, 46-item Service Leadership Attitude (SLA) Scale; SLA-SF-46-F1: SLA Factor 1 "Vision and competence"; SLA-SF-46-F2: SLA Factor 2 "People orientation"; SLA-SF-46-F3: SLA Factor 3"Caring disposition"; SLA-SF-46-F4: SLA Factor 4 "Ethical role model"; SLA-SF-46-F5: SLA Factor 5 "Social competence"; SLA-SF-46-F6: SLA Factor 6 "Self-understanding and reflection"; SLA-SF-46-F7: SLA Factor 7 "Positive view about human beings"; SLA-SF-46-F8: SLA Factor 8 "Unchangeable and dark human nature."

DISCUSSION

Utilizing a large sample of Hong Kong undergraduates, the present study attempted to validate the Short-Form Service Leadership Behavior Scale. The findings underlined the excellent reliability amongst the items. Results of the EFA suggested a six-factor solution which was demonstrated to be stable across sub-samples, hence providing support for the factorial validity of the 48-item Service Leadership Behavior Scale (SLB-SF-48). Besides, the six subscales were found to correlate significantly and positively with all external criterion measures. The SLB-SF-48 and subscales, which recorded excellent internal consistencies, were also demonstrated to correlate positively and significantly with the two other Serviced Leadership scales. These results provide support for the convergent validity of SLB-SF-48. Taken together, the present analyses lend support to the legitimacy of SLB-SF-48 as a valid and reliable rubric to judge whether someone demonstrated qualities of a good Service Leader.

There are several contributions of the present chapter. First, in view of the lack of leadership assessment tools in the Chinese context, this is an important addition to the literature. As Chinese people constitute roughly one-fifth of the world's population, objective leadership scales for Chinese people need to be developed. Second, the present findings are important for the Service Leadership literature. As the ever-expanding global economy becomes more service-oriented, this is a timely effort to develop objective tools in this area. Third, the scale permits an objective assessment of Service Leadership behavior which is important for personnel decisions. Employers may wish to employ workers capable of exhibiting Service Leadership behaviors. Fourth, the scale can be used by researchers to evaluate the effectiveness of Service Leadership training programs. Basically, if a training program works, the trainees should show positive changes after completion of the program. Finally, the scale can enable an individual to understand oneself more regarding his/her attributes in Service Leadership.

While the current chapter may have underscored the psychometric soundness and factorial stability of SLB-SF-48, there are still aspects which warrant addressing. First, this chapter focuses only on the exploratory side of the dimensionality assessment of the behavior scale. While an interpretable and stable initial factorial solution has been established, to further quantify and accordingly, ascertain the absolute and relative agreement (i.e., the fit indices) of this six-factor solution with the response data, it is imperative that a confirmatory factor analysis (CFA) be administered (38). Due to the limitation of word count in this book, the present article is unable to also report the CFA which had been conducted as part of this large-scale validation study. As reiterated throughout this chapter, the findings of the CFA would be detailedly discussed in another paper under preparation.

Second, the *Knowledge-Behavior* link ($r = 0.17$) was noticeably weaker compared to the *Attitude-Behavior* association ($r = 0.56$), implying a disconnect between one's *understanding* and propensity to *practice* in relation to the SLAM curriculum. This may be attributable to the varying nature of different Service Leadership surveys. Unlike the knowledge scale which has a "correct" answer for every item, the behavior and attitude scales are more like an opinion poll. It is, therefore, conceivable that respondents in behavior and attitude scales may respond according to their *personal* or *normative theory* rather than their *genuine stances* on the matter (39). Social desirability responding may also come into the equation (40). In other words, instead of indicating whether he/she had previously demonstrated a certain behavioral quality of a Service Leader, a participant may have responded based on what he/she believes a Service Leader *should* do in this situation, or alternatively, he/she may have tried to rate in a particular fashion that presents him/her in a favorable light (41).

In spite of all these shortcomings, this chapter does not only evidence the internal consistency and convergent validity of the SLB-SF-65, but also informs the "rightsizing" of the scale (accordingly forming the SLB-SF-48) which has been well-documented to promote response rate and minimize response burden (see 42 for a review). As systematic evaluation research in the context of Service Leadership education remains scanty (7, 12), the present chapter constitutes a valuable addition to the literature by presenting a pioneer assessment tool in behavioral qualities of Service Leadership which was demonstrated to be valid and reliable.

ACKNOWLEDGMENTS

The validation project is financially supported by the Victor and William Fung Foundation. The preparation for this chapter is supported by the Foundation and the Endowed Professorship in Service Leadership Education at The Hong Kong Polytechnic University.

REFERENCES

[1] Hoshmand AR. The role of service leadership in the university's GE curriculum: The HKBU experience. In: Shek DTL, Chung PPY, eds. Promoting Service Leadership qualities in university students: The case of Hong Kong. Singapore: Springer, 2015:17-28.

[2] Snell RS, Chan MYL, Zou TXP. Key practices of leadership for service in Hong Kong. In: Shek DTL, Chung PPY, Lin L, Merrick J, eds. Service Leadership education for university students. New York: Nova Science, 2017:127-38.

[3] Chung PPY. Service reborn: The knowledge, skills, and attitudes of service companies, 1st ed. New York: Lexingford, 2012.

[4] Shek DTL, Chung PPY, Leung H. Manufacturing economy vs. service economy: Implications for Service Leadership. Int J Disabil Hum Dev 2015;14:205-15.

[5] Shek DTL, Lin L, Leung H, Yu L, Ma CMS, Li X. Development and validation of the Service Leadership Knowledge Scale in a Chinese context. In: Shek DTL, Chung PPY, Lin L, Merrick J, eds. Service leadership education for university students. New York: Nova Science, 2017:163-88.

[6] Census and Statistics Department. Hong Kong monthly digest of statistics: The four key industries and other selected industries in the Hong Kong economy. Hong Kong: Census and Statistics Department, 2017.

[7] Shek DTL, Chung PPY, eds. Promoting service leadership qualities in university students: The case of Hong Kong. Singapore: Springer, 2015.

[8] Chung PPY, Bell AH. 25 Principles of service leadership, 1st ed. New York: Lexingford, 2015.

[9] Chung PPY, Elfassy R. The 12 dimensions of a service leader, 1st ed. New York: Lexingford, 2016.

[10] Shek DTL, Yu L, Ma CMS, Sun RCF, Liu TT. Development of a credit-bearing service leadership subject for university students in Hong Kong. Int J Adolesc Med Health 2013;25:353-61.

[11] Shek DTL, Lin L. Evaluating Service Leadership programs with multiple strategies. In: Shek DTL, Chung PPY, eds. Promoting Service Leadership qualities in university students: The case of Hong Kong. Singapore: Springer, 2015:197-211.

[12] Shek DTL, Lin L. Validation of the Service Leadership Knowledge Scale: Criterion-related validity. In: Shek DTL, Chung PPY, Lin L, Merrick J, eds. Service leadership education for university students. New York: Nova Science, 2017:189-204.

[13] Grant AM, Franklin J, Langford P. The self-reflection and insight scale: A new measure of private self-consciousness. Soc Behav Pers 2002;30:821-35.

[14] Page D, Wong PTP. A conceptual framework for measuring servant leadership. In: Adjibolooso SBSK, ed. The human factor in shaping the course of history and development. Lanham, MD: University Press of America, 2000:69-110.

[15] Wielkiewicz RM. The Leadership Attitudes and Beliefs Scale: An instrument for evaluating college students' thinking about leadership and organizations. J Coll Stud Dev 2000;41:335-47.

[16] Greenleaf RK. Servant leadership: A journey into the nature of legitimate power and greatness. New York: Paulist Press, 1977.

[17] Davis MH. Measuring individual differences in empathy: Evidence for a multidimensional approach. J Pers Soc Psychol 1983;44:113-26.

[18] Cheng CHK. The Chinese Adolescent Self-Esteem Scales (CASES): A user manual. Hong Kong: City University of Hong Kong Press, 2005.

[19] Chemers MM, Watson CB, May ST. Dispositional affect and leadership effectiveness: A comparison of self-esteem, optimism, and efficacy. Pers Soc Psychol Bull 2000;26:267-77.

[20] Murphy SE. The contribution of leadership experience and self-efficacy to group performance under evaluation apprehension. Dissertation. Seattle: WA: University of Washington, 1992.

[21] Mullin EM. Scale development: Heterosexist attitudes in women's collegiate athletics. Meas Phys Educ Exerc Sci 2013;17:1-21.

[22] Field A. Discovering statistics using IBM SPSS statistics, 4th ed. London: SAGE, 2013.

[23] King DB, DeCicco TL. A viable model and self-report measure of spiritual intelligence. Int J Transpersonal Stud 2009;28:68-85.

[24] Wong PTP, Page D. Servant leadership: An opponent-process model and the Revised Servant Leadership Profile. Virginia Beach, VA: Regent University, 2003.

[25] Shek DTL, Lin L. Core beliefs in the service leadership model proposed by the Hong Kong Institute of Service Leadership and Management. Int J Disabil Hum Dev 2015;14:233-42.

[26] de Corte K, Buysse A, Verhofstadt LL, Roeyers H, Ponnet K, Davis MH. Measuring empathic tendencies: Reliability and validity of the Dutch version of the Interpersonal Reactivity Index. Psychol Belg 2007;47:235-60.

[27] Fernandez AM, Dufey M, Kramp U. Testing the psychometric properties of the Interpersonal Reactivity Index (IRI) in Chile: Empathy in a different cultural context. Eur J Psychol Assess 2011;27:179-85.

[28] Siu AMH, Shek DTL. Validation of the Interpersonal Reactivity Index in a Chinese context. Res Soc Work Pract 2005;15:118-26.

[29] Shamay-Tsoory SG, Aharon-Peretz J, Perry D. Two systems for empathy: A double dissociation between emotional and cognitive empathy in inferior frontal gyrus versus ventromedial prefrontal lesions. Brain 2009;132:617-27.

[30] Shek DTL, Yu L. General University Requirements and holistic development in university students in Hong Kong. Int J Adolesc Med Health 2017;29:41-8.

[31] Armenakis AA, Feild HS, Wilmoth JN. An algorithm for assessing factor structure congruence. Educ Psychol Meas 1977;37:213-4.

[32] Lorenzo-Seva U, ten Berge JMF. Tucker's congruence coefficient as a meaningful index of factor similarity. Methodology (Gott) 2006;2:57-64.

[33] Shek DTL, Yu L. Factorial validity of a subjective outcome evaluation tool for implementers of a positive youth development program. J Pediatr Adolesc Gynecol 2014;27:S32-42.

[34] Jamal AAA, Ramlan WK, Karim MRA, Mohidin R, Osman Z. The effects of social influence and financial literacy on savings behavior: A study on students of higher learning institutions in Kota Kinabalu, Sabah. Int J Bus Manag Soc Res 2015;6:110-9.

[35] Milan GS, da Silva MBC, Bebber S. Analysis of attributes and dimensions of the built environment quality from the perspective of employees from furniture companies. Braz Bus Rev 2015;12:66-86.

[36] Diedenhofen B, Musch J. cocor: A comprehensive solution for the statistical comparison of correlations. PLoS ONE 2015;10:e0121945. doi:10.1371/journal.pone.0121945.

[37] Steiger JH. Tests for comparing elements of a correlation matrix. Psychol Bull 1980;87:245-51.

[38] Cohen RJ, Swerdlik ME. Psychological testing and assessment: An introduction to tests and measurement, 6th ed. New York: McGraw-Hill, 2005.

[39] Weiner B, Russell D, Lerman D. The cognition-emotion process in achievement-related contexts. J Pers Soc Psychol 1979;37:1211-20.

[40] van de Mortel TF. Faking it: Social desirability response bias in self-report research. Aust J Adv Nurs 2008;25:40-8.

[41] Shek DTL, Leung JTY, Ma LK, Lin L, Wu FKY. Training of potential program implementers for the Tin Ka Ping P.A.T.H.S. Project in China: Subjective outcome evaluation findings. Int J Child Adolesc Health, in press.

[42] Edwards P, Roberts I, Clarke M, DiGuiseppi C, Pratap S, Wentz R, et al. Increasing response rates to postal questionnaires: Systematic review. BMJ 2002;324:1183-5.

In: Service Leadership
Editors: Daniel TL Shek, Xiaoqin Zhu, Li Lin et al.
ISBN: 978-1-53614-852-7

Chapter 11

THE SERVICE LEADERSHIP KNOWLEDGE SCALE: NORMS AND PSYCHOLOGICAL CORRELATES

Daniel TL Shek*[1-6,*]*, PhD, FHKPS, BBS, SBS, JP,
Xiaoqin Zhu*[1]*, PhD and Samson Tse*[7]*, PhD
[1]Department of Applied Social Sciences,
The Hong Kong Polytechnic University, Hong Kong, PR China
[2]Centre for Innovative Programmes for Adolescents and Families,
The Hong Kong Polytechnic University, Hong Kong, PR China
[3]Department of Social Work, East China Normal University, Shanghai, PR China
[4]Kiang Wu Nursing College of Macau, Macau, PR China
[5]Hong Kong Institute of Service Leadership and Management Limited,
Hong Kong, PR China
[6]Division of Adolescent Medicine, Department of Pediatrics,
Kentucky Children's Hospital, University of Kentucky School of Medicine,
Lexington, Kentucky, US
[7]Faculty of Social Sciences, The University of Hong Kong, Hong Kong, PR China

ABSTRACT

Guided by the Service Leadership Theory, substantial effort has been devoted to service leadership education in Hong Kong. In contrast, scientific instruments that assess the basic concepts of service leadership are non-existent. As such, we developed three scales pertinent to the notion of service leadership, including knowledge, attitude, and behavior

---

* Correspondence: Daniel TL Shek, PhD, FHKPS, BBS, SBS, JP, Associate Vice President (Undergraduate Programme), Chair Professor of Applied Social Sciences and Li and Fung Professor in Service Leadership Education, Department of Applied Social Sciences, The Hong Kong Polytechnic University, Hung Hom, Hong Kong, PR China. E-mail: daniel.shek@polyu.edu.hk.

scales. The present study reported the development of norms and psychological correlates of the Service Leadership Knowledge Scale consisting of 40 multiple-choice questions (i.e., SLK-SF-40). Based on a large and representative sample (N = 4,486) of university students recruited from the eight University Grants Committee (UGC)-funded universities in Hong Kong, the results showed that the female students had a significantly higher level of service leadership knowledge than did the male students, resulting in the separate norms for the two groups. While age did not show significant influence on the students' knowledge score, the students' grade point average (GPA), leadership training experience, and experience of taking leadership roles in university organizations were all positively associated with their service leadership knowledge scores, but the effect size was small. The percentile norms of this knowledge scale developed in this study provide a useful tool for designing, implementing, and evaluating service leadership education programs.

INTRODUCTION

With the growing globalization and rapid technology development which have intensified international economic competition, skilled human capital is deemed vital to sustaining a nation's competitiveness and long-term prosperity (1, 2). Regarding the list of desirable attributes, leadership is among the most frequently cited ones. As Ewing, Bruce and Ricketts (3) stated, "the future success of local communities, states, and the country is tied to the development of quality leaders" (p. 119).

The increasing need for leadership qualities comes with a great emphasis on leadership education. In particular, higher education institutions have incorporated leadership into their mission statements and included leadership as one of the important student learning outcomes (4-6). To cultivate leadership qualities among the university students, a vast number of leadership programs in different forms (e.g., curriculum, course, workshop and outdoor training) have been offered to them (7-9). For instance, with the financial support of the Victor and William Fung Foundation, a large-scale leadership project was launched in eight public universities funded by the University Grants Committee (UGC) in Hong Kong to satisfy the needs of predominant service economy by nurturing "service leaders" (10).

Despite the divergent patterns, common themes of learning goals can be identified for these leadership programs, such as improving leadership knowledge and nurturing a diverse range of leadership attributes (11, 12). From the perspective of evidence-based practice (13), it is essential to carry out systematic evaluation studies to examine whether these intended learning outcomes are achieved and whether the related leadership education is effective. Unfortunately, rigorously designed evaluation research for leadership education is scarce, particularly in the Chinese culture. One possible reason has to do with the severe lack of valid tools to assess Chinese people's leadership attributes in the dimensions of leadership knowledge, attitudes and behavior.

Service leadership education and evaluation in Hong Kong

With specific reference to Hong Kong, the economic structure has shifted from the manufacturing economy to the service economy which calls for leaders with a service mindset (14). To facilitate leadership education in the service era, Chung (15) proposed the Service Leadership Theory which defines service leadership as to "satisfy needs by consistently providing quality personal service to everyone one comes into contact with, including one's self, others, groups, communities, systems, and environments" (p. 5). To elaborate, service leadership highlights service orientation and manifest itself in three realms—self, others, and systems (15, 16). Furthermore, it is believed that effective service leadership is determined by three key elements: leadership competency including intra- and inter-personal competencies, moral character, and caring disposition (15).

Guided by the Service Leadership Theory and with the financial support of the Victor and William Fung Foundation, the eight UGC-funded universities in Hong Kong have designed and implemented their own service leadership programs, which incorporate knowledge and beliefs of service leadership and aim to nurture critical service leadership qualities (i.e., leadership competency, caring disposition, and moral character) in the university students (10). For instance, at The Hong Kong Polytechnic University (PolyU), both credit-bearing service leadership subjects embedded in the general education curriculum and the non-credit bearing programs have been offered to the students since the 2012/2013 academic year (17). In addition, PolyU and other universities in mainland China jointly organized several intensive service leadership training programs for their students. While evaluation findings have consistently shown that the participants were highly satisfied with these service leadership education programs and they showed improvements in self-perceived service leadership attributes (18-20), the participants' actual gain in service leadership knowledge remains unknown.

Evaluation on knowledge gain and Service Leadership Knowledge Scale

Acquisition and application of leadership knowledge are among the desirable outcomes of leadership education (12, 17). This learning outcome can be regarded as the foundation of service leadership education, which endeavors to promote a new leadership philosophy. To illustrate, without mastering service leadership knowledge, for example, what does service leadership emphasize and what qualities an effective service leader should develop, it is quite difficult, if not impossible, for the participants to adapt for the leadership beliefs and optimize their leadership practice. In this sense, it is indispensable to evaluate the participants' knowledge gained through a service leadership program so as to portray a full picture of the program effectiveness.

In leadership education, it is not uncommon to examine what the participants have learned from the program. However, due to the dearth of validated leadership knowledge scales, most studies examined self-perceived knowledge instead of objectively assessed knowledge. For instance, in an evaluation study conducted by Stedman, Rutherford, Rosser, and Elbert (21), the participants were asked to evaluate their own capacity in defining authentic leadership, character, relationship building stages, and other related knowledge points after a 5-day leadership conference. While measuring self-perceived knowledge seems to have advantages (e.g., easy and efficient), this approach has potential shortcomings. For example, the participants may overestimate their own knowledge level due to social desirability bias (22). Besides, the trainees' self-ratings are likely to be affected by their subjective experience in the training. As argued by Sitzmann, Ely, Brown, and Bauer (23), "self-assessed knowledge is generally more useful as an indicator of how learners feel about a course than as an indicator of how much they learned from it" (p. 180).

Concerning these potential issues of measuring subjective leadership knowledge, it can be argued that a validated objective knowledge scale is a prerequisite for rigorously assessing the participants' improvement of knowledge in a leadership program. Unfortunately, such objective leadership knowledge assessment tools are virtually non-existent in the Chinese communities. To fill this research gap as well as facilitating the evaluation of service leadership education in Hong Kong, we have developed a 200-item long-form Service Leadership Knowledge Scale (SLK-LF-200), which is able to assess individuals' actual understanding of service leadership. The scale primarily covered the knowledge points of the aforementioned Service Leadership Theory and associated publications of Chung, Shek and collaborators (e.g., 24, 25). The details of the content of the SLK-LF-200 have been reported elsewhere (26).

The SLK-LF-200's content-validity and criterion-related validity were found to be good (26, 27). More specifically, the criterion-related validation study compared an experimental group (i.e., 67 students who took the "Service Leadership" subject at PolyU) with a control group (i.e., 94 students who had never received any service leadership education) regarding their scores on the SLK-LF-200. In the study, 63 out of the initial 200 items were identified as being able to significantly differentiate the two groups (27). A further item screening procedure was conducted and another 13 items were discarded concerning face validity or item duplication issues. As a result, a 50-item short-form Service Leadership Knowledge Scale (SLK-SF-50) was formed, constituting a fundamental assessment tool for evaluating service leadership education.

Norms and correlates of the Knowledge Scale

While the content validity and criteria-related validity of the long-form Service Leadership Knowledge Scale (i.e., SLK-LF-200) have been supported, psychometric properties such as the convergent and divergent validity of the 50-item scale (i.e., SLK-SF-50) are unknown. Besides, the norms, as well as the potential correlates of the knowledge scale, are also important issues to be considered. As such, the eight UGC-funded universities in Hong Kong jointly organized a large-scale online survey to validate and finalize the service leadership assessment tools including the knowledge scale. Using the SLK-SF-50, the validation study yielded a final version of the Service Leadership Knowledge Scale which consists of 40 items (i.e., SLK-SF-40). While the procedure of obtaining the SLK-SF-40 as well as the scale's convergent and construct validity is reported in another article of this issue, the norms and the possible psychological correlates of university students' scores on SLK-SF-40 are the foci of the current chapter.

The norms of the service leadership knowledge are important because it serves as a benchmark to assist educators and researchers in developing, implementing, and evaluating effective service leadership programs for the purpose of helping students become knowledgeable service leaders. First, the established norms can be used to identify the standing of the target group's knowledge level in the normative population, based on which training needs can be determined and tailored training programs can be designed. Second, with the norms, participants' progress during training can be monitored by examining changes of their rank in the normative population. Likewise, the norms can be applied to evaluate the training effectiveness.

Normative data can be presented in terms of means and standard deviations of the raw score (28). In using this type of normative data, one's standing on the assessment can be estimated through using a standardized score (i.e., z score), which can be further referred to a table of areas under the normal curve. While this method assumes normative data to be normally distributed, the reality is that normative data will often depart significantly from a normal distribution. Under this circumstance, an alternative, maybe a better choice is percentile norms, which may consist of a full presentation of the percentile rank for each raw score, or it may simply present some of the raw scores corresponding to several landmark percentiles (e.g., the 1st, 5th, 10th, 50th percentile etc.). Various examples of the use of percentile norms can be found in the extant literature (29-31).

Apart from its usefulness when normative data are not normally distributed, a further advantage of percentile norms is simplicity. While a standardized score needs to be interpreted by mapping it on to percentile rank through a look-up table developed by the researcher or an external conversion table (28), the percentile norms can tell us directly the relative position of an individual's test score in the normative population. Percentile norms are easy to understand even for lay people, as the meaning of percentiles is apparently unequivocal (32). In view of the above positive features of percentile norms, the current study utilized this method to develop norms for the Service Leadership Knowledge Scale using university students in Hong Kong as the normative population.

To determine whether there is a need to develop separate norms for sub-groups, the present study considered two demographic characteristics: gender and age. For gender, in the previous studies, women were found to be more cooperative, relational, empathetic and caring as compared with men (33-37). Possessing these characteristics which are related to service leadership qualities, women may be more aware of the demands of service leaders in today's service economy and have a better understanding of the philosophy and concepts of service leadership. Therefore, we expected that female students would have a higher level of service leadership knowledge as compared to male students (Hypothesis 1). For the influence of age, very little evidence can be identified in the existing literature. Besides, for the target population (i.e., university students) in the present study, variability in age is generally very small. Thus, we did not expect a significant influence of age on the participants' service leadership knowledge score.

The current study also considered the participants' academic achievement indexed by grade point average (i.e., GPA), the experience of receiving leadership training and experience of being a leader as another three potential correlates of service leadership knowledge score. A high GPA generally indicates an individual's success in course assignments thus could in part represent one's cognitive ability (38). Based on the prior studies which consistently showed a positive relationship between leadership and intelligence observers including GPA (38, 39), we expected a positive association between GPA and service leadership knowledge (Hypothesis 2).

Although leadership training received by university students may not be directly related to the notion of service leadership, some overlapped knowledge points might be covered, such as the required leadership competency (e.g., problem solving and emotional competence). As a result, it is quite reasonable to expect that one's leadership training experience, regardless of its form and content, will be positively associated with one's service leadership knowledge score (Hypothesis 3). For student leadership experience, we argue that being a leader in a student organization will allow a student to understand what is demanded by such a position and how he or she can better serve other students. Indeed, previous research found that years of being in a leadership role increased a leader's servant leader behaviors such as altruistic and empathetic behaviors (35). As such, we hypothesized that the experience of being a leader would positively correlate with service leadership knowledge score as well (Hypothesis 4).

The present study

In March 2017, an online-survey project was initiated in the eight UGC-funded institutions in Hong Kong to validate measures assessing the qualities of service leaders as outlined by the Service Leadership Theory. The eight universities include The Hong Kong Polytechnic University (PolyU), The Chinese University of Hong Kong, The Education University of Hong Kong, Hong Kong Baptist University, City University of Hong Kong, Lingnan University, The University of Hong Kong, and Hong Kong University of Science and Technology. Ethics approval for the validation study was obtained from the Human Subjects Ethics Sub-committee of PolyU, which served as the lead institution of the project. The project aimed at validating three scales including knowledge, attitude, and behavior scales, among which the knowledge scale was the focus of the present study. Specifically, the present study outlined the norms and psychological correlates of the final version of the Service Leadership Knowledge Scale (i.e., SLK-SF-40).

OUR STUDY

The online survey was launched simultaneously in eight higher education institutions in Hong Kong. While the research team at PolyU prepared the questionnaire and set up the online survey, each participating university recruited their undergraduate students as participants by distributing the link of the online survey. The participants were well informed the principles of voluntary, anonymity, and freedom to withdraw from the study at any time. The students' consent was sought and each was given a supermarket voucher of 100 Hong Kong dollars as a token of appreciation upon completion of the survey.

The data collection lasted for approximately four months from March to June in 2017. Cases having at least one of the following issues were excluded from further analyses: 1) the participants did not provide consent as indicated by their selection of the option "I decline" on the consent form page, 2) the case was identified as repeated completion due to its same student ID as that of another case, and 3) the participants who claimed to be postgraduate students by themselves. After removing these invalid cases ($n = 69$), the final sample consisted of 4,486 participants, among whom 1,517 (33.82%) were male and 2,969 (66.18%) were female. The participating students' age range was between 15 to 34 years ($M = 20.47$, $SD = 1.67$), with 1,344 (29.96%) aged between 15 to 19 years and 3,142 (70.04%) aged 20 years or above. Table 1 summarizes the demographic characteristics of the participants in each university based on age and gender.

Table 1. Demographic characteristics of the sample

University	1	2	3	4	5	6	7	8	Total
No. of participants	1,000	505	500	517	464	500	500	500	4,486
Percentage	22.29%	11.26%	11.15%	11.52%	10.34%	11.15%	11.15%	11.15%	100%
Age range	18-27	17-29	17-34	15-28	18-34	18-29	17-28	16-28	15-34
Age (Mean/SD)	20.46/1.65	20.08/1.55	21.05/1.75	20.79/1.67	20.63/1.77	20.54/1.55	20.38/1.67	19.85/1.50	20.47/1.67
Age group (15-19) (*n*/%)	297/29.70	193/38.22	95/19.00	117/22.63	112/24.14	133/26.60	173/34.60	224/44.80	1,344/29.96
Age group (≥ 20) (*n*/%)	703/70.30	312/61.78	405/81.00	400/77.37	352/75.86	367/73.40	327/65.40	276/55.2	3,142/70.04
Male students (*n*/%)	409/40.90	130/25.74	98/19.60	122/23.60	128/27.59	148/29.60	151/30.20	331/66.20	1,517/33.82
Female students (*n*/%)	591/59.10	375/74.26	402/80.40	395/76.40	336/72.41	352/70.40	349/69.80	169/33.80	2,969/66.18

Measures

The validation project included a wide array of measurements including the three service leadership scales, external criterion scales such as Moral Self Concept, demographic measures, and potential correlates. The present study focused on the Service Leadership Knowledge Scale, and its demographic and other potential correlates.

Service Leadership Knowledge Scale

The knowledge scale (i.e., SLK-SF-50) administrated in the present project consisted of 50 multiple-choice questions generated based on the Service Leadership Theory proposed by Chung (15). The scale had a holistic coverage of the service leadership knowledge points pertaining to different domains such as the general description and the three realms of service leadership, service leadership competency, moral character, caring disposition, the core belief "everyone can be a leader," and so on. Detail description of each knowledge domain has been reported elsewhere (26).

In the present study, 10 items in the SLK-SF-50 were discarded due to their low item-total correlations (i.e., below .30; see another chapter in this book). The retained 40 items formed the final scale (i.e., SLK-SF-40) which covered the same knowledge domains as did the original scale. The final scale possessed a one-factor structure with good overall goodness-of-fit indices (e.g., $\chi^2_{(740)} = 3,492.44$, $p < .001$; CFI = .98; TLI = .99; RMSEA = .03). The validation procedure and related validation indicators of the SLK-SF-40 are reported in another article in this issue. The present study was based on the final 40-item scale, which showed good internal reliability (i.e., Cronbach Alpha = .94). Each participant's answer on each item was coded as "1" or "0" to indicate a correct or incorrect answer, respectively. A total score across the 40 items was computed as the service leadership knowledge score for each participant. In the present study, the participants' knowledge score ranged from 2 to 40 ($M = 22.55$, $SD = 10.46$).

Demographic and other potential correlates

The demographic characteristics concerned in the present study included age and gender. Other potential correlates included grade point average (i.e., GPA), the experience of leadership training and experience of being in a leadership role.

For GPA, while four participating universities adopted a system with 4.00 as the maximum score, other three universities had different maximum GPA scores (e.g., 4.5). Thus, for participants coming from these three universities, their raw GPA scores were converted to new scores using the formula: new GPA score = raw GPA score × 4/the maximum GPA score in the university. After this adjustment, the participants' GPA ranged between 0 and 4 ($M = 2.89$, $SD = .45$).

Furthermore, the participants reported whether they had ever taken any leadership course or training including that related to service leadership (0 = No, 1 = Yes), and whether they had served in any leadership position in an organization such as student association (0 = No, 1 = Yes).

Data analyses

First, a multiple regression analysis was performed to examine whether gender (1 = Male, 2 = Female) and age significantly influenced participants' knowledge score. The results were used to decide whether there was a need to create separate norms for sub-groups. For example, if male students' knowledge scores significantly differ from that of their female counterparts, norms will be constructed separately for male and female students.

Second, we run normality tests to see whether knowledge scores are normally distributed. If the data are normally distributed, we will calculate standardized scores as well as percentile norms, and percentiles will be constructed only if the data are not normally distributed.

When constructing percentile norms, we first mapped raw scores to each percentile from 1 to 100. As several students gained the same knowledge score, one raw score can have several percentile rank scores, which may cause difficulties in interpreting the norms. Therefore, we further calculated a unique percentile for each raw score. As strongly recommend by Crawford et al. (28), we defined the unique percentile of raw scores as the percentage including those fall below as well as half of those obtaining the score of interest. This calculation method can be presented by the formula below:

$$\text{Percentile rank of a given raw score} = 100 \times (m + 0.5k)/N,$$

where m means the number of participants scoring below the given raw score, k is the number of participants obtaining the given score, and N represents the overall size of the normative sample considered. This method is adopted as it takes the discrepancy between a test score and the real-valued score into account (28). After this calculation procedure, we further rounded off the figures to present the integer values.

Third, correlational analyses were utilized to investigate associations between other potential correlates (e.g., GPA and leadership training experience) and the participants' knowledge score.

OUR FINDINGS

While age did not show significant predicting effect on the knowledge score ($\beta = -.0003$, $p = .99$), gender significantly predicted the participants' knowledge score ($\beta = .17$, $p < .001$; Cohen's $f^2 = .03$), with female students ($M = 23.85$, $SD = 10.10$) having significantly higher knowledge scores than male students ($M = 20.02$, $SD = 10.70$). Thus, Hypothesis 1 was supported.

Table 2. Percentiles and related raw scores for Service Leadership Knowledge Scale (SLK-SF-40) by gender

Percentile (1-50)	Raw Score				Percentile (51-99)	Raw Score		
	Male (N = 1,517)	Female (N = 2,969)	Total sample (N = 4,486)			Male (N = 1,517)	Female (N = 2,969)	Total sample (N = 4,486)
1	≤ 4.00	≤ 5.00	≤ 5.00		51	18.00	27.00	24.00
2	5.00	6.00	6.00		52	19.00	27.00	25.00
3	6.00	7.00	6.00		53	19.00	27.00	25.00
4	6.00	7.00	6.00		54	20.00	28.00	26.00
5	6.00	7.00	7.00		55	20.00	28.00	26.00
6	6.00	8.00	7.00		56	21.00	28.00	27.00
7	7.00	8.00	7.00		57	22.00	29.00	27.00
8	7.00	9.00	8.00		58	23.00	29.00	28.00
9	7.00	9.00	8.00		59	23.00	29.00	28.00
10	7.00	9.00	8.00		60	24.00	30.00	28.00
11	7.00	10.00	9.00		61	24.00	30.00	29.00
12	8.00	10.00	9.00		62	25.00	30.00	29.00
13	8.00	10.00	9.00		63	26.00	30.00	29.00
14	8.00	10.00	9.00		64	26.00	31.00	30.00
15	8.00	11.00	10.00		65	27.00	31.00	30.00
16	8.00	11.00	10.00		66	27.00	31.00	30.00
17	9.00	11.00	10.00		67	28.00	31.00	30.00
18	9.00	12.00	10.00		68	28.00	31.00	31.00
19	9.00	12.00	11.00		69	28.42	32.00	31.00

Percentile (1-50)	Raw Score			Percentile (51-99)	Raw Score		
	Male (*N* = 1,517)	Female (*N* = 2,969)	Total sample (*N* = 4,486)		Male (*N* = 1,517)	Female (*N* = 2,969)	Total sample (*N* = 4,486)
20	9.00	12.00	11.00	70	29.00	32.00	31.00
21	9.00	13.00	11.00	71	29.00	32.00	31.00
22	9.96	13.00	12.00	72	30.00	32.00	32.00
23	10.00	13.00	12.00	73	30.00	32.00	32.00
24	10.00	14.00	12.00	74	30.00	33.00	32.00
25	10.00	14.00	12.00	75	31.00	33.00	32.00
26	10.00	14.00	13.00	76	31.00	33.00	33.00
27	10.00	15.00	13.00	77	31.00	33.00	33.00
28	11.00	15.00	13.00	78	32.00	33.60	33.00
29	11.00	16.00	14.00	79	32.00	34.00	33.00
30	11.00	16.00	14.00	80	32.00	34.00	33.00
31	12.00	17.00	14.00	81	32.00	34.00	34.00
32	12.00	17.00	15.00	82	33.00	34.00	34.00
33	12.00	18.00	15.00	83	33.00	34.00	34.00
34	12.00	18.00	15.00	84	33.00	35.00	34.00
35	13.00	19.00	16.00	85	34.00	35.00	35.00
36	13.00	19.00	16.00	86	34.00	35.00	35.00
37	13.00	20.00	17.00	87	34.00	35.00	35.00
38	13.00	20.00	17.00	88	35.00	35.00	35.00
39	13.00	21.00	18.00	89	35.00	36.00	35.00
40	14.00	21.00	18.00	90	35.00	36.00	36.00
41	14.00	22.00	19.00	91	35.00	36.00	36.00
42	14.00	23.00	19.00	92	36.00	36.00	36.00
43	15.00	23.00	20.00	93	36.00	36.00	36.00
44	15.00	23.00	20.00	94	36.00	37.00	36.00
45	15.00	24.00	21.00	95	36.00	37.00	37.00
46	16.00	24.00	22.00	96	37.00	37.00	37.00
47	16.00	25.00	22.00	97	37.00	38.00	37.00
48	16.64	25.00	23.00	98	38.00	38.00	38.00
49	17.00	26.00	23.00	99	38.82	39.00	39.00
50	17.00	26.00	24.00	100	39.00	40.00	40.00

Then we performed normality tests for female and male groups separately. A Shapiro-Wilk's test ($p < .001$) (40, 41) showed that the knowledge scores were not normally distributed for both males and females, with a skewness of .22 (SE = .06, z-value = 3.67, $p < .001$) and a kurtosis of –1.43 (SE = .13, z-value = –11, $p < .001$) for the male participants, and a skewness of –.30 (SE = .04, z-value = –7.5, $p <.001$) and a kurtosis of –1.31 (SE = .09, z-value = –14.56, $p < .001$) for the female group (42-44). A further visual inspection of their histograms revealed a bimodal distribution for both groups. As such, only percentile norms were built separately for both male and female students. (see Table 2 and Table 3).

Table 3. Raw scores and related percentiles for Service Leadership Knowledge Scale (SLK-SF-40)

Raw score	Percentiles		
	Male (N = 1,517)	Female (N = 2,969)	Total sample (N = 4,486)
1	0.0	0.0	0.0
2	0.0	0.0	0.0
3	0.0	0.0	0.0
4	1.0	0.0	0.0
5	2.0	1.0	1.0
6	5.0	2.0	3.0
7	9.0	4.0	6.0
8	14.0	6.0	9.0
9	19.0	9.0	12.0
10	25.0	12.0	17.0
11	29.0	16.0	20.0
12	33.0	19.0	24.0
13	37.0	22.0	27.0
14	41.0	25.0	30.0
15	44.0	27.0	33.0
16	47.0	30.0	35.0
17	49.0	32.0	38.0
18	51.0	34.0	40.0
19	53.0	36.0	41.0
20	55.0	37.0	43.0
21	56.0	39.0	45.0
22	57.0	41.0	47.0
23	59.0	43.0	48.0
24	60.0	45.0	50.0
25	62.0	48.0	52.0
26	64.0	50.0	54.0
27	66.0	52.0	57.0
28	68.0	55.0	59.0
29	70.0	58.0	62.0
30	73.0	62.0	66.0
31	76.0	66.0	70.0
32	80.0	71.0	74.0
33	83.0	76.0	78.0
34	86.0	81.0	83.0
35	90.0	86.0	87.0
36	94.0	91.0	92.0
37	97.0	95.0	96.0
38	98.0	98.0	98.0
39	100.0	99.0	99.0
40	100.0	100.0	100.0

Correlates of knowledge score

Results of correlational analysis showed that the participants' service leadership score was significantly correlated with their GPA ($r = .20$, $p < .001$; $r^2 = .04$), experience of taking leadership course or training ($r = .07$, $p < .001$; $r^2 = .005$), and experience of being a leader ($r = .12$, $p < .001$; $r^2 = .014$), meaning that students with higher GPA, having experience of taking leadership course or training, or having experience of being a leader before were likely to have a better understanding of service leadership knowledge. Hence, Hypotheses 2 to 4 were also supported. However, it is noteworthy that the effect size involved was small.

Discussion

The present study outlined percentile norms and potential psychological correlates of the Service Leadership Knowledge Scale (SLK-SF-40). As a pioneering attempt to develop and validate objective knowledge scale pertinent to service leadership, the present study is a timely response to the lack of assessment tools measuring individuals' leadership knowledge in the Chinese context. Concerning the fact that substantial effort has been taken on promoting service leadership education in Hong Kong while little research has articulated the effectiveness, the present study also makes an important progress in addressing the issue of evaluation. In particular, the established norms will serve as a useful instrument not only to assess individuals' standing in a normative population regarding the fundamental knowledge of service leadership but also to track the improvement of the participants' relative standing during and after receiving service leadership education.

Noteworthy, the current study has two methodological strengths. First, we developed the norms based on a large and representative sample of university students coming from multiple higher education institutions in Hong Kong. Therefore, we believe that the generalizability of the findings is good. Second, we used an objective knowledge scale where the items were derived from a solid leadership framework. In addition, the validity and other psychometric properties of the scale have been proved to be good. Thus, the norms can be regarded as reliable and valid in delineating university students' service leadership knowledge level.

Apart from the norms, our study adds to the extant literature on the potential correlates of university students' comprehension of service leadership. Three notable observations from the present findings could be highlighted. First, as expected, the university students' service leadership knowledge scores were not significantly associated with their age. This result indicates that the students will not gain a better understanding of the service leadership concepts automatically as time goes by. Instead, leadership training could be an effective means for knowledge acquisition. Indeed, previous studies suggest that leadership development among youth is closely related to their involvement in leadership training programs (45, 46). The present study also found that overall leadership training experience was positively correlated to service leadership knowledge score, supporting the utility of conducting leadership training for youth. Nevertheless, the effect size of the correlation between leadership training experience and service leadership knowledge was not large. This may be because we did not specify the focus of leadership training. Although leadership training programs, regardless of their focus, may cover some common knowledge points which are also useful for increasing the understanding of service leadership, those training programs specifically focusing on service leadership may be more effective.

Second, also in line with our hypothesis, the female students demonstrated a higher knowledge level than did the male students. This is understandable because women are more service-oriented than men in nature, as evidenced by research findings showing that women tended to be more caring, relationship-oriented and empathetic than men (34-36). These qualities fit the demands of the service economy at the first place and help women better understand the service leadership concepts than men. Given this gender difference, two separate norms were established for female and male students. One practical implication of this finding is that gender effect should be considered when implementing and evaluating service leadership education programs.

Third, the participants' GPA was positively correlated with their service leadership knowledge score. For GPA, a better score usually indicates a student's better cognitive ability such as reasoning and problem solving skills (38), which may better enable them to infer what kind of leadership qualities can fulfill the needs of service economy. Fourth, we found that the experience of being a leader in a student organization was associated with a higher service leadership knowledge score. This result also echoes the previous findings which suggested that serving in leadership roles in university exerts positive impacts on diverse student learning outcomes such as leadership efficacy (47). It is believed that student leadership in college embody a wide range of elements such as helping people, building relationship and working as a team (48), all of which are related to service leadership concepts, directly or indirectly.

Although the present study represents a pioneering effort to construct percentile norms and identify potential psychological correlates for service leadership knowledge, it has three limitations. First, we only investigated university students which may limit the generalizability of the findings to other populations. Future research will certainly benefit from employing a more heterogeneous sample of potential service leaders including employees in different economic sectors and constructing norms of service leadership knowledge accordingly. Second, we did not collect data in other Chinese communities. As service economy grows rapidly as well in mainland China where there is also a need to launch service leadership education programs, it is also necessary to build norms among mainland Chinese people for evaluation purpose. Thus, future research could go further by collecting data and comparing knowledge levels in different Chinese communities. The final limitation is related to the limited number of potential correlates considered in the present study. For example, we did not examine the influence of students' undergraduate major. As some of the knowledge points are not unique to service leadership, it is thus possible that students in certain majors can learn the knowledge from their own major subjects such as social work or psychology. Future studies could include students' major and other individual traits such as personality to examine and compare the relationships between these factors and service leadership knowledge level.

ACKNOWLEDGMENTS

The validation project is financially supported by the Victor and William Fung Foundation. The preparation for this paper is supported by the Foundation and the Endowed Professorship in Service Leadership Education at The Hong Kong Polytechnic University. This chapter is an updated version of a publication in the special issue "Development and validation of assessment tools on service leadership knowledge, attitude and behavior" edited by Daniel TL Shek, Xiaoqin Zhu and Joav Merrick published in the International Journal of Child and Adolescent Health, 2018;11(4).

REFERENCES

[1] Hong Kong Education Commission. Learning for life, learning through life: Report proposals for the education system in Hong Kong. 2000. URL: http://www.e-c.edu.hk/doc/en/publications_and_related_documents/education_reform/Edu-reform-eng.pdf.

[2] Partnership for 21st Century Skills. 21st Century skills, education and competitiveness: A resource and policy guide. Tucson, AZ: Partnership for 21st Century Skills, 2008.

[3] Ewing JC, Bruce JA, Ricketts KG. Effective leadership development for undergraduates: How important is active participation in collegiate organizations. J Leadersh Educ 2009;7(3):118-32.

[4] Ho SP, Odom SF. Mindsets of leadership education undergraduates: An approach to program assessment. J Leadersh Educ 2015;14(1):92-106. DOI: 1012806/V14/I1/R6.

[5] Jackling B, De Lange P. Do accounting graduates' skills meet the expectations of employers? A matter of convergence or divergence. Acc Educ 2009;18(4-5):369-85. DOI: 10.1080/09639280902719341.

[6] Keeling RP. Learning reconsidered: A campus-wide focus on the student experience. Washington, DC: National Association of Student Personnel Administrators and American College Personnel Association, 2004.

[7] Riggio RE, Ciulla J, Sorenson G. Leadership education at the undergraduate level: A liberal arts approach to leadership development. In: Murphy SE, Riggio RE, eds. The future of leadership development. Mahwah, NJ: Lawrence Erlbaum, 2003: 223-36.

[8] Sessa VI, Matos C, Hopkins CA. Evaluating a college leadership course: What do students learn in a leadership course with a service-learning component and how deeply do they learn it. J Leadersh Educ 2009;7(3):167-200.

[9] Komives SR, Dugan JP, Owen JE, Slack C, Wagner W, eds. The handbook for student leadership development. 2nd ed. San Francisco, CA: Jossey-Bass, 2011.
[10] Shek DTL, Chung PPY, eds. Promoting service leadership qualities in university students. Singapore: Springer, 2015.
[11] Cress CM, Astin HS, Zimmerman-Oster K, Burkhardt JC. Developmental outcomes of college students' involvement in leadership activities. J Coll Student Dev 2001;42(1):15-27.
[12] Seemiller C, Murray T. The common language of leadership. J Leadersh Stud 2013;7(1):33-45. DOI: 10.1002/jls.21277.
[13] Shek DTL. Evaluation of the Project P.A.T.H.S. using multiple evaluation strategies. In: Shek DTL, Sun RCF, eds. Development and evaluation of Positive Adolescent Training through Holistic Social Programs (PATHS). Singapore: Springer, 2013:53-67.
[14] Shek DTL, Chung PPY, Leung H. Manufacturing economy vs. service economy: Implications for service leadership. Int J Disabil Hum Dev 2015;14(3):205-15. DOI: 10.1515/ijdhd-2015-0402.
[15] Chung PPY. Hong Kong Institute of Service Leadership and Management curriculum framework. Hong Kong: Hong Kong Institute of Service Leadership and Management 2011. URL: http://hki-slam.org/index.php?r=article&catid=1&aid=11.
[16] Shek DTL, Chung PPY, Leung H. How unique is the service leadership model? A comparison with contemporary leadership approaches. Int J Disabil Hum Dev 2015;14(3):217-31. DOI: 10.1515/ijdhd-2015-0403.
[17] Shek DTL, Yu L, Ma CMS, Sun RCF, Liu TT. Development of a credit-bearing service leadership subject for university students in Hong Kong. Int J Adolesc Med Health 2013;25(4):353-61. DOI: 10.1515/ijamh-2013-0033.
[18] Shek DTL, Li X. Nurturing students to be caring service leaders. Int J Disabil Hum Dev 2015;14(4):361-9. DOI: 10.1515/ijdhd-2015-0457.
[19] Shek DTL, Lin L, Liu TT. Service leadership education for university students in Hong Kong: Subjective outcome evaluation. Int J Disabil Hum Dev 2014;13(4):513-21. DOI: 10.1515/ijdhd-2014-0349.
[20] Shek DTL, Zhu X, Lin L. Evaluation of an intensive service leadership course in mainland China. Int J Child Adolesc Health 2017;10(2):223-31.
[21] Stedman NL, Rutherford TA, Rosser MH, Elbert C. When leadership counts: Engaging youth through the Washington Leadership Conference. J Agric Educ 2009;50(1):92-104.
[22] Chiaburu DS, Huang JL, Hutchins HM, Gardner RG. Trainees' perceived knowledge gain unrelated to the training domain: The joint action of impression management and motives. Int J Train Dev 2014;18(1):37-52. DOI: 10.1111/ijtd.12021.
[23] Sitzmann T, Ely K, Brown KG, Bauer KN. Self-assessment of knowledge: A cognitive learning or affective measure? Acad Manag Learn Edu 2010;9(2):169-91.
[24] Chung PPY, Bell A. Service reborn: The knowledge, skills and attitudes of service companies. New York: Lexingford Publishing, 2012.
[25] Shek DTL, Chung PPY, Yu L, Merrick J. Service leadership education for university students: the Hong Kong experience. Int J Disabil Hum Dev 2015;14(3):203-4. DOI: 10.1515/ijdhd-2015-0401.
[26] Shek DTL, Lin L, Leung H, Yu L, Ma CMS, Li X. Development and validation of the service leadership knowledge scale in a Chinese context. In: Shek DTL, Chung PPY, Lin L, Merrick J, eds. Service Leadership Education for University Students New York: Nova Science, 2017:163-88.
[27] Shek DTL, Lin L. Validation of the service leadership knowledge scale: Criterion-related validity. In: Shek DTL, Chung PPY, Lin L, Merrick J, eds. Service leadership education for university students. New York: Nova Science, 2017:189-204.
[28] Crawford JR, Garthwaite PH, Slick DJ. On percentile norms in neuropsychology: Proposed reporting standards and methods for quantifying the uncertainty over the percentile ranks of test scores. Clin Neuropsychol 2009;23(7):1173-95. DOI: 10.1080/13854040902795018.

[29] Hilbert A, Baldofski S, Zenger M, Löwe B, Kersting A, Braehler E. Weight Bias Internalization Scale: Psychometric properties and population norms. PLoS One 2014;9(1):e86303. DOI: 10.1371/journal.pone.0086303.

[30] Crawford J, Cayley C, Lovibond PF, Wilson PH, Hartley C. Percentile norms and accompanying interval estimates from an Australian general adult population sample for self-report mood scales (BAI, BDI, CRSD, CES-D, DASS, DASS-21, STAI-X, STAI-Y, SRDS, and SRAS). Aust Psychol 2011;46(1):3-14. DOI: 10.1111/j.1742-9544.2010.00003.x.

[31] Hasbrouck J, Tindal GA. Oral reading fluency norms: A valuable assessment tool for reading teachers. Read Teach 2006;59(7):636-44. DOI: 10.1598/RT.59.7.3.

[32] Lezak MD, Howieson DB, Loring DW, Hannay HJ, Fischer JS. Neuropsychological assessment, 4th ed. New York: Oxford University Press, 2004.

[33] Eagly AH, Johannesen-Schmidt MC. The leadership styles of women and men. J Soc Iss 2001;57(4):781-97. DOI: 10.1111/0022-4537.00241.

[34] Eagly AH, Johannesen-Schmidt MC, Van Engen ML. Transformational, transactional, and laissez-faire leadership styles: A meta-analysis comparing women and men. Psychol Bull 2003;129(4):569-91. DOI: 10.1037/0033-2909.129.4.569.

[35] Beck CD. Antecedents of servant leadership: A mixed methods study. J Leadersh Organ Stud 2014;21(3):299-314. DOI: 10.1177/1548051814529993.

[36] Gleichgerrcht E, Decety J. Empathy in clinical practice: How individual dispositions, gender, and experience moderate empathic concern, burnout, and emotional distress in physicians. PLoS One 2013;8(4):e61526. DOI: 10.1371/journal.pone.0061526.

[37] Ye R, Wang X-H, Wendt JH, Wu J, Euwema MC. Gender and managerial coaching across cultures: female managers are coaching more. Int J Hum Resour Manag 2016;27(16):1791-812. DOI: 10.1080/09585192.2015.1075570.

[38] Kellett JB, Humphrey RH, Sleeth RG. Empathy and complex task performance: Two routes to leadership. Leadersh Q 2002;13(5):523-44. DOI: 10.1016/S1048-9843(02)00142-X.

[39] Mumford MD, Zaccaro SJ, Harding FD, Jacobs TO, Fleishman EA. Leadership skills for a changing world: Solving complex social problems. Leadersh Q 2000;11(1):11-35. DOI: 10.1016/S1048-9843(99)00041-7.

[40] Razali NM, Wah YB. Power comparisons of shapiro-wilk, kolmogorov-smirnov, lilliefors and anderson-darling tests. J Stat Modeling Analytics 2011;2(1):21-33.

[41] Shapiro SS, Wilk MB. An analysis of variance test for normality (complete samples). Biometrika 1965;52(3/4):591-611. DOI: 10.2307/2333709.

[42] Cramer D. Fundamental statistics for social research. London: Routledge, 1998.

[43] Cramer D, Howitt DL. The SAGE dictionary of statistics: A practical resource for students in the social sciences. London: Sage, 2004.

[44] Doane DP, Seward LE. Measuring skewness: A forgotten statistic. J Stat Educ 2011;19(2):1-18.

[45] Posner BZ. A longitudinal study examining changes in students' leadership behavior. J Coll Student Dev 2009;50(5):551-63. DOI: 10.1353/csd.0.0091.

[46] Fischer DV, Wielkiewicz RM, Stelzner SP, Overland M, Meuwissen AS. Changes in leadership attitudes and beliefs associated with the college experience: A longitudinal study. J Leadersh Educ 2015; 14(1):14-32. DOI: 1012806/V14/I1/R2.

[47] Dugan JP, Komives SR. Developing leadership capacity in college students: Findings from a national study. College Park, MD: National Clearinghouse for Leadership Programs, 2007.

[48] Logue CT, Hutchens TA, Hector MA. Student leadership: A phenomenological exploration of postsecondary experiences. J Coll Student Dev 2005;46(4):393-408. DOI: 10.1353/csd.2005.0039.

In: Service Leadership
Editors: Daniel TL Shek, Xiaoqin Zhu, Li Lin et al.
ISBN: 978-1-53614-852-7

Chapter 12

THE SERVICE LEADERSHIP ATTITUDE SCALE: NORMATIVE DATA AND PERSONAL CORRELATES IN CHINESE UNIVERSITY STUDENTS

Daniel TL Shek[1-6,*], PhD, FHKPS, BBS, SBS, JP, Jing Wu[1], PhD and Ben YB Chan[7], PhD

[1]Department of Applied Social Sciences, The Hong Kong Polytechnic University, Hong Kong, PR China
[2]Centre for Innovative Programmes for Adolescents and Families, The Hong Kong Polytechnic University, Hong Kong, PR China
[3]Department of Social Work, East China Normal University, Shanghai, PR China
[4]Kiang Wu Nursing College of Macau, Macau, PR China
[5]Hong Kong Institute of Service Leadership and Management, Hong Kong, PR China
[6]Division of Adolescent Medicine, Department of Pediatrics, Kentucky Children's Hospital, University of Kentucky School of Medicine, Lexington, Kentucky, US
[7]Center for Engineering Education Innovation, The Hong Kong University of Science and Technology, Hong Kong, PR China

[*] Correspondence: Daniel TL Shek, PhD, FHKPS, BBS, SBS, JP, Associate Vice President (Undergraduate Programme), Chair Professor of Applied Social Sciences and Li and Fung Professor in Service Leadership Education, Department of Applied Social Sciences, The Hong Kong Polytechnic University, Hung Hom, Hong Kong, PR China. E-mail: daniel.shek@polyu.edu.hk.

Abstract

As there are few validated measures of service leadership in the Chinese contexts, there is a need to develop and validate scientific instruments to assess service leadership attitudes and beliefs of Hong Kong university students. In this chapter, we present normative findings for the 46-item Service Leadership Attitude Scale (SLA-SF-46) and explore the potential personal correlates in a large university sample (N = 4,486) recruited from eight universities in Hong Kong. Results showed that while female students scored significantly higher on the SLA-SF-46 compared to male students, no age-related differences were observed. Hence, separate norm tables for both gender groups were constructed. With regard to the potential personal correlates, students' grade point average (GPA), previous leadership training, and experiences of being a leader were all positively correlated with their SLA-SF-46 scores, although the effect sizes were not large. The creation of the percentile norms helps educators and practitioners to understand the service leadership attributes of individuals.

Introduction

Hong Kong has experienced a drastic reform of the economic system from an industrial era to a post-industrial era since the 1970s. The service sector, represented by traditional key industrials (such as trading, tourism, and financial services) and emerging industries (such as medical services, education services, and creative industries), has replaced manufacturing and become the engine of economic development in Hong Kong. The core assets of the modern society are intangible human capitals (e.g., knowledge, intelligence, and skills) beyond tangible physical assets (e.g., the real estate or the machinery). Leadership, as a core determinant for the operation of contemporary business enterprises, has different meanings in every era and every society (1). For the traditional manufacturing economy, top-down and bureaucratic paradigms of leadership models are notably effective as they are product-oriented and task-focused. However, those paradigms are no longer well suited for the modern service-oriented and knowledge-based economy (2). As commented by Manville and Ober in the "Harvard Business Review," "we're in a knowledge economy, but our managerial and governance systems are stuck in the Industrial Era. It's time for a whole new model" (3). Unfortunately, we find very few explicit discussions of leadership models for the knowledge era with regard to Hong Kong. Against this background, Chung (4) advocated the notion of service leadership and refined the idea with the Service Leadership and Management (SLAM) model. According to him, service leadership "is about satisfying needs by consistently providing quality personal service to everyone one comes into contact with, including one's self, others, groups, communities, systems, and environments" (4).

Classic leadership models proposed that leaders shall possess specific genetic traits, which was much based on the belief that leaders are born and not made (5). In contrast, service leadership theory begins with the basic assumption that leadership could be learned and everyone can be a leader (6). Therefore, the call for leadership is for everyone. Particularly, for students in tertiary institutions, leadership development is viewed as one of the most prominent themes and objectives as they will become pillars of the society in the foreseeable future (7). Although there are leadership courses and programs targeting young people, several limitations merit attention. First, most of the existing leadership development programs in the business world are usually expensive and still aim for "elitists" solely (8). Second, only "hard" skills (such as knowledge and management skills) of a leader are emphasized in most leadership development programs (9), whereas "soft" skills (such as interpersonal and intrapersonal competences) are overlooked. Third, there is a lack of systematic evaluation of leadership training programs (9).

Service leadership education in Hong Kong

Effective leadership courses or programs designed for university students are rare in Hong Kong. As such, with the theoretical groundwork of the Hong Kong Institute of Service Leadership and Management (HKI-SLAM) and financial support of the Victor and William Fung Foundation, the Fung Service Leadership Initiative was launched in 2012 and a series of service leadership projects were subsequently conducted in eight institutions that funded by the University Grants Committee (UGC). These projects included both credit-bearing subjects and non-credit bearing programs aiming to nurture leaders with the fundamental service leadership qualities, including competences, characters, and caring dispositions (4). To date, findings from many evaluation studies suggested that service leadership training had received favorable responses from different stakeholders. Taking The Hong Kong Polytechnic University (PolyU) as an example, participants indicated their satisfaction with the service leadership programs and showed great improvements in service leadership attributes (such as intrapersonal competences) based on multiple evaluation strategies (10-12).

One important dimension of leadership training is leadership attitudes and beliefs such as whether a leader believes the followers are changeable. It is not rare to measure leadership attitudes and beliefs with respect to a particular leadership model. For instance, Fleishman (13) developed the Leadership Opinion Questionnaire (LOQ) to assess leadership attitudes in the industry setting from the perspective of the Leadership Skills Model that mainly focused on the competences of leaders, such as problem-solving skills and social judgment skills. Wielkiewicz (14) also developed a Leadership Attitudes and Beliefs Scale (LABS) based on the assumption that leadership could be understood through organizational success rather than individual actions. Unfortunately, none of the extant leadership attitude scales is suitable for examining individuals' understanding of the service leadership theory. In contrast to these existing theories, Service Leadership theory adopts a more systematic and comprehensive approach. As service leadership training programs have been designed and organized in different institutions, it is imperative for researchers and educators to have a standardized tool assessing service leadership attitude.

Under this premise, the Research Team at PolyU endeavored to develop and validate scales on service leadership knowledge, attitude, and behavior. With regard to the Service Leadership Attitude Scale (SLA), a 132-item long form (i.e., SLA-LF-132), was initially developed on the grounds of the SLAM framework (4) with relevant publications authored by Chung, Shek, and collaborators (15-17). The previous study demonstrated that SLA-LF-132 had good content validity (18). Results of an initial exploratory factor analysis (EFA) based on 200 sets of questionnaires suggested a 5-factor solution with 73 items (i.e., SLA-SF-73), which showed good reliability and significant correlation with the 50-item short-form Service Leadership Knowledge Scale (i.e., SLK-SF-50). Based on the SLA-SF-73, further EFA and confirmatory factor analysis (CFA) based on larger samples ($N = 2{,}246$ and 2,240, respectively) informed a finalized solution with 46 items (i.e., SLA-SF-46), which demonstrated good fit indices ($CFI = 0.93$; $NNFI = 0.92$; $RMSEA = 0.041$). Results showed that the SLA-SF-46 covered dimensions of vision and competence, people orientation, caring disposition, ethical role model, social competence, self-understanding and reflection, positive view about human beings, and unchangeable and dark human nature. The findings are reported in a chapter in this book. In the current study, all the results were based on the final version Service Leadership Attitude Scale (i.e., SLA-SF-46).

Normative data for the Service Leadership Attitude Scale

Normative data for the Service Leadership Attitude Scale is fundamental to the development and implementation of the service leadership education. The use of normative data is common in psychological assessment. In the field of leadership study, there has been relatively little research concerning the norms of leadership (19), not to mention in different Chinese contexts. Accordingly, the development of normative data for SLA-SF-46 is an important addition to the literature. First, normative data provides a yardstick to measure, rank, and compare individuals' level of service leadership attitudes and beliefs. Second, with the help of normative data, educators could detect students' current beliefs and blind spots on service leadership. Then targeted curriculum and teaching could be offered and developed. Third, a straightforward and convenient norm table provides a very useful research tool that could objectively assess program effectiveness.

The literature on normative data suggested different ways of explaining the means and standard deviations of raw scores (20). For normative distributions, standardized Z scores could be calculated for estimation. The normal curve could indicate the corresponding area with the given Z score. However, the distributions in real life are usually non-normal. In such situations, another alternative but complementary approach to describe normative data is percentile norms (21), which provides a full and concise picture of the correspondence between a raw score and its percentile rank. Furthermore, percentile norm is convenient to use, even for non-professionals. As such, the overarching objective of this chapter was to provide the estimates of percentile ranks corresponding to raw scores on the SLA-SF-46.

Personal correlates of Service Leadership Attitude

For sub-groups of a population, separate norms would be needed if they demonstrate notable differences. Gender and age were the principal demographic factors covered in the current study. Societies always have discrepant gender role expectations, which influence individuals' leadership attitudes and beliefs. Across cultures, females are still underrepresented in leadership positions in comparison to males (22). In previous literature, there was an incongruity in the association of gender and leadership attitude. According to Wielkiewicz et al. (23), a greater percentage of male first-year college students was located in the Low Hierarchical/Low Systemic category of leadership beliefs, which was associated with effective ecological leadership. Based on this finding, it was hypothesized that male college students in Hong Kong would possess a higher level of service leadership attitude than female college students (Hypothesis 1a). Nevertheless, multiple empirical studies demonstrated that women leaders were better at emotional balance and control, more expressive, and cooperative than men (24, 25). Hence, it could also be assumed that female college students in Hong Kong would possess a higher level of service leadership attitude compared with male college students (Hypothesis 1b). The primary goal of this study was to test these two competing hypotheses, and preliminarily explore the gender differences issue in service leadership.

Although a body of research has tried to shed light on the age-related differences in leadership over the last decades, there is no solid conclusion (26). Existing findings on age-leadership linkages are scare and contradictory. For example, Barbuto et al. (27) found that age positively predicted transformational leadership and individualized consideration. Other studies, in contrast, observed that older leaders demonstrated less mastery of teamwork knowledge (28), less delegating and considerate behaviors (29). Besides, other studies have reported non-significant relationships between leaders' age and their task-oriented behaviors (27, 30) or leadership styles (31). Considering the inconclusive findings of the relationship between age and leadership, and the narrow span in age for the targeted population (i.e., university students), we did not put up any specific hypothesis on the relationship between age and service leadership attitude.

Other personal factors were assumed to be associated with service leadership attitude in the current study, which included participants' grade point average (i.e., GPA), their leadership training experience, and the previous experience of being a leader. GPA has been regarded as a good predictor of the performance of solving complex tasks, which was closely associated with favorable leadership attributes (32). Besides, studies have observed that university students' GPA was positively correlated with their life-long learning attitude, self-rated leadership abilities, and disagreement with hierarchical leadership thinking (33). Therefore, the current study attempted to examine this GPA-leadership linkage and expected a positive correlation between participants' GPA and service leadership attitude (Hypothesis 2).

Multifarious leadership training programs in and out of campus are not uncommon for university students. Empirical studies have investigated the benefits of such education efforts. According to a longitudinal study that assessed the outcomes of 31 leadership development programs in ten institutions in the United States (34), participation in leadership programs had a positive impact on college students' personal development, multi-cultural awareness, and values understanding ability. Although the philosophy and concepts of other leadership programs would not perfectly match service leadership theory, some could share the similar attitudes or beliefs. As inspired by previous studies, it was expected that one's leadership training experiences would be positively related to the service leadership attitude (Hypothesis 3).

Apart from the leadership training experiences, college students nowadays have abundant opportunities to serve as a leader. Qualitative findings showed that college students' practices in leadership roles brought about positive experiences in the aspects of skills-building and interacting personality (35). Accordingly, it was expected that being a leader previously would be positively associated with service leadership attitude (Hypothesis 4).

OUR RESEARCH

An online survey was adopted in the present study. A total of 4,555 university students were recruited using snowball sampling from the eight UGC-funded universities in Hong Kong, including The Hong Kong Polytechnic University (PolyU), The University of Hong Kong (HKU), The Chinese University of Hong Kong (CUHK), Hong Kong Baptist University (HKBU), City University of Hong Kong (CityU), The Education University of Hong Kong (EdUHK), Lingnan University (LU), and Hong Kong University of Science and Technology (HKUST). Each institution recruited at least 500 full-time undergraduate students to complete the survey via the PolyU "mySurvey" online survey platform (https://www.polyu.edu.hk/mysurvey/).

Table 1. Socio-demographic profiles of participants ($N = 4486$)

	N (%)
Gender	
Male	1,517 (33.82%)
Female	2,969 (66.18%)
Age	
15-19 years	1,344 (29.96%)
20-24 years	3,070 (68.44%)
25-29 years	69 (1.54%)
30 years or above	3 (0.07%)
University	
PolyU	1,000 (22.29%)
CUHK	505 (11.26%)
EdUHK	500 (11.15%)
HKBU	517 (11.52%)
CityU	464 (10.34%)
LU	500 (11.15%)
HKU	500 (11.15%)
HKUST	500 (11.15%)

Note. PolyU = The Hong Kong Polytechnic University; CUHK = The Chinese University of Hong Kong; EdUHK = The Education University of Hong Kong; HKBU = Hong Kong Baptist University; CityU = City University of Hong Kong; LU = Lingnan University; HKU = The University of Hong Kong; HKUST = Hong Kong University of Science and Technology.

Website link of the survey was provided for interested participants, where they were able to electronically sign a consent form before the survey started. Students were informed about the confidentiality of their responses and the rights to withdraw from this study at any time. Each participant would be given $HK100 as a token of appreciation upon completion of the survey. The online survey hosted at each university with links between March to June 2017. Among all the 4,555 respondents, six students were excluded as they declined to complete the questionnaire. In the next step, thirty-three cases who completed the questionnaire for multiple times were also removed. Other thirty more cases were deleted due to the ineligibility of participants (e.g., mismatching in the institution and the questionnaire version, as well as those postgraduate students who accidentally completed the questionnaire). In the end, the sample of this study consisted of 4,486 university students between the age of 15 and 34 years ($M_{age} = 20.47$, $SD_{age} = 1.67$), including 1,517 (33.82%) males and 2,969 (66.18%) females. Table 1 summarizes the socio-demographic characteristics of the participants.

Instruments

The online survey consisted of demographics, the composite Service Leadership Scale, and several well-validated leadership or personality measurements (e.g., Leadership Efficacy

Scale; Interpersonal Reactivity Index) (36-38) serving as external criteria. The composite Service Leadership Scales measured Service Leadership Attitude, Service Leadership Knowledge, and Service Leadership Behavior. This chapter only focused on Service Leadership Attitude Scale and its potential personal correlates.

Service Leadership Attitude Scale

The 46-item final version SLA-SF-46 was developed and validated by the first author of the current study (18) on the basis of the SLAM framework and relevant literature on service leadership theory (9, 39). Details for the scale validation procedure shall be documented in another article in this book.

The scale aims to assess individuals' views and beliefs about the role of leader or desirable leadership practices/qualities. Scores for each item range from 1 (very dissimilar to me) to 6 (very similar to me). Eight subscales are incorporated in the SLA-SF-46, including vision and competence (10 items), people orientation (8 items), caring disposition (7 items), ethical role model (5 items), social competence (4 items), self-understanding and reflection (5 items), positive view about human beings (2 items), and unchangeable and dark human nature (5 items). A raw score of SLA is yielded by summing scores of all 46 items. The SLA-SF-46 was found to be internally consistent in this study ($\alpha = .94$ for the full scale; $\alpha = .70$ to .90 for all subscales).

Personal correlates

The demographic profile in the survey covered participants' age ($M_{age} = 20.47$, $SD = 1.67$) and gender (0 = Female, 1 = Male). Other potential correlates concerned their learning experiences in leadership-related courses/programs, leadership experience, and grade point average (GPA) in University. Specifically, participating students reported whether they had ever taken any leadership (including but not limited to service leadership) course or program (0 = No, 1 = Yes), whether they had ever served in any leadership position in an organization (0 = No, 1 = Yes), and their recent GPA (ranged between 0 and 4 after standardization).

Data analyses

All statistical analyses were performed using SPSS for Windows, version 23.0 (IBM-SPSS Inc, Chicago, Illinois, USA). First of all, to decide if there was a need to create separate SLA-SF-46 norms for different sub-groups, differences originated from gender and age were firstly assessed utilizing a multiple regression analysis.

Before creating the percentile norms, we ran normality tests to make sure whether SLA-SF-46 total scores were normally distributed or not. If the test scores of the sample are normally distributed, the raw scores should be standardized to Z scores based on the means and SDs. Then a parametric method (40) could be adopted to provide an interval estimate of the percentile rank. If not normally distributed, the interval cannot be estimated and only the percentiles for raw scores would be constructed.

To sketch the percentile norms, we listed all raw scores to each percentile from 1 to 100. Because of the granularity of raw scores, a given raw score could match more than one percentile. As suggested in the article of Crawford, Garthwaite, and Slick (20), in such situations, if the number of test items is modest, the user would be suggested to calculate the unique percentile rank for each raw score based on the standard formula (41): *Percentile Rank* = $(m + 0.5k)/N \times 100$. Among which, m stands for the number of individuals who scored lower than that specific raw score, k means the number of individuals who scored that specific raw score, while N indicates the total number of the norm sample. The calculated percentile ranks were then rounded to integers from 1st to 99th percentiles.

Last, correlational analyses were carried out to assess other potential correlates (i.e., training experience in leadership courses/programs; experiences of being a leader; and GPA).

FINDINGS

Multiple regression analysis (Cohen's f^2 = .02) showed that age did not significantly contribute to the variances of participants' SLA-SF-46 score ($\beta = -.01$, $p = .41$). Generally speaking, gender significantly predicted participants' SLA-SF-46 score ($\beta = -.14$, $p < .001$), with higher SLA-SF-46 total scores for female students ($M = 217.29$, $SD = 19.49$) compared with male students ($M = 210.79$, $SD = 24.07$). Univariate analysis showed gender differences for all dimensions of SLA, with female students obtaining higher scores than male students ($F = 14.60 \sim 96.39$, $ps < .001$, $\eta^2 = .005 \sim .021$). Therefore, Hypothesis 1b was supported while Hypothesis 1a rejected. Separate norm tables were subsequently created for different genders.

The normality tests showed that the SLA-SF-46 scores for both female and male groups were negatively skewed with a skewness of -.67 for females and -1.07 for males, and a kurtosis of 3.58 for females and 3.90 for males. Kolmogorov-Smirnov tests confirmed that the distributions deviated highly significantly from a normal distribution (D = .071 and .076 respectively for female and male groups, $ps < .001$). Hence, percentiles for raw scores, instead of standardized Z scores, were calculated due to the non-normalized distributions. The tabulation method was adopted to display the corresponding raw score for each percentile rank (Table 2). Meanwhile, another lookup table demonstrated the corresponding percentile for each raw score (Table 3). The normative data were stratified by gender as gender influenced SLA-SF-46 scores appreciably.

Correlational analyses showed that the participants' SLA-SF-46 scores were significantly correlated with their leadership training experience ($r = .09$, $p < .001$; $r^2 =$

.008), leadership position experience ($r = .09$, $p < .001$; $r^2 = .008$), and GPA ($r = .15$, $p < .001$; $r^2 = .02$). As such, Hypotheses 2 to 4 were all supported. However, the findings should be interpreted with caution, as the effect sizes were limited.

Table 2. Percentiles and related raw scores for Service Leadership Attitude Scale (SLA-SF-46) by gender

Percentile (1-50)	Raw Score				Percentile (51-99)	Raw Score		
	Male (*N* = 1,517)	Female (*N* = 2,969)	Total sample (*N* = 4,486)			Male (*N* = 1,517)	Female (*N* = 2,969)	Total sample (*N* = 4,486)
1	≤ 136.36	≤ 163.70	≤ 155.00		51	214.00	218.00	216.37
2	155.00	173.40	165.74		52	214.00	218.00	217.00
3	161.54	179.00	172.00		53	215.00	219.00	217.00
4	167.00	182.00	176.48		54	215.00	219.00	218.00
5	172.00	185.00	179.00		55	215.00	219.00	218.00
6	174.00	187.00	182.00		56	215.00	220.00	218.00
7	176.00	190.00	184.00		57	216.00	220.00	219.00
8	178.00	191.00	186.00		58	216.00	220.00	219.00
9	179.00	193.00	188.00		59	217.00	221.00	220.00
10	181.00	194.00	190.00		60	217.00	221.00	220.00
11	182.00	195.70	191.00		61	218.00	221.00	220.00
12	184.00	197.00	192.00		62	218.00	222.00	221.00
13	186.00	198.00	194.00		63	219.00	222.00	221.00
14	187.00	199.00	195.00		64	219.00	223.00	222.00
15	188.00	200.00	196.00		65	220.00	223.00	222.00
16	190.00	201.00	197.00		66	220.00	224.00	222.00
17	191.00	202.00	198.00		67	221.00	224.00	223.00
18	192.00	203.00	199.00		68	221.00	225.00	223.00
19	193.00	203.00	200.00		69	222.00	225.00	224.00
20	194.00	204.00	201.00		70	222.00	226.00	224.00
21	195.00	205.00	202.00		71	223.00	226.00	225.00
22	196.00	206.00	203.00		72	223.00	227.00	226.00
23	197.00	207.00	203.00		73	224.00	227.00	226.00
24	197.32	207.00	204.00		74	224.00	228.00	227.00
25	198.00	207.00	205.00		75	225.00	228.00	227.00
26	199.00	208.00	205.00		76	226.00	229.00	228.00
27	200.00	209.00	206.00		77	226.00	229.00	228.00
28	201.00	209.00	207.00		78	227.00	230.00	229.00
29	202.00	210.00	207.00		79	228.00	231.00	230.00
30	203.00	210.00	208.00		80	228.00	231.00	230.00
31	203.00	210.00	209.00		81	229.00	232.00	231.00
32	204.00	211.00	209.00		82	229.00	233.00	232.00
33	204.00	211.00	209.00		83	230.00	233.00	232.00
34	205.00	212.00	210.00		84	231.00	234.00	233.00
35	206.00	212.00	210.45		85	232.00	235.00	234.00
36	206.00	213.00	211.00		86	234.00	236.00	235.00
37	207.00	213.00	211.00		87	235.00	237.00	236.00
38	207.00	213.00	212.00		88	236.00	239.00	237.56
39	208.00	214.00	212.00		89	237.00	240.00	239.00

Percentile (1-50)	Raw Score			Percentile (51-99)	Raw Score		
	Male (*N* = 1,517)	Female (*N* = 2,969)	Total sample (*N* = 4,486)		Male (*N* = 1,517)	Female (*N* = 2,969)	Total sample (*N* = 4,486)
40	209.00	214.00	213.00	90	238.00	242.00	240.00
41	209.00	214.00	213.00	91	239.00	243.70	242.00
42	210.00	215.00	213.00	92	241.00	246.00	244.00
43	211.00	215.00	214.00	93	243.00	247.00	246.00
44	211.00	215.00	214.00	94	245.00	248.80	248.00
45	212.00	215.00	214.00	95	247.10	250.00	249.00
46	212.00	216.00	215.00	96	251.00	252.00	251.00
47	212.00	216.00	215.00	97	252.00	254.00	253.00
48	213.00	217.00	215.00	98	255.00	257.00	256.00
49	213.00	217.00	216.00	99	259.00	261.00	261.00
50	214.00	217.00	216.00	100	≥ 271.00	≥ 272.00	≥ 272.00

Table 3. Raw scores and related percentiles for Service Leadership Attitude Scale (SLA-SF-46)

Raw score	Percentiles		
	Male (*N* = 1517)	Female (*N* = 2969)	Total sample (*N* = 4486)
≤ 136	1.0	1.0	1.0
137	2.0	1.0	1.0
138	2.0	1.0	1.0
139	2.0	1.0	1.0
140	2.0	1.0	1.0
141	2.0	1.0	1.0
142	2.0	1.0	1.0
143	2.0	1.0	1.0
144	2.0	1.0	1.0
145	2.0	1.0	1.0
146	2.0	1.0	1.0
147	2.0	1.0	1.0
148	2.0	1.0	1.0
149	2.0	1.0	1.0
150	2.0	1.0	1.0
151	2.0	1.0	1.0
152	2.0	1.0	1.0
153	2.0	1.0	1.0
154	2.0	1.0	1.0
155	2.0	1.0	1.0
156	3.0	1.0	2.0
157	3.0	1.0	2.0
158	3.0	1.0	2.0
159	3.0	1.0	2.0
160	3.0	1.0	2.0
161	3.0	1.0	2.0
162	4.0	1.0	2.0
163	4.0	1.0	2.0
164	4.0	1.0	2.0
165	4.0	2.0	2.0
166	4.0	2.0	2.0

Table 3. (Continued)

Raw score	Percentiles		
	Male (N = 1517)	Female (N = 2969)	Total sample (N = 4486)
167	4.0	2.0	3.0
168	5.0	2.0	3.0
169	5.0	2.0	3.0
170	5.0	2.0	3.0
171	5.0	2.0	3.0
172	5.0	2.0	3.0
173	6.0	2.0	4.0
174	6.0	3.0	4.0
175	7.0	3.0	4.0
176	7.0	3.0	4.0
177	8.0	3.0	5.0
178	8.0	3.0	5.0
179	9.0	3.0	5.0
180	10.0	4.0	6.0
181	10.0	4.0	6.0
182	11.0	4.0	6.0
183	12.0	5.0	7.0
184	12.0	5.0	7.0
185	13.0	5.0	8.0
186	13.0	6.0	8.0
187	14.0	6.0	9.0
188	15.0	7.0	9.0
189	16.0	7.0	10.0
190	16.0	7.0	10.0
191	17.0	8.0	11.0
192	18.0	9.0	12.0
193	19.0	9.0	13.0
194	20.0	10.0	13.0
195	21.0	11.0	14.0
196	22.0	11.0	15.0
197	24.0	12.0	16.0
198	25.0	13.0	17.0
199	26.0	14.0	18.0
200	27.0	15.0	19.0
201	28.0	16.0	20.0
202	29.0	17.0	21.0
203	31.0	19.0	23.0
204	33.0	20.0	24.0
205	34.0	21.0	26.0
206	36.0	22.0	27.0
207	38.0	24.0	29.0
208	39.0	26.0	30.0
209	41.0	28.0	32.0
210	42.0	30.0	35.0
211	44.0	33.0	37.0
212	46.0	35.0	39.0
213	49.0	37.0	41.0
214	51.0	40.0	44.0

Raw score	Percentiles		
	Male (*N* = 1517)	Female (*N* = 2969)	Total sample (*N* = 4486)
215	55.0	44.0	47.0
216	58.0	47.0	50.0
217	60.0	49.0	53.0
218	62.0	52.0	55.0
219	64.0	54.0	58.0
220	66.0	57.0	60.0
221	68.0	60.0	63.0
222	70.0	63.0	65.0
223	72.0	65.0	68.0
224	74.0	67.0	70.0
225	75.0	69.0	71.0
226	77.0	71.0	73.0
227	78.0	73.0	75.0
228	80.0	75.0	77.0
229	82.0	77.0	78.0
230	83.0	78.0	80.0
231	84.0	80.0	81.0
232	85.0	81.0	83.0
233	86.0	83.0	84.0
234	86.0	84.0	85.0
235	87.0	85.0	86.0
236	88.0	86.0	87.0
237	89.0	87.0	88.0
238	90.0	88.0	88.0
239	91.0	88.0	89.0
240	92.0	89.0	90.0
241	92.0	90.0	91.0
242	93.0	90.0	91.0
243	93.0	91.0	92.0
244	94.0	91.0	92.0
245	94.0	92.0	93.0
246	95.0	92.0	93.0
247	95.0	93.0	94.0
248	96.0	94.0	94.0
249	96.0	94.0	95.0
250	96.0	95.0	96.0
251	96.0	96.0	96.0
252	97.0	96.0	97.0
253	98.0	97.0	97.0
254	98.0	97.0	98.0
255	98.0	98.0	98.0
256	99.0	98.0	98.0
257	99.0	98.0	99.0
258	99.0	99.0	99.0
259	99.0	99.0	99.0
260	99.0	99.0	99.0
261	99.0	99.0	99.0
262	99.0	99.0	99.0
263	99.0	99.0	99.0
264	99.0	99.0	99.0

Table 3. (Continued)

Raw score	Percentiles		
	Male (N = 1517)	Female (N = 2969)	Total sample (N = 4486)
265	99.0	99.0	99.0
266	99.0	99.0	99.0
267	99.0	99.0	99.0
268	99.0	99.0	99.0
269	99.0	99.0	99.0
270	99.0	99.0	99.0
271	100.0	99.0	100.0
272	100.0	100.0	100.0
273	100.0	100.0	100.0
274	100.0	100.0	100.0
275	100.0	100.0	100.0
276	100.0	100.0	100.0

DISCUSSION

To address the issue of evaluation and assess objective changes in attitudes and beliefs in Service Leadership education program, a validated measurement is indispensable. To fill this gap, the current study presents findings on the percentile norms and personal correlates of the Service Leadership Attitude Scale with a large university sample (N = 4,486) in a Chinese context. The constructed norms shall serve as a reference to rank and compare individuals' service leadership attitude among a particular population, as well as a useful resource for educators and practitioners to detect the changes before and after receiving service leadership courses or programs.

The present study contributes to the future service leadership research and practices in two ways. First, a multi-institutional sample of Hong Kong university students helps to develop the normative profile, which can assist the interpretations of the raw scores. Second, the scale that originated from the SLAM framework provides some insight into the content of the service leadership theory.

Beyond the norms, the examination of individual differences and potential personal correlates broadens researchers and educational practitioners' understanding of university students' attitudes and beliefs towards service leadership. First, the current study revealed that female college students in Hong Kong possessed a higher level of service leadership attitude compared with male students. Although leadership has been traditionally viewed as a masculine activity (42), some studies have identified females' strengths being as leaders (23-25). One factor that contributes to gender differences in service leadership attitude owes to the features of service leaders. A service-oriented economy requires service leaders to be caring and interpersonal-oriented, which have been viewed as the unique features of femininity.

Second, no age-related difference was observed in the service leadership attitude, echoing prior scholars' arguments that non-significant relationship exists between leaders' age and their leadership behaviors (27, 30). Meanwhile, leadership training experiences turned out to be positively associated with the service leadership attitude in the current study. The findings imply the importance of service leadership education that one's service leadership attitudes and beliefs could be acquired through training and learning.

Third, participants' service leadership attitude scores were positively associated with their GPA, leadership training experiences, and the experience of being a leader. These findings can be attributed to the fact that students with higher GPA usually perform better in solving cognitively complex tasks (32), which may promote their understanding of service leadership attitude. On the other hand, experiences of receiving leadership training and opportunities being a leader were believed to positively impact university students' service leadership attitude. It is consistent with previous studies (43) that student leadership in universities creates positive impacts on building their skills and characters.

Although our study is pioneering in the field of leadership, it is not without limitations. First, the sample recruited in the current study was limited to Hong Kong university students. Hence, it restricts the generalizability of the findings to other populations or the same population in other regions. To follow up the pioneering work of this study, future research shall employ other heterogeneous populations to create corresponding norm tables, as well as test the possible personal correlates. To this end, the service leadership theory should be tested in various professions and industries. The second limitation pertains to the investigation of possible personal correlates. On the one hand, although the correlations were significant, the effect sizes were not large. A possible explanation for this might be the undetected intermediate effects, which should be further explored in the future. Hence, future studies should take possible correlates, such as students' majors and personalities, into account. Despite these limitations, this study constitutes a good progress for the area of service leadership measurement.

ACKNOWLEDGMENTS

The validation project is financially supported by the Victor and William Fung Foundation. The preparation for this paper is supported by the Foundation and the Endowed Professorship in Service Leadership Education at The Hong Kong Polytechnic University. This chapter is an updated version of a publication in the special issue "Development and validation of assessment tools on service leadership knowledge, attitude and behavior" edited by Daniel TL Shek, Xiaoqin Zhu and Joav Merrick published in the International Journal of Child and Adolescent Health, 2018;11(4).

REFERENCES

[1] Northouse PG. Leadership: Theory and practice, 7th edition. Thousand Oaks, CA: Sage, 2015.

[2] Uhl-Bien M, Marion R, McKelvey B. Complexity leadership theory: Shifting leadership from the industrial age to the knowledge era. Leadersh Q 2007;18(4):298-318.

[3] Manville B, Ober J. Beyond empowerment: Building a company of citizens. Harv Bus Rev 2003;81(1):48-53.

[4] Chung PPY. Hong Kong Institute of Service Leadership and Management curriculum framework. Hong Kong Institute of Service Leadership and Management, 2011. URL: http://hki-slam.org/index.php?r=article&catid=1&aid=11.

[5] Zaccaro SJ. Trait-based perspectives of leadership. Am Psychol 2007;62(1):6-16.

[6] Shek DTL, Lin L. Core beliefs in the service leadership model proposed by the Hong Kong Institute of Service Leadership and Management. Int J Disabil Hum Dev 2015;14(3):233-42.

[7] Amirianzadeh M, Jaafari P, Ghourchian N, Jowkar B. College student leadership competencies development: A model. Int J Cross-Disciplinary Subj Educ 2010;1(3):168-72.

[8] Day DV. Leadership development: A review in context. Leadersh Q 2000;11(4):581-613.

[9] Shek DTL, Chung PPY, Yu L, Merrick J. Service leadership curriculum and higher education reform in Hong Kong. Int J Disabil Hum Dev 2015;14(4):297-8.

[10] Shek DTL, Lin L. Evaluating service leadership programs with multiple strategies. In: Shek DTL, Chung PPY, eds. Promoting service leadership qualities in university students. Singapore: Springer, 2015:197-211.

[11] Shek DTL, Wu J, Lin L, Pu EXP. Qualitative evaluation of a service leadership subject in a Chinese context. Int J Disabil Hum Dev 2017;16(4):433-41.

[12] Shek DTL, Law MYM. Evaluation of a subject on leadership and intrapersonal development: Views of the students based on qualitative evaluation. In: Shek DTL, Siu AMH, Merrick J, eds. Tomorrow's leaders: Service leadership and holistic development in Chinese university students. New York: Nova Science, 2015:43-54.

[13] Fleishman EA. The measurement of leadership attitudes in industry. J Appl Psychol 1953;37(3):153-8.

[14] Wielkiewicz RM. The Leadership Attitudes and Beliefs Scale: An instrument for evaluating college students' thinking about leadership and organizations. J Coll Stud Dev 2000;41(3):335-47.

[15] Chung PPY, Bell AH. The 25 principles of service leadership. New York: Lexingford Publishing, 2015.

[16] Shek DTL, Sun RCF, Liu TT. Evolution and realms of service leadership and leadership models. Int J Disabil Hum Dev 2015;14(3):243-54.

[17] Chung PPY, Bell A. Service reborn: The knowledge, skills and attitudes of service companies. New York: Lexingford Publishing, 2012.

[18] Shek DTL, Lin L, Leung H, Yu L, Ma CMS, Li X. Content validation of the Service Leadership Attitudes Scale. In: Shek DTL, Chung PPY, Lin L, Merrick J, eds. Service leadership education for university students. New York: Nova Science, 2017:205-26.

[19] Dugan JP. Involvement and leadership: A descriptive analysis of socially responsible leadership. J Coll Stud Dev 2006;47(3):335-43.

[20] Crawford JR, Garthwaite PH, Slick DJ. On percentile norms in neuropsychology: Proposed reporting standards and methods for quantifying the uncertainty over the percentile ranks of test scores. Clin Neuropsychol 2010;23(7):1173-95.

[21] Crawford JR, Garthwaite PH, Lawrie CJ, Henry JD, MacDonald MA, Sutherland J, Sinha P. A convenient method of obtaining percentile norms and accompanying interval estimates for self-report mood scales (DASS, DASS-21, HADS, PANAS, and sAD). Br J Clin Psychol 2009;48(2):163-80. DOI:10.1348/014466508X377757.

[22] Sczesny S, Bosak J, Neff D, Schyns B. Gender stereotypes and the attribution of leadership traits: A cross-cultural comparison. Sex Roles 2004;51(11/12):631-45.
[23] Wielkiewicz RM, Fischer DV, Stelzner SP, Overland M, Sinner AM. Leadership attitudes and beliefs of incoming first-year college students: A multi-institutional study of gender differences. J Leadersh Educ 2012;11(2):1-25.
[24] Eagly AH, Johannesen-Schmidt MC. The leadership styles of women and men. J Soc Issues 2001;57(4):781-97.
[25] Eagly AH. Female leadership advantage and disadvantage: Resolving the contradictions. Psychol Women Q 2007;31(1):1-12.
[26] Walter F, Scheibe S. A literature review and emotion-based model of age and leadership: New directions for the trait approach. Leadersh Q 2013;24(6):882-901.
[27] Barbuto JEJ, Fritz SM, Matkin GS, Marx DB. Effects of gender, education, and age upon leaders' use of influence tactics and full range leadership behaviors. Sex Roles 2007;56(1-2):71-83. DOI: 10.1007/s11199-006-9152-6.
[28] Hirschfeld RR, Thomas CH. Age- and gender-based role incongruence: Implications for knowledge mastery and observed leadership potential among personnel in a leadership development program. Pers Psychol 2011;64(3):661-92.
[29] Gilbert GR, Collins RW, Brenner R. Age and leadership effectiveness: From the perceptions of the follower. Hum Resour Manage 1990;29(2):187-96.
[30] Ng ES, Sears GJ. CEO leadership styles and the implementation of organizational diversity practices: Moderating effects of social values and age. J Bus Ethics 2012;105(1):41-52. DOI: 10.1007/s10551-011-0933-7.
[31] Oshagbemi T. Age influences on the leadership styles and behaviour of managers. Employee Relat 2004;26(1):14-29.
[32] Kellett JB, Humphrey RH, Sleeth RG. Empathy and complex task performance: Two routes to leadership. Leadersh Q 2002;13(5):523-44.
[33] Wielkiewicz RM, Prom CL, Loos S. Relationships of the leadership attitudes and beliefs scale with student types, study habits, life-long learning, and GPA. Coll Stud J 2005;39(1):31-44.
[34] Cress CM, Astin HS, Zimmerman-Oster K, Burkhardt JC. Developmental outcomes of college students' involvement in leadership activities. J Coll Stud Dev 2001;42(1):15-27.
[35] Logue CT, Hutchens TA, Hector MA. Student leadership: A phenomenological exploration of postsecondary experiences. J Coll Stud Dev 2005;46(4):393-408.
[36] Chemers MM, Watson CB, May ST. Dispositional affect and leadership effectiveness: A comparison of self-esteem, optimism, and efficacy. Pers Soc Psychol Bull 2000;26(3):267-77.
[37] Murphy SE. The contribution of leadership experience and self-efficacy to group performance under evaluation apprehension. Dissertation. Seattle, WA: University of Washington, 1992.
[38] Davis MH. Measuring individual differences in empathy: Evidence for a multidimensional approach. J Pers Soc Psychol 1983;44(1):113-26.
[39] Shek DTL, Chung PPY, Yu L, Merrick J. Service leadership education for university students: The Hong Kong experience. Int J Disabil Hum Dev 2015;14(3):203-4.
[40] Crawford JR, Garthwaite PH. Investigation of the single case in neuropsychology: Confidence limits on the abnormality of test scores and test score differences. Neuropsychologia 2002;40(8):1196-208.
[41] Ley P. Quantitative aspects of psychological assessment: An introduction. London: Duckworth, 1972.
[42] Bass BM. Bass & Stogdill's handbook of leadership: Theory, research and managerial applications, 3rd ed. New York: Free Press, 1990.
[43] Fischer DV, Wielkiewicz RM, Stelzner SP, Overland M, Meuwissen AS. Changes in leadership attitudes and beliefs associated with the college experience: A longitudinal study. J Leadersh Educ 2015;14(1):14-32.

In: Service Leadership
Editors: Daniel TL Shek, Xiaoqin Zhu, Li Lin et al.
ISBN: 978-1-53614-852-7

Chapter 13

THE SERVICE LEADERSHIP BEHAVIOR SCALE: NORMS AND PERSONAL CORRELATES

Daniel TL Shek[1-6,*], PhD, FHKPS, BBS, SBS, JP, Diya Dou[1], PhD and Robin S Snell[7], PhD

[1]Department of Applied Social Sciences,
The Hong Kong Polytechnic University, Hong Kong, PR China
[2]Centre for Innovative Programmes for Adolescents and Families,
The Hong Kong Polytechnic University, Hong Kong, PR China
[3]Department of Social Work, East China Normal University, Shanghai, PR China
[4]Kiang Wu Nursing College of Macau, Macau, PR China
[5]Hong Kong Institute of Service Leadership and Management, Hong Kong, PR China
[6]Division of Adolescent Medicine, Department of Pediatrics,
Kentucky Children's Hospital, University of Kentucky School of Medicine,
Lexington, Kentucky, US
[7]Department of Management, Lingnan University, Hong Kong, PR China

ABSTRACT

The shift from industrial society to service society calls for effective service leaders who can unite and motive people to work together effectively. However, valid scales assessing important leadership qualities required by service economy are rare. To fill this gap, three scales were developed based on the Service Leadership Theory to measure leadership qualities. In this chapter we present findings on the norms and personal correlates of the

* Correspondence: Daniel TL Shek, PhD, FHKPS, BBS, SBS, JP, Associate Vice President (Undergraduate Programme), Chair Professor of Applied Social Sciences, and Li and Fung Endowed Professor in Service Leadership Education, Department of Applied Social Sciences, The Hong Kong Polytechnic University, Hung Hom, Hong Kong, PR China. E-mail: daniel.shek@polyu.edu.hk.

Service Leadership Behavior Scale using data collected from an online questionnaire administered to 4,486 students from eight University Grants Committee (UGC) funded universities in Hong Kong. As significant gender differences were found, two norms were developed separately for female and male participants. No significant influence of age on leadership behaviors was noted. For other personal correlates, students' grade point average (GPA), experience in leadership training, and experience of being a leader were associated with the leadership behavior scores, though the effect size was small. Limitations and implications of the present findings are discussed.

INTRODUCTION

The economic growth in the twenty-first century is shown by the transition from the manufacturing economy into service economy (1). This transition, characterized by the provision of service rather than goods, has transformed global economies on a massive scale. As service is essentially delivered through people to people, strong service leadership that helps people work together effectively has become the key to organization success.

The era of service economy calls for effective leaders. Growing leadership training programs in higher education sectors have been developed to improve university students' leadership qualities, which can better prepare them for the challenges in the service economy. For example, supported by the Victor and William Fung Foundation, a leadership program entitled "Fung Service Leadership Initiative" was developed and launched in eight public universities funded by the University Grants Committee (UGC) in Hong Kong, aiming at nurturing students' development in leadership knowledge, attitude and behavior (2).

To improve program effectiveness, objective outcome evaluation is essential as it provides evidence of the program's contribution to students' leadership development and the knowledge base. However, scales specifically designed to measure leadership qualities required by service economy are rare. In the following sections, the "Fung Service Leadership Initiative" in Hong Kong and the development of the Service Leadership Behavior Scale are described.

Service leadership education and evaluation in Hong Kong

The economy of Hong Kong is very service-oriented (3). The share of the service sector has almost reached 93% of the Gross Domestic Product (GDP) in Hong Kong in 2007, and remained around that level in the recent decade (4). Chung has thoroughly discussed the contemporary service society in Hong Kong and proposed the Service Leadership Theory (5–7). According to Chung (8), service leadership is to "satisfy needs by consistently providing quality personal service to everyone one comes into contact with, including one's self, others, groups, communities, systems, and environments". Service Leadership Theory highlights three essential qualities underlying effective service leadership, which include competence, character and care. All of these three qualities are indispensable to effective leadership. In other words, a lack of any of three fundamental characteristics may lead to ineffectiveness, dysfunction, and even the dark side of leadership (9).

The Service Leadership Theory serves as the cornerstone of the leadership education program of eight UGC-funded universities in Hong Kong. Supported by the Victor and William Fung Foundation, these universities have developed service leadership education programs to enrich students' knowledge about service leadership, shape their attitude of being service leaders, and improve their leadership behavior in practice (2). For example, in The Hong Kong Polytechnic University (PolyU), education programs have been provided in different forms, including credit-bearing and non-credit-bearing courses, as well as short-term workshops (10). These programs have been carefully designed to help students improve the three fundamental service leadership qualities, namely competence, character and care. Previous studies have showed that students reported a high level of satisfaction towards the programs, and the programs were perceived to be effective (11–13).

Development of the Service Leadership Behavior Scale (SLBS)

Many leadership theories have focused on behavior of leaders (14). A number of leadership models have been developed in the postindustrial era to understand the role of leadership behavior in employees' engagement and organization effectiveness (15). Recent leadership literature has increasingly moved the focus from highlighting leaders' competences (e.g., charismatic leadership) towards an emphasis on shared, ethical, people-centered leadership styles (e.g., servant leadership and ethical leadership) (16, 17). For example, servant leadership highlights the personal growth of followers (16). Ethical leadership focuses on normatively appropriate conduct demonstrated by leaders (17).

The above-mentioned models capture many key elements of leadership skills and behaviors, but are not sufficient to measure service leadership behavior in specific cultural contexts. First, most models solely measure leadership competences, and only a few theories specifically focus on leaders' character and care. However, almost none of these theories has considered competence, character and care three indispensable elements of effective service leadership (18). In other words, a model integrating these three leadership qualities required by service economy is missing. Second, though it is widely agreed that culture and local contexts are important to leadership research, assessment tools of leadership behavior seldom take cultural contexts into accounts. As Tsui advocated, to develop contextual measurement to deepen leadership research in China is "not only desirable, but essential" (19).

To fill the above gaps, the research team at The Hong Kong Polytechnic University (PolyU) designed a long-form Service Leadership Behavior Scale (SLB-LF-97) guided by the Service Leadership Theory. The SLB-LF-97 contains 97 items, aiming to measure the behavioral characteristics of a service leader (20). The initial validation of SLB-LF-97 was conducted in a study involving 231 PolyU undergraduate students as part of the "Development and validation of measures based on the Service Leadership Model" project. The reliability of the SLB-LF-97 was excellent ($\alpha = 0.97$). Exploratory factor analysis (EFA) suggested the removal of 32 items with multiple or low loadings. A short-form of the Service Leadership Behavior Scale (SLB-SF-65) containing 65 items was formed. The results of the initial validation of the SLB-LF-97 were reported in another article prepared by Shek, Ma and Lin in this book. Generally speaking, the refined scale (i.e., SLB-SF-65) reflected good internal consistency and convergent validity. The SLB-SF-65 was further validated in a large-scale project, which resulted in the final version of the scale including 38 items (SLB-SF-38). Details can be seen in another chapter prepared by Shek and Ma in this book as well as in the User Manual.

Norms and correlates of the Service Leadership Behavior Scale

The present study aims to provide norm data of the Service Leadership Behavior Scale to better interpret students' leadership behavior scores. Besides, potential personal correlates between gender, age, academic achievement, experience in leadership training, experience of being a leader and students' service leadership behavior scores were examined.

Norm data of a scale provide the necessary frame of reference to aid test administrators, educators and researchers to interpret the scores of individuals. For the test data that are normally distributed, standardized scores are commonly used to represent an individual's performance level (21). For the non-normative sample, however, percentile rank is often used as an alternative option. Compared with standardized score, percentile rank provides the ranking position of individual's score among the population, and directly shows the intrinsic meaning which the standardized scores do not (22). The norms can consist the tables including all percentile ranks for each raw score, or only including some landmark percentiles and the corresponding raw scores (22). The norms are useful source that helps improve the effectiveness of leadership educational programs. On the one hand, identifying the benchmarks of behavior performance for different populations helps better design these programs for populations with specific needs. On the other hand, changes in percentile rank for an individual can be tracked, implying that the effectiveness of the leadership program at the individual level can be evaluated.

As the norm data may differ among populations, gender and age are two important demographic characteristics that were taken into account in the present study. Several reviews have thoroughly discussed gender difference in leadership styles and behaviors (23-25). For example, Mandell and Pherwani (24) examined gender difference in emotional intelligence and transformational leadership style. The results suggested that female leaders managed their own and others' emotions better than their counterparts did. In addition, using 40 data sets drawn from 28 studies in research of gender and instructional leadership, Hallinger and his colleagues (23) concluded that compared with male principals, female principals tended to engage in more active instructional leadership. However, gender difference in leadership behavior remains inconclusive. For example, Oshabemi and Gill (25) collected data from leaders in UK and found no significant gender difference in leadership styles.

Despite the different results drawn from statistical comparison, many studies have suggested that female leadership are often characterized by strong interactive, transformational and cooperative management. Rosener (26) pointed out that women tend to adopt a transformational style through providing care to others. This argument was supported by Carless (27), who argued that women were naturally socialized towards skills in participative leadership, collaborative group management, and quality interpersonal relations. Therefore, in the present study, we hypothesized that female participants' service leadership behavior scores would be higher than those of male participants (Hypothesis 1). As to age, some studies have suggested that the elder leaders may present stronger leadership as both their leadership experience and social relationship would be developed as time goes on (28), but the associations were often found to be weak (29). In addition, given that the participants were all university students in this study, the variation in age was small. Therefore, we included age as a demographic characteristic in the analysis, but did not anticipate that age would significantly influence service leadership behavior scores.

The present study also took participants' academic achievement, experience of receiving leadership training and experience of being a leader into account. Grade Point Average (GPA) has been commonly used to define participants' academic achievement. Though the direct relationship between university students' GPA and their leadership remains unclear (30), many studies have revealed that GPA is closely related to some important abilities that can strongly predict leadership. For example, Kellett, Humphrey and Sleeth (31) found that GPA was a strong predictor to complex task choice, and these two factors showed a combined positive influence on leadership perceptions. In addition, studies in the Chinese context also observed similar correlations (32). As such, we hypothesized that there would be a positive correlation between GPA and leadership behavior scores (Hypothesis 2).

As to the potential correlation between leadership training experience and behavior, research has highlighted the benefits of service and experiential learning to students' leadership development (33). Many leadership programs often provide a variety of activities to construct the connection between students' own experience and reflection, which can effectively engage students in learning process. We hypothesized that leadership training experience would be positively related to students' service leadership behavior (Hypothesis 3).

Regarding the experience of being a leader, it is argued that students with relevant experience may have a deeper understanding of how to lead, motivate, unite, and serve others (28). Therefore, we hypothesized that the experience of being a leader would show positive correlation with service leadership behavior (Hypothesis 4).

OUR STUDY

The data were collected from an online questionnaire administered to undergraduate students from eight UGC-funded universities in Hong Kong in March 2017, which included The Hong Kong Polytechnic University (PolyU), The Chinese University of Hong Kong (CUHK), The Education University of Hong Kong (EdUHK), Hong Kong Baptist University (HKBU), City University of Hong Kong (CityU), Lingnan University (LU), The University of Hong Kong (HKU), and Hong Kong University of Science and Technology (HKUST). The research team in PolyU developed the questionnaire and set up the online survey. The local researchers in each university distributed the link to students. The participants were informed of the purpose of the study, and were assured that the data would be analyzed anonymously, and all information would be kept confidential. In addition, they were encouraged to response honestly based on their knowledge and impression about themselves. Each participant received a supermarket voucher of HK$100 as a token of appreciation for completing the survey.

Data collection lasted for around four months from March till June 2017. A total of 4,555 participants completed the survey. Sixty-nine responses were excluded from the following analyses due to a denial of consent form, duplicated responses, and the responses completed by non-targeted group (e.g., graduates). After removing the invalid responses, the final sample consisted of 4,486 participants, including 2,969 females (66.2%) and 1,517 males (33.8%). The age of the participants ranged from 15 to 34 years old ($M = 20.47$, $SD = 1.67$). The demographic characteristics of the participants are showed in Table 1.

Table 1. Demographic characteristics of the participants

University	PolyU	CUHK	EdUHK	HKBU	CityU	LU	HKU	HKUST	Total
Participants (n/%)	1000/22.29	505/11.26	500/11.15	517/11.52	464/10.34	500/11.15	500/11.15	500/11.15	4486/100
Age range	18-27	17-29	17-34	15-28	18-34	18-29	17-28	16-28	15-34
Age (Mean/SD)	20.46/1.65	20.08/1.55	21.05/1.75	20.79/1.67	20.63/1.77	20.54/1.55	20.38/1.67	19.85/1.50	20.47/1.67
15-19 (*n*/%)	297/29.70	193/38.22	95/19.00	117/22.63	112/24.14	133/26.60	173/34.60	224/44.80	1,344/29.96
≥ 20 (*n*/%)	703/70.30	312/61.78	405/81.00	400/77.37	352/75.86	367/73.40	327/65.40	276/55.2	3,142/70.04
Males (*n*/%)	409/40.90	130/25.74	98/19.60	122/23.60	128/27.59	148/29.60	151/30.20	331/66.20	1,517/33.82
Females (*n*/%)	591/59.10	375/74.26	402/80.40	395/76.40	336/72.41	352/70.40	349/69.80	169/33.80	2,969/66.18

Note. PolyU = The Hong Kong Polytechnic University; CUHK = The Chinese University of Hong Kong; EdUHK = The Education University of Hong Kong; HKBU = Hong Kong Baptist University; CityU = City University of Hong Kong; LU = Lingnan University; HKU = The University of Hong Kong; HKUST = Hong Kong University of Science and Technology.

Measures

Based on the literature on the service leadership, the Service Leadership Behavior Scale was developed to measure the extent to which the participants demonstrate behaviors that are representative of a service leader. The SLB-SF-65 is measured on a 6-point Likert scale (1 = strongly disagree; 2 = disagree; 3 = slightly disagree; 4 = slightly agree; 5 = agree; 6 = strongly agree). Some sample items include: "I constantly seek to improve my personality," "I strive to take care of other people regardless of their positions," "when there is a problem, I can solve it quickly," and "I am able to develop positive relationships with my friends."

In the large-scale validation study, the SLB-SF-65 was refined based on exploratory factor analysis (EFA) and confirmatory factor analysis (CFA). Two subsets were randomly generated from the entire dataset (*N subset A* = 2,246; *N subset B* = 2,240). EFA was conducted on subset A to examine the factorial structure of the SLB-SF-65 by applying the principal component analysis. A trimmed scale (SLB-SF-48) containing 48 items was formed. Six factors were extracted, including self-improvement and self-reflection, people and principles orientation, resilience, social competence, problem-solving and mentorship. Details of the formation of SLB-SF-48 based on the EFA can be found in another article prepared by Shek and Ma in this book. CFA was performed on subset B using Maximum Likelihood estimation to evaluate the factorial structure. After removing ten items reflecting unsatisfactory factor loadings, and allowing the residual covariance for three pairs of parameters, we observed a significant improvement in goodness-of-fit. The resultant 38-item scale (SLB-SF-38) reflected a good fit (CFI = .92; NNFI = .91; RMSEA = .055), which met the benchmarks suggested by Hu and Bentler (34). The SLB-SF-38 reflected the same factorial structure and labeling as the SLB-SF-48 did. In addition, the SLB-SF-38 showed good internal reliability (Cronbach Alpha = .96). The detailed information of CFA and indicators of the SLB-SF-38 are reported in another article submitted for the consideration of publication as well as in the User Manual. In the present study, the final data generated by CFA were used to develop norm tables and personal correlates.

Demographic characteristics and personal correlates

Age and gender were two important demographic characteristics included in the present study. In addition, students' academic achievement, experiences of participating leadership training program, and being a leader were taken into account. Following previous research, we also used GPA to represent participants' academic achievement. The GPA systems in eight universities were adjusted and the GPA scores were standardized. Students were asked to report their recent GPA (ranging from 0-4), whether they have ever participated any leadership course or program (0 = No, 1 = Yes), and whether they have served in any leadership position in any organization (0 = No, 1 = Yes).

Data analyses

We performed multiple regression analyses to examine the influence of gender and age on participants' behavior scores with SPSS version 23. If the behavior scores were significantly predicted by gender, separate percentiles norms should be provided for female and male groups.

Normality tests were conducted for selecting the way to present norms. If the sample was normatively distributed, both the standardized scores and percentile norms would be presented. If the sample is non-normatively distributed, only the percentile norms would be provided.

When producing the norm data, we first presented the raw scores corresponding to the percentiles from 0 to 100. Second, the full tables presenting the percentiles for each raw score were provided. By doing so, the individual's score can be positioned precisely, which is useful for proper interpretation of the results. Crawford and colleagues (22) have suggested that though the behavior score is discrete, the underlying leadership ability is considered a continuous index. Thus, a given score x is actually a point estimate of the real valued behavior ability ranging from x - 0.5 (inclusive) to x + 0.5 (exclusive). In other words, given that the population distribution is unknown, the best estimation would be that the ability of half of the participants scoring x is actually below x and half above (22). Thus, we followed Crawford et al.'s suggestion on the definition of a percentile rank: the percentage of scores that fall below the score of interest and half of those obtaining the score of interest (22). The calculation formula is showed as follows:

$$\text{Percentile rank} = \left(\frac{m + .5\,k}{N}\right) \times 100$$

In this formula, m refers to the number of participants scoring below a given raw score, k represents the number of participants that obtain a given raw score, and N means the entire normative sample size. The percentile ranks were calculated and rounded to integer.

For GPA, experience of leadership training and experience of being a leader, correlation analyses were applied to examine the potential relations between these factors and students' behavior scores with SPSS 23.

Table 2. Percentiles and corresponding raw scores of Service Leadership Behavior Scale (SLB-SF-38) by gender

Percentile (1-50)	Raw Score			Percentile (51-99)	Raw Score		
	Male (N = 1,517)	Female (N = 2,969)	Total sample (N = 4,486)		Male (N = 1,517)	Female (N = 2,969)	Total sample (N = 4,486)
1	≤ 94.36	≤ 112.70	≤ 107.00	51	173.00	174.00	174.00
2	112.36	123.00	119.74	52	173.00	175.00	174.00
3	121.00	131.00	128.00	53	174.00	175.00	175.00
4	126.00	135.00	131.00	54	175.00	176.00	175.00
5	129.00	137.00	134.00	55	175.00	176.00	176.00
6	131.00	139.00	136.00	56	176.00	177.00	177.00
7	133.00	142.00	138.00	57	177.00	177.00	177.00
8	135.00	143.00	141.00	58	177.00	178.00	178.00
9	137.00	145.00	142.00	59	178.00	178.00	178.00
10	139.00	146.00	144.00	60	178.00	179.00	179.00
11	141.00	147.00	145.00	61	179.00	179.00	179.00
12	142.00	148.00	146.00	62	180.00	180.00	180.00
13	143.00	149.00	147.00	63	180.34	180.00	180.00
14	144.00	150.00	148.00	64	181.00	181.00	181.00
15	146.00	151.00	149.00	65	182.00	181.00	181.00
16	147.00	152.00	150.00	66	182.00	182.00	182.00
17	148.00	152.00	151.00	67	183.00	182.00	183.00
18	149.00	152.60	152.00	68	183.00	183.00	183.00
19	150.00	154.00	152.00	69	184.00	183.00	183.00
20	151.00	154.00	153.00	70	184.00	184.00	184.00
21	152.00	155.00	154.00	71	185.00	184.00	185.00
22	152.00	156.00	154.00	72	186.00	185.00	185.00
23	152.00	156.00	155.00	73	186.00	185.00	186.00
24	153.00	157.00	156.00	74	187.00	186.00	186.00
25	154.00	158.00	157.00	75	188.00	186.00	187.00
26	155.00	159.00	157.00	76	188.00	187.00	187.00
27	155.00	160.00	158.00	77	189.00	187.00	188.00
28	156.00	160.00	159.00	78	190.00	188.00	188.00
29	157.00	161.00	160.00	79	190.00	188.00	189.00
30	158.00	162.00	160.10	80	190.00	189.00	189.00
31	158.00	162.70	161.00	81	190.00	189.00	190.00
32	159.00	163.00	162.00	82	191.00	190.00	190.00
33	160.00	164.00	163.00	83	191.00	190.00	191.00
34	161.00	165.00	163.00	84	192.00	191.00	191.00
35	162.00	165.00	164.00	85	193.00	191.50	192.00
36	162.00	166.00	165.00	86	194.00	192.00	193.00
37	163.00	167.00	165.00	87	195.00	193.00	194.00
38	164.00	167.00	166.00	88	196.00	194.00	195.00
39	164.00	168.00	167.00	89	197.00	195.00	196.00
40	165.00	168.00	167.00	90	198.00	197.00	197.00
41	165.00	169.00	168.00	91	199.00	198.00	199.00
42	166.00	169.00	168.00	92	201.00	200.00	200.00

Percentile (1-50)	Raw Score			Percentile (51-99)	Raw Score		
	Male (N = 1,517)	Female (N = 2,969)	Total sample (N = 4,486)		Male (N = 1,517)	Female (N = 2,969)	Total sample (N = 4,486)
43	167.00	170.00	169.00	93	202.00	201.00	201.00
44	167.00	171.00	170.00	94	204.00	202.00	203.00
45	168.00	171.00	170.00	95	207.00	205.00	205.00
46	169.00	172.00	171.00	96	208.00	207.20	208.00
47	169.00	172.00	171.00	97	212.00	211.00	212.00
48	171.00	173.00	172.00	98	217.00	215.00	216.00
49	171.00	173.00	173.00	99	222.82	221.30	222.00
50	172.00	174.00	173.00	100	≥ 228.00	≥ 228.00	≥ 228.00

FINDINGS

The results of multiple regression analyses suggested that students' behavior scores were significantly predicted by gender, though the effect size was small (β = .049, $p < .001$; Cohen's f^2 = .002). In particular, female students obtained higher behavior scores (*Mean* = 172.02, *SD* = 21.49) than male students did (*Mean* = 169.69, *SD* = 25.15). Hypothesis 1 was supported. The influence of age on behavior scores was not statistically significant.

Tests for normality were conducted separately on female and male groups. The results of Shapiro-Wilk's test indicated that the distribution of behavior scores was non-normative for both female and male groups ($p < .001$) (35). Field has suggested that the Shapiro-Wilk's test for large samples can be significant though the scores are only slightly different from a normal distribution (35). Therefore, we also checked the histograms and the values of skew and kurtosis. The histograms showed a left-skewed and leptokurtic distribution for both female and male groups. In particular, the behavior scores yielded a skewness of -0.78 for male participants (SE = .06, z-value = -12.37, p < .001) and a skewness of -0.54 for female participants (SE = .04, z-value = –11.99, p <.001). In terms of kurtosis, the results showed a peaked distribution with positive kurtosis for both male (kurtosis = 2.23, SE = .13, z-value = 17.79, p < .001) and female groups (kurtosis = 1.76, SE = .09, z-value = – 19.61, p < .001) (35). According to the results of multiple regression and normality tests, we presented separate percentile norms for male and female participants (see Table 2 and Table 3).

Personal correlates of Service Leadership Behavior Score

The results of correlation analysis suggested that the behavior scores were significantly correlated with GPA (r = .10, $p < .001$; r^2 = .01), experience of taking leadership course or training (r = .13, $p < .001$; r^2 = .036), and experience of being a leader (r = .14, $p < .001$;

r^2 = .028). Students achieving higher GPA, having experience of taking leadership course or training, or having experience of being a leader were likely to have a better understanding of service leadership behavior. The results supported Hypotheses 2, 3 and 4, though the effect size of the correlates was low.

Table 3. Raw scores and corresponding percentiles of Service Leadership Behavior Scale (SLB-SF-38)

Raw score	Percentiles		
	Male (N = 1,517)	Female (N = 2,969)	Total sample (N = 4,486)
≤ 78	0.0	0.0	0.0
79	1.0	0.0	0.0
80	1.0	0.0	0.0
81	1.0	0.0	0.0
82	1.0	0.0	0.0
83	1.0	0.0	0.0
84	1.0	0.0	0.0
85	1.0	0.0	0.0
86	1.0	0.0	0.0
87	1.0	0.0	0.0
88	1.0	0.0	0.0
89	1.0	0.0	0.0
90	1.0	0.0	0.0
91	1.0	0.0	0.0
92	1.0	0.0	0.0
93	1.0	0.0	1.0
94	1.0	0.0	1.0
95	1.0	0.0	1.0
96	1.0	0.0	1.0
97	1.0	0.0	1.0
98	1.0	0.0	1.0
99	1.0	0.0	1.0
100	1.0	0.0	1.0
101	1.0	0.0	1.0
102	1.0	0.0	1.0
103	1.0	1.0	1.0
104	1.0	1.0	1.0
105	1.0	1.0	1.0
106	1.0	1.0	1.0
107	1.0	1.0	1.0
108	2.0	1.0	1.0
109	2.0	1.0	1.0
110	2.0	1.0	1.0
111	2.0	1.0	1.0
112	2.0	1.0	1.0
113	2.0	1.0	1.0
114	2.0	1.0	1.0

Raw score	Percentiles		
	Male (*N* = 1,517)	Female (*N* = 2,969)	Total sample (*N* = 4,486)
115	2.0	1.0	2.0
116	2.0	1.0	2.0
117	2.0	1.0	2.0
118	2.0	1.0	2.0
119	3.0	1.0	2.0
120	3.0	2.0	2.0
121	3.0	2.0	2.0
122	3.0	2.0	2.0
123	3.0	2.0	2.0
124	4.0	2.0	3.0
125	4.0	2.0	3.0
126	4.0	2.0	3.0
127	4.0	2.0	3.0
128	4.0	2.0	3.0
129	5.0	2.0	3.0
130	5.0	3.0	4.0
131	6.0	3.0	4.0
132	6.0	3.0	4.0
133	7.0	3.0	5.0
134	7.0	4.0	5.0
135	8.0	4.0	5.0
136	8.0	5.0	6.0
137	9.0	5.0	6.0
138	9.0	5.0	7.0
139	10.0	6.0	7.0
140	10.0	6.0	8.0
141	11.0	7.0	8.0
142	12.0	7.0	9.0
143	13.0	8.0	9.0
144	14.0	8.0	10.0
145	14.0	9.0	11.0
146	15.0	10.0	12.0
147	16.0	11.0	13.0
148	17.0	12.0	14.0
149	18.0	13.0	15.0
150	19.0	14.0	16.0
151	20.0	15.0	17.0
152	22.0	17.0	19.0
153	24.0	18.0	20.0
154	25.0	20.0	22.0
155	26.0	21.0	23.0
156	28.0	22.0	24.0
157	29.0	24.0	25.0
158	30.0	25.0	27.0
159	32.0	26.0	28.0
160	33.0	27.0	29.0

Table 3. (Continued)

Raw score	Percentiles		
	Male (N = 1,517)	Female (N = 2,969)	Total sample (N = 4,486)
161	34.0	29.0	31.0
162	35.0	30.0	32.0
163	37.0	32.0	34.0
164	38.0	33.0	35.0
165	40.0	35.0	37.0
166	42.0	36.0	38.0
167	44.0	38.0	40.0
168	45.0	39.0	41.0
169	46.0	41.0	43.0
170	47.0	43.0	45.0
171	49.0	45.0	46.0
172	50.0	47.0	48.0
173	52.0	49.0	50.0
174	53.0	51.0	51.0
175	55.0	53.0	53.0
176	56.0	55.0	55.0
177	58.0	57.0	57.0
178	59.0	59.0	59.0
179	61.0	61.0	61.0
180	62.0	62.0	62.0
181	64.0	64.0	64.0
182	66.0	66.0	66.0
183	67.0	68.0	68.0
184	69.0	70.0	70.0
185	71.0	72.0	72.0
186	73.0	74.0	74.0
187	74.0	76.0	76.0
188	76.0	78.0	77.0
189	77.0	80.0	79.0
190	80.0	82.0	82.0
191	83.0	84.0	84.0
192	84.0	86.0	85.0
193	85.0	87.0	86.0
194	86.0	88.0	87.0
195	87.0	89.0	88.0
196	88.0	89.0	89.0
197	89.0	90.0	90.0
198	90.0	91.0	91.0
199	91.0	92.0	91.0
200	92.0	92.0	92.0
201	92.0	93.0	93.0
202	93.0	94.0	93.0
203	94.0	94.0	94.0
204	94.0	95.0	95.0

Raw score	Percentiles		
	Male ($N = 1{,}517$)	Female ($N = 2{,}969$)	Total sample ($N = 4{,}486$)
205	94.0	95.0	95.0
206	95.0	96.0	95.0
207	95.0	96.0	96.0
208	96.0	96.0	96.0
209	96.0	96.0	96.0
210	96.0	97.0	97.0
211	97.0	97.0	97.0
212	97.0	97.0	97.0
213	97.0	97.0	97.0
214	97.0	98.0	98.0
215	98.0	98.0	98.0
216	98.0	98.0	98.0
217	98.0	98.0	98.0
218	98.0	99.0	98.0
219	98.0	99.0	99.0
220	99.0	99.0	99.0
221	99.0	99.0	99.0
222	99.0	99.0	99.0
223	99.0	99.0	99.0
224	99.0	99.0	99.0
225	99.0	99.0	99.0
226	99.0	99.0	99.0
227	100.0	99.0	100.0
228	100.0	100.0	100.0

DISCUSSION

Using data collected through a survey carried out in eight UGC-funded universities in Hong Kong ($N = 4{,}486$), the present study examined percentile norms and important correlates of the service leadership behavior scores. This study responded the call for valid assessment tool evaluating university students' leadership behavior in a Chinese context.

Results showed that female students achieved higher behavior scores than male students did, which was in line with previous research (27,29). Though men are often perceived as having stronger leadership qualifications (36), females were found to perform better in building relationship with others, showing care and empathy, and leading in a transformational way. The development of service economy provides females more opportunities in professional development, which will improve gender equity in organizational leadership roles.

Our results also indicated that students who have attended leadership training course or have acted as a leader tended to perceive themselves having a higher level of leadership behavior. This implies the value of training programs in improving students' leadership, as the related training may enrich their knowledge and provide opportunities from them to reflect and practice leadership behavior. Similarly, acting as a leader directly provides specific task and contexts that students need to make decisions, coordinate, solve problems, and even handle conflicts, which will reinforce their leadership development. In addition, students' GPA was also positively correlated with their leadership behavior score. As GPA has been often used as an indicator of cognitive ability, students achieving high GPA may know how to choose learning strategies and possess the ability to work well with others in group projects, which will facilitate their learning process in relation to leadership development.

There are several theoretical, methodological, and practical implications. As stated earlier, numerous programs have been developed to respond the call for effective leaders in service economies. However, valid measurements are limited. This study tried to contribute to the literature by presenting the norms and correlates of service leadership scores. A main methodological strength of this study is the development and validation of a measurement based on large sample size and confirmatory factor analyses. The findings also clarify the conceptual dimensions underlying the concept of service leadership behavior, which include self-improvement and self-reflection, people and principles orientation, resilience, social competence, problem-solving and mentorship dimensions revealed by the scale. This study also provides some practical implications for practitioners. The gender difference in service leadership behavior scores implies that more efforts should be made to improve male students' leadership performance.

Although we believe that our study has an addition to the Service Leadership Theory literature and leadership program evaluation, some limitations should be noted. More research variables can be included in the analysis to better understand the leadership behavior scores and variance. For example, students' major can have an influence on their service leadership behavior scores. It is possible that students majoring in helping professions, such as nursing, psychological counseling, education and social work, may possess a higher level of service leadership skills. As to the research sample, the present study was conducted solely in eight universities in Hong Kong, implying that some results may be difficult to be generalized to other contexts. For example, some idiosyncratic characteristics of Hong Kong, such as its long-standing service economy, can have an influence on the norm data. In addition, as one of our research aims was to evaluate leadership programs in higher education, only university students were involved in our study. Special attention should be paid to this issue when using the Service Leadership Behavior Scale in other populations. Despite these limitations, the present study contributes to the current literature by providing norm data of Service Leadership Behavior Scale to evaluate individual's leadership behavior and monitor their improvements.

ACKNOWLEDGMENTS

The validation project is financially supported by the Victor and William Fung Foundation. The preparation for this paper is supported by the Foundation and the Endowed Professorship in Service Leadership Education at The Hong Kong Polytechnic University. This chapter is an updated version of a publication in the special issue "Development and validation of assessment tools on service leadership knowledge, attitude and behavior" edited by Daniel TL Shek, Xiaoqin Zhu and Joav Merrick published in the International Journal of Child and Adolescent Health, 2018;11(4).

REFERENCES

[1] Shek DTL, Chung PPY, Leung H. Manufacturing economy vs. service economy: Implications for service leadership. Int J Disabil Hum Dev 2015;14(3):205-15.
[2] Shek DTL, Chung PPY, eds. Promoting service leadership qualities in university students: The case of Hong Kong. Quality of life in Asia, vol 6. Singapore: Springer, 2015.
[3] Information Services Department. Hong Kong as a service economy. Hong Kong: Information Services Department, 2015. URL: http://www.gov.hk/en/about/abouthk/factsheets/docs/service_economy.pdf.
[4] The World Bank. Services, etc., value added (% of GDP). The World Bank, 2016. URL: https://data.worldbank.org/indicator/NV.SRV.TOTL.ZS.
[5] Chung PPY, Bell AH. 25 principles of service leadership. Grandville, MI: Lexingford, 2015.
[6] Chung PPY, Elfassy R. The 12 dimensions of a service leader. Grandville, MI: Lexingford, 2016.
[7] Chung PPY. Service reborn: The knowledge, skills and attitudes of service companies. New York: Lexingford, 2012.
[8] Chung PPY. Hong Kong Institute of Service Leadership and Management (HKI-SLAM) curriculum framework. Hong Kong: Hong Kong Institute of Service Leadership and Management, 2011. URL: http://hki-slam.org/index.php?r=article&catid=1&aid=11.
[9] Shek DTL, Chung PPY, Dou D. The dark side of leadership. In: Alvinius A, ed. Dark sides of organizational behavior and leadership. Rijeka, Croatia: InTech Open, in press.
[10] Shek DTL, Yu L, Ma CMS, Liu TT, Sun RCF. Development of a credit-bearing service leadership subject for university students in Hong Kong. Int J Adolesc Med Health 2013;25(4):353-61.
[11] Shek DTL, Liang J, Zhu X. Subjective outcome evaluation of a service leadership subject for university students in Hong Kong. Int J Child Health Hum Dev 2016;9(2):225-32.
[12] Shek DTL, Lin. L, Xie Q. Service leadership education for university students in Hong Kong: A qualitative evaluation study. Int J Child Adolesc Health 2016;9(2):235-43.
[13] Shek DTL, Lin L. Changes in university students after joining a service leadership program in China. J Leadersh Educ 2016;15(1):96-109.
[14] Weller LD, Weller SJ. Leadership knowledge and skills: The essentials for effectiveness. In: The assistant principal: Essentials for effective school leadership. Thousand Oaks, CA: Corwin Press, 2002:1-28.
[15] Avolio BJ, Walumbwa FO, Weber TJ. Leadership: Current theories, research, and future directions. Annu Rev Psychol 2009;60:421-49.
[16] van Dierendonck D. Servant leadership: A review and synthesis. J Manage 2011;37(4):1228-61.

[17] Brown ME, Treviño LK. Ethical leadership: A review and future directions. Leadersh Q 2006;17(6):595-616.
[18] Shek DTL, Chung PPY, Leung H. How unique is the service leadership model? A comparison with contemporary leadership approaches. Int J Disabil Hum Dev 2015;14(3):217-31.
[19] Tsui AS. Contextualization in Chinese management research. Manage Organ Rev 2006;2(1):1-13.
[20] Shek DTL, Lin L, Leung H, Yu L, Ma CMS, Li X. Development and validation of the Service Leadership Knowledge Scale in a Chinese context. In: Shek DTL, Chung PPY, Li L, Merrick J, eds. Service Leadership education for university students. New York: Nova Science, 2017:163-88.
[21] Crawford JR. Psychometric foundations of neuropsychological assessment. In: Goldstein LH, McNeil JE, eds. Clinical neuropsychology: A practical guide to assessment and management for clinicians. Chichester, UK: Wiley, 2004:121-40.
[22] Crawford JR, Garthwaite PH, Slick DJ. On percentile norms in neuropsychology: Proposed reporting standards and methods for quantifying the uncertainty over the percentile ranks of test scores. Clin Neuropsychol 2009;23(7):1173-95.
[23] Hallinger P, Li D, Wang WC. Gender differences in instructional leadership: A meta-analytic review of studies using the Principal Instructional Management Rating Scale. Educ Adm Q 2016;52(4):567-601.
[24] Mandell B, Pherwani S. Relationship between emotional intelligence and transformational leadership style: A gender comparison. J Bus Psychol 2003;17(3):387-404.
[25] Oshagbemi T, Gill R. Gender differences and similarities in the leadership styles and behaviour of UK managers. Women Manage Rev 2003;18(6):288-98.
[26] Rosener JB. Ways women lead. Harv Bus Rev 1990;68(6):119-25.
[27] Carless SA. Gender differences in transformational leadership: An examination of superior, leader, and subordinate perspectives. Sex Roles 1998;39(11-12):887-902.
[28] Beck CD. Antecedents of servant leadership: A mixed methods study. J Leadersh Organ Stud 2014;21(3):299-314.
[29] Barbudo JE, Fritz SM, Matkin GS, Marx DB. Effects of gender, education, and age upon leaders' use of influence tactics and full range leadership behaviors. Sex Roles 2007;56(1-2):70-83.
[30] Thompson MD. Student leadership development and orientation: Contributing resources within the liberal arts. Am J Educ Res 2013;1(1):1-5.
[31] Kellett JB, Humphrey RH, Sleeth RG. Empathy and complex task performance: Two routes to leadership. Leadersh Q 2002;13(5):523-44.
[32] Liang F, Zheng W, Zhao J. Study of influencing factors and training pattern of college students' leadership - Take Shanghai Jiao Tong University as an example. Theory Pract Educ 2015;35(30):9-11. [Chinese]
[33] Eich D. A grounded theory of high-quality leadership programs: Perspectives from student leadership development programs in higher education. J Leadersh Organ Stud 2008;15(2):176-87.
[34] Hu L, Bentler PM. Evaluating model fit. In: Hoyle RH ed. Structural equation modeling: Concepts, issues, and applications. Thousand Oaks, CA: Sage, 1995:76-99.
[35] Field A. Discovering statistics using SPSS, 3rd ed. London, UK: Sage Publications, 2009.
[36] Stelter NZ. Gender differences in leadership: Current social issues and future organizational implications. J Leadersh Stud 2002;8(4):88-99.

SECTION THREE: MANUAL

In: Service Leadership
Editors: Daniel TL Shek, Xiaoqin Zhu, Li Lin et al.
ISBN: 978-1-53614-852-7

Chapter 14

A USER MANUAL FOR THE SERVICE LEADERSHIP KNOWLEDGE SCALE

Daniel TL Shek[1-6,*], PhD, FHKPS, BBS, SBS, JP, Lawrence K Ma[1], PhD, Siew Shen Low[1], MSc, Xiaoqin Zhu[1], PhD and Diya Dou[1], PhD

[1]Department of Applied Social Sciences, The Hong Kong Polytechnic University, Hong Kong, PR China,
[2]Centre for Innovative Programmes for Adolescents and Families, The Hong Kong Polytechnic University, Hong Kong, PR China,
[3]Department of Social Work, East China Normal University, Shanghai, PR China,
[4]Kiang Wu Nursing College of Macau, Macau, PR China,
[5]Hong Kong Institute of Service Leadership and Management Limited, Hong Kong, PR China
[6]Division of Adolescent Medicine, Department of Pediatrics, Kentucky Children's Hospital, University of Kentucky School of Medicine, Lexington, Kentucky, US

ABSTRACT

With a strong evidence base linking leadership knowledge to leadership practices, the Service Leadership Knowledge Scale was developed as an objective assessment tool to assess an individual's knowledge pertaining to Service Leadership based on the Service Leadership Theory. With an initial item pool of 200 items, the final Service Leadership Knowledge Scale consists of 40 items which demonstrated robust psychometric properties. In this chapter, a brief introduction of the development of the Service Leadership Knowledge Scale as well as its conceptual framework is attempted. The validation process,

[*] Correspondence: daniel.shek@polyu.edu.hk.

norm statistics, administration notes, and guidelines for scale score interpretation are also discussed.

INTRODUCTION

Owing to the transformation in economic composition amongst capitalist societies across the globe, Hong Kong, as a cosmopolitan Asian financial hub, has transitioned from the once manufacturing-dominant economy to a service-driven economy (1-3). According to the Information Services Department (4), nearly 90% of jobs in Hong Kong are currently service-oriented. This shift in the economic structure has huge implications on what constitutes good leadership practices in this age (2, 5). Po Chung, the co-founder of DHL International and the incumbent chairperson of the Hong Kong Institute of Service Leadership and Management Limited (HKI-SLAM), asserted that a corresponding evolution to a service mentality, which stresses nurturance of human assets, autonomy, and innovation (2), is the key to leadership success in this Service era (6).

Obviously, such an evolution cannot be taken for granted. As stated by Shek et al. (3), there is still a noticeable incompatibility between what is valued amongst the potential employers vis-à-vis the graduates or the employees in certain service sectors. Such a discrepancy does not only engender mismatch in recruitment and under-utilization of talents (8) but also deterioration in employees' job satisfaction as well as mental and physical well-being (9). In view of such a backdrop, the Service Leadership and Management (SLAM) framework was put forth by HKI-SLAM, with the vision to educate a new generation of service leaders who can thrive in the contemporary service economy by possessing task-specific competences, a caring disposition, and capability to make morally correct decisions (3, 10).

According to the SLAM framework, effective leadership is conceptualized as a "service aimed at ethically satisfying the needs of self, others, groups, communities, systems, and environments" (11, p. 233). To put this in the context of leadership education, Chung and Bell (12) proposed 25 defining principles of effective Service Leadership which are subsumed under seven Core Beliefs (see Table 1).

Furthermore, Chung and Elfassy (6) highlighted 12 areas of personal qualities instrumental to Service Leadership. These include Expertise, Character, Compassion, Relationship, Daily Management, Happiness, Intellectual, Inspirational, Health, Security, Follower, and Maturation dimensions. As Chung and colleagues (12, 13) astutely pointed out, these 12 dimensions boil down to three core features of an effective Service Leader, which are Competence (i.e., "doing things right"), Character (i.e., "doing the right things"), and Caring (i.e., "serving with an unselfish intent"). In a nutshell, both the seven core beliefs and the 3-Cs of Service Leadership outline the theoretical foundation of the model of Service Leadership education (i.e., 14, 15).

Table 1. The seven core beliefs of the SLAM framework (HKI-SLAM, n.d.)

Core Beliefs (CB)
CB1: Leadership is a service aimed at ethically satisfying the needs of self, others, groups, communities, systems, and environments.
CB2: Everyday, every human occupies a position of leadership and possesses the potential to improve his or her leadership quality and effectiveness.
CB3: Leadership effectiveness and service satisfaction are dependent on a leader or service provider possessing relevant situational task *competences* plus being judged by superiors, peers, and subordinates as possessing *character* and exhibiting *care*.
CB4: Service includes self-development efforts aimed at ethically improving one's competences, abilities, and willingness to help satisfy the needs of others.
CB5: Service Leadership is about creating appropriate personal service prepositions in real time and constantly striving to provide the highest quality service one afford to everyone one comes into contact with and whose lives are affected by one's actions or leadership.
CB6: Service Leadership is the world's oldest, most competitive, and longest surviving business model.
CB7: Now and in the future, high-paying, high-status positions and management promotions will go to people who have domain-specific knowledge and skills plus Service Leadership competences, appropriate character strengths and a caring social disposition.

Note. Adapted from Shek and Lin (2015).

With the objective of nurturing and developing future leader with service mindset and key Service Leadership qualities the Victor and William Fung Foundation financed the "Fung Service Leadership Initiative" (FSI) in eight government-funded Hong Kong universities from 2012 to 2015. To assess one's attitude, knowledge, and behavior in an objective manner, three assessment tools were developed and subsequently validated (3).

This manual outlines the development and validation of the Service Leadership Knowledge Scale (SLK-SF-40), including its conceptual framework, item development, psychometric properties, and potential use. Validity and reliability of the finalized scale are provided to corroborate its effectiveness on measuring knowledge of Service Leadership. Administration guidelines and interpretation on raw scores are also included for scale users to have a better understanding when using the scale.

CONCEPTUAL FRAMEWORK

On the basis of the SLAM framework (10), 25 Principles of Service Leadership (12), the 12 Dimensions of a Service Leader (6), and related literature (e.g., 16, 17), the initial item pool containing a total of 200 multiple-choice items was developed covering seven crucial domains of knowledge points pertaining to the Service Leadership paradigm. These included a) General description of Service Leadership, b) Three realms of Service Leadership, c) Principle "E (Effective Leadership) = 3Cs (i.e., **C**ompetence, **C**aring Disposition, and Moral **C**haracter)", d) Manufacturing vs. service economies and current societal status, e) Distinction of Service Leadership and other leadership theories, and f) other knowledge points in SLAM framework. Table 1 provides an overview of all the above-mentioned domains and the coverage for each of them. Detailed description regarding each domain are documented in the previously published work (e.g., 3, 7).

DIFFERENT STAGES OF THE VALIDATION PROCESS

The Long-Form Service Leadership Knowledge Scale (i.e., SLK-LF-200) including 200 English items was developed by Shek et al. (3) with the primary purpose of examining the "essential knowledge points of Service Leadership in the format of multiple-choice questions" (3, p.164).

Following the initial development of the item pool, the knowledge scale was subjected to multiple stages of the validation process. The following steps below summarizes the three validation studies which ultimately led to the trimming of the initial 200-item knowledge scale to the final version that contained roughly one-fifth of the items in the initial item pool:

Stage 1: A content validation study was conducted to exam the 200-item SLK-LF-200. A group of experts who were previously involved in the development of the SLAM curriculum evaluated the 200 items based on three criteria, including relevance, clarity, and representativeness. The analyses revealed that the SLK-LF-200 demonstrated meritorious content validity on both the individual item and the scale levels (3, 7).

Stage 2: The SLK-LF-200 was administered to 160 PolyU students in a criterion-related validation study. Amongst them, 67 took a three-credit course "Service Leadership" before served as the experimental group, while the remaining 93 students who had not taken the course served as the control group. Analyses revealed that the experimental group performed significantly better in all component scores as well as the composite score for the SLK-LF-200, indicating good criterion validity of the scale. Additionally, analyses on the individual item revealed that the experimental group outperformed the control group on 63 items. These 63 items were subjected to further screening, resulting in the removal of 13 items based on item duplication and face validity concern (18). Eventually, these 50 items constituted the Short-Form Service Leadership Knowledge Scale (i.e., SLK-SF-50) which were utilized in a large-scale validation study involving 4,486 university students (18, 19).

Stage 3: The SLK-SF-50 was administered to 4,486 undergraduates from eight government-funded universities in Hong Kong. Initial inspection of reliability informed the deletion of ten items due to low item-total correlations (i.e., < 0.30). Consequently, a single-factor, 40-item factorial solution (i.e., SLK-SF-40) was subjected to confirmatory factor analysis (CFA) using the robust weighted least squares (WLSMV) estimation (18).

Overall, the goodness-of-fit statistics, which were detailed in Section 5 of the present manual, underscored the factorial validity of the proposed SLK-SF-40. Aside from recording good internal consistency, the SLK-SF-40 also exhibited robust convergent validity as evidenced by its significant correlations with different constructs theorized to be relevant to the SLAM curriculum.

DESIGN AND USE OF THE SCALE

As abovementioned, the original item pool of the SLK-LF-200 was developed based on the SLAM framework and other related publications from the Service Leadership literature. These items, written in English and taking the form of multiple-choice questions, were created with the objective to measure respondents' "understanding of the fundamental knowledge points that a Service Leader is expected to obtain" (3, p. 166). The final version of the scale (i.e., SLK-SF-40) is comprised of 40 items (see Table 2 for three sample items) assessing mastery of key knowledge points in Service Leadership as a unidimensional construct (see 18). For each item, there is a correct answer, where "1" ("0") point is scored for each correct (incorrect) answer. A higher total score (out of 40) is indicative of the acquisition of more key knowledge points of Service Leadership (3, 18). The final 40-item version of the Service Leadership Knowledge Scale (SLK-SF-40) was revised based on findings from the psychometric analyses.

Table 2. Three sample items of the SLK-SF-40

Items	Options	Model Answers
6. A manager under the service economy plans to hire someone. Based on the Service Leadership model, which of the following advice would you give him/her?	A. Hire for qualifications, train for character B. Hire for character, train for skills C. Hire for attitude, train for character D. Hire for efficiency, train for mindset	B

Table 2. (Continued)

Items	Options	Model Answers
28. Which of the below attributes constitutes one of the three key components of Caring Disposition according to the Service Leadership and Management (SLAM) model?	A. Responsibility B. Conscientiousness C. Empathy D. Warmth	C
39. According to the 25 Principles of Service Leadership, which of the below statements is most appropriate?	A. It is not the Service Leaders' responsibility to predict and avoid errors that are costly to one's service reputation. B. Service Leaders should hide the errors that are costly to one's service reputation. C. Service Leaders can easily make amends for errors detrimental to one's service reputation. D. Service Leaders have to try to predict and avoid errors that are costly to one's service reputation.	D

Note. These sample items were slightly re-worded to minimize familiarity effect.

Target respondents

The SLK-SF-40 was targeted at the undergraduate and adult population in Hong Kong and other Chinese communities (i.e., Taiwan and mainland China). Norms based on other populations may be needed when the scale is used elsewhere because the normative data reported in this manual were based on university students in Hong Kong.

Instructions

The SLK-SF-40 is administered in a self-report manner in English. A standardized set of instructions is provided as illustrated in Figure 1, while slight modifications in wordings may be acceptable. A cover page including a) the objective of the survey, b) the emphasis on voluntary participation and data confidentiality, c) compensation (in terms of credit or pecuniary interest if applicable), d) contact details of the administrators or the researchers, and e) options for potential respondents to agree or refuse to join the study should be included. While no time limit is explicitly specified, the normal completion time for SLK-SF-40 is around 30 minutes.

Information on the personal particulars of respondents may be sought (see Figure 2). Additional items may be included depending on the test administrators' needs (e.g., whether a repeated/pretest/posttest design is utilized) as well as the characteristics of the target sample (e.g., an undergraduate sample or a group of adult trainees signed up to certain training course in Service Leadership).

Please read each question carefully and select the best option to your understanding about leadership. The following questions are about Service Leadership and Management (SLAM) Model. No matter whether or not you have learned anything about this model, please respond to the questions based on what you know as of this moment.

Figure 1. A sample introductory note.

The below contains questions on personal particulars of yours. Please select or write down your answers in the space provided. *Please delete as appropriate 1. Your 8-digit student ID: 2. Your Gender: *Male/Female 3. Age: 4. Have you taken any of the following credit-bearing Service Leadership courses (You may select multiple answers)? 5. Have you ever participated in any of the below non-credit bearing Service Leadership programs organized by your university (You may select multiple answers)? 6. Have you ever taken any other leadership training (e.g., any extra-curricular activities that warrant applications of your leadership competence)? *Yes/No 7. How much do you think you know about "Service Leadership"? **No* Knowledge/*Little* Knowledge/*Some* Knowledge/*A Lot of* Knowledge/*All* the Knowledge 8. Have you worked before (You may select multiple answers)? *No Work Experience (*single* choice only)/Full-Time Work/Part-Time Work/Internship

Figure 2. Sample questions on respondents' personal information.

Administration guidelines

While users are at liberty to customize the cover page, introductory notes, the personal information sheet as well as the mode of administration (i.e., electronic or paper-based) according to their needs, the following points should be strictly observed:

1. The full title of the test "Service Leadership Knowledge Scale" should not appear or be explicitly announced anywhere in the introductory note
2. Even though the SLK-SF-40 was constructed as a knowledge test pertaining to the SLAM curriculum, it can still be utilized to gauge the individual's "baseline" knowledge concerning Service Leadership before the start of any training programs or workshops. Specifically, upon administration to respondents who are untrained in Service Leadership, the users may remind the respondents to just respond to the items based on their current knowledge
3. The scale must be completed by the participant on his/her own. No discussion or collaboration with fellow participants should be permitted. Furthermore, the scale must be administered in a closed-book fashion, meaning that participants are not allowed to search for answers from the Internet, lecture notes and/or other relevant materials (e.g., books or journal articles) throughout the test. The test administrator, however, may

offer explanations for certain specific terms (e.g., decentralized, formalized, etc.) when participants express difficulties in comprehending those terminologies. While no specific time limit is stipulated, the normal time of completion of the SLK-SF-40 is approximately 30 minutes

4. It is advisable that the SLK-SF-40 be administered by trained personnel including, but not limited to teachers, psychologists or social workers, or self-administered in the presence of such qualified users on an individual or a group basis. Under normal circumstances, the scale should be completed in ONE setting. Should the paper-based version be utilized, the questionnaire ought to be collected by the test administrators immediately upon completion.

RELIABILITY AND VALIDITY

Normative sample in this manual was derived through a large-scale validation study involving 4,486 university students in Hong Kong. All analyses presented in this chapter are based on the normative sample data.

Internal consistency

Analyses revealed that the SLK-SF-40 possesses excellent internal consistency, with the Kuder-Richardson 20 (KR-20) coefficient = 0.94. To inspect the internal consistency of the SLK-SF-40 across gender and various age groups, KR-20 coefficients and mean inter-item correlations were also computed for each gender and age group (see Tables 3 and 4, respectively). The KR-20 coefficients, as shown in tables 3 and 4, were over 0.90 across gender and different age groups. Additionally, the mean inter-item correlations for all four sub-groups were within the optimal range (i.e., 0.20 to 0.40) defined by Briggs and Cheek (20). Taken together, the SLK-SF-40 demonstrates excellent internal consistency in the present sample.

Table 3. Reliability indices by gender

Reliability indices	Male (N = 1,517)	Female (N = 2,969)	Total (N = 4,486)
Kuder-Richardson 20	0.94	0.94	0.94
Mean inter-item correlations	0.28	0.27	0.28

Table 4. Internal consistency Kuder-Richardson 20 coefficients by age groups

Reliability indices	15-19 (N = 1,344)	≥ 20 (N = 3,142)	Total (N = 4,486)
Kuder-Richardson 20	0.94	0.94	0.94
Mean inter-item correlations	0.28	0.28	0.28

Table 5. Correlations between SLK-SF-40 and the adopted external criterion scales

Correlations with the external criterion scales (and subscales)			Z-scores of difference between *r*s with SLK-SF-40:				
	□□(MITC)	*r*	MSC	LEF	IRI	IRI-EC	IRI-PT
1. RSLP	0.94 (0.46)	0.200***	-16.17***	4.83***	-16.92***	-14.15***	-10.09***
2. MSC	0.83 (0.44)	0.361***	—	15.11***	-6.25***	-4.31***	1.12
3. LEF	0.72 (0.25)	0.125***	—	—	-18.83***	-16.76***	-13.09***
4. IRI	0.74 (0.17)	0.438***	—	—	—	2.97**	12.91***
4a. IRI- EC	0.62 (0.19)	0.419***	—	—	—	—	5.64***
4b. IRI- PT	0.58 (0.19)	0.346***	—	—	—	—	—

Note. $^{**}p$ <.01 (two-tailed). $^{***}p$ <.001 (two-tailed). MITC: Mean inter-item correlations. RSLP: Revised Servant Leadership Profile; MSC: Moral Self-Concept; LEF: Leadership Efficacy; IRI: Interpersonal Reactivity Index; IRI-EC: Subscale "Empathic Concern"; IRI: PT: Subscale "Perspective Taking".

Concurrent validity

Aside from the strong internal consistency, the SLK-SF-40 was demonstrated to be valid as it was associated with various measures of theoretically-relevant constructs, including empathy and servant leadership. As detailed in Table 5, the composite score of SLK-SF-40, which was calculated via summing each participant's correct response to every item, was positively and significantly (all *p*s <. 001, two-tailed) correlated to well-established external measures of Servant Leadership (r = 0.20), Moral Self-Concept (r = 0.36), Leadership Efficacy (r = 0.13), and Empathy (i.e., Interpersonal Reactivity Index, $r_{composite}$ = 0.44, $r_{empathic\ concern}$ = 0.42, and $r_{perspective\ taking}$ = 0.35). Notably, comparisons (21, 22) revealed that the SLK-SF-40 was correlated most strongly with the empathy measure while least correlated with the leadership efficacy measure (see Table 6).

The concurrent validity of the SLK-SF-40 was further supported by its correlations with the final versions of the two other measures of Service Leadership. As demonstrated in Table 6, the SLK-SF-40 was positively and significantly correlated with both the 38-item Service Leadership Behavior Scale (SLB-SF-38, r = 0.18) as well as the 46-item Service Leadership Attitude Scale (SLA-SF-46, r = 0.38). The SLK-SF-40 was also positively and significantly correlated with most of the subscales of the SLB-SF-38 and SLA-SF-46 (see Table 6). Additionally, comparison of the strengths of correlation (21, 22) revealed that the SLK-SF-40 was significantly more strongly linked to the SLA-SF-46 than to the SLB-SF-38 (see Table 6).

In short, findings from the correlational analyses provided a solid convergent evidence base for the construct validity of SLK-SF-38. Besides recording significant and positive correlations with constructs theorized to underpin the SLAM curriculum (10), the SLK-SF-40 also demonstrated significant correlation with the two separate objective assessment tools of Service Leadership.

Table 6. Correlations between SLK-SF-40 and other Service Leadership scales (and subscales) under validation

Correlations with other Service Leadership Scales under validation	α (MITC)	r	Z-scores of difference between rs with SLK-SF-40[a]														
			SLB-SF-38-F2	SLB-SF-38-F3	SLB-SF-38-F4	SLB-SF-38-F5	SLB-SF-38-F6	SLB-SF-38-Total	SLA-SF-46-F1	SLA-SF-46-F2	SLA-SF-46-F3	SLA-SF-46-F4	SLA-SF-46-F5	SLA-SF-46-F6	SLA-SF-46-F7	SLA-SF-46-F8	SLA-SF-46-Total
1.SLB-SF-38-F1	0.91 (0.53)	0.203***	-5.93	12.03	-0.20[n.s.]	6.39	21.47	3.32	-7.57	-8.78	3.06	8.76	-11.35	-2.05	8.91	-10.53	-12.44
2.SLB-SF-38-F2	0.87 (0.42)	0.269***	—	16.39	5.56	10.44	26.85	11.54	-3.36	-5.08	8.01	13.51	-7.81	2.31	13.37	-7.42	-8.87
3.SLB-SF-38-F3	0.87 (0.50)	0.047**	—	—	-12.57	-5.26	9.64	-14.88	-16.03	-17.07	-6.42	-0.48[n.s.]	-18.95	-10.93	0.53[n.s.]	-17.40	-20.59
4.SLB-SF-38-F4	0.86 (0.55)	0.205***	—	—	—	6.06	20.81	2.92	-7.19	-8.71	3.18	8.77	-11.25	-1.82[n.s.]	9.17	-10.59	-12.14
5.SLB-SF-38-F5	0.87 (0.56)	0.117***	—	—	—	—	13.36	-5.80	-12.20	-13.09	-2.22	3.35	-15.34	-7.05	4.06	-14.54	-16.32
6.SLB-SF-38-F6	0.85 (0.65)	-0.097***	—	—	—	—	—	-25.32	-23.05	-24.12	-15.34	-9.03	-25.78	-18.11	-7.35	-23.05	-28.03
7.SLB-SF-38-Total	0.96 (0.37)	0.178***	—	—	—	—	—	—	-9.59	-10.91	1.61[n.s.]	7.67	-13.46	-3.74	7.92	-11.54	-15.12
8.SLA-SF-46-F1	0.90 (0.46)	0.315***	—	—	—	—	—	—	—	-2.35	12.83	18.20	-5.98	6.73	15.51	-4.97	-8.93
9.SLA-SF-46-F2	0.87 (0.47)	0.337***	—	—	—	—	—	—	—	—	14.30	18.90	-3.52	7.80	17.93	-3.96	-5.44
10.SLA-SF-46-F3	0.86 (0.47)	0.155***	—	—	—	—	—	—	—	—	—	8.28	-17.20	-5.85	7.01	-12.12	-24.59
11.SLA-SF-46-F4	0.85 (0.53)	0.055***	—	—	—	—	—	—	—	—	—	—	-21.46	-11.92	1.05[n.s.]	-16.15	-27.97

Correlations with other Service Leadership Scales under validation			Z-scores of difference between *r*s with SLK-SF-40[a]														
	α (MITC)	*r*	SLB-SF-38-F2	SLB-SF-38-F3	SLB-SF-38-F4	SLB-SF-38-F5	SLB-SF-38-F6	SLB-SF-38-Total	SLA-SF-46-F1	SLA-SF-46-F2	SLA-SF-46-F3	SLA-SF-46-F4	SLA-SF-46-F5	SLA-SF-46-F6	SLA-SF-46-F7	SLA-SF-46-F8	SLA-SF-46-Total
12.SLA-SF-46-F5	0.83 (0.56)	0.373***	—	—	—	—	—	—	—	—	—	—	—	11.05	19.00	-2.09	$-0.54^{n.s.}$
13.SLA-SF-46-F6	0.82 (0.49)	0.235***	—	—	—	—	—	—	—	—	—	—	—	—	10.41	-8.53	-13.48
14.SLA-SF-46-F7	0.70 (0.54)	0.037***	—	—	—	—	—	—	—	—	—	—	—	—	—	-18.97	-22.18
15.SLA-SF-46-F8	0.79 (0.42)	0.411***	—	—	—	—	—	—	—	—	—	—	—	—	—	—	$1.92^{n.s.}$
16.SLA-SF-46-Total	0.93 (0.28)	0.377***	—	—	—	—	—	—	—	—	—	—	—	—	—	—	—

Note. [a]Unless otherwise specified by the superscript "n.s." which denotes statistical non-significance, all other Z-scores of difference were significant at p <.05 (two-tailed) (i.e., |Z-score| > 1.96). ** p <.01 (two-tailed). *** p <.001 (two-tailed). MITC: Mean inter-item correlations. SLB-SF-38-Total: Scale score of the six-factor, 38-item Service Leadership Behavior (SLB) Scale; SLA-SF-46-Total: Scale score of the eight-factor, 46-item Service Leadership Attitude (SLA) Scale; SLB-SF-38-F1: SLB Factor 1 "Self-improvement and self-reflection"; SLB-SF-38-F2: SLB Factor 2 "People and principles orientation"; SLB-SF-38-F3: SLB Factor 3 "Resilience"; SLB-SF-38-F4: SLB Factor 4 "Social competence"; SLB-SF-38-F5: SLB Factor 5 "Problem-solving"; SLB-SF-38-F6: SLB Factor 6 "Mentorship"; SLA-SF-46-F1: SLA Factor 1 "Vision and competence"; SLA-SF-46-F2: SLA Factor 2 "People orientation"; SLA-SF-46-F3: SLA Factor 3 "Caring disposition"; SLA-SF-46-F4: SLA Factor 4 "Ethical role model"; SLA-SF-46-F5: SLA Factor 5 "Social competence"; SLA-SF-46-F6: SLA Factor 6 "Self-understanding and reflection"; SLA-SF-46-F7: SLA Factor 7 "Positive view about human beings"; SLA-SF-46-F8: SLA Factor 8 "Unchangeable and dark human nature".

Factorial validity

We subjected the proposed one-factor structure of the SLK-SF-40 to a Confirmatory Factor Analysis (CFA) using Mplus version 6.12 (23). Overall, the goodness-of-fit statistics (e.g., CFI, NNFI, and RMSEA) strongly supported the unidimensional structure of the SLK-SF-40 (see Table 7). Almost all indices, with the exception of WRMR, met the well-established criteria of adequate fit according to the literature (24). Besides, as indicated in Table 8, the standardized factor loadings of all 40 items ranged from moderate to strong (i.e., 0.32 to 0.90) and were statistically significant ($p < .001$, two-tailed). In short, the present study supports the unidimensionality of the SLK-SF-40 (18).

Table 7. Model fit indices of the one-factor SLK-SF-40

Model Tested	χ^2	df	WRMR	NNFI	CFI	RMSEA (pclose)	RMSEA (90% CI)
One-factor	3,492.44	740	1.725	0.985	0.984	0.029 (1.00)	0.028/0.030
Criterion for goodness-of-fit	-	-	≤ 0.90	≥ 0.95	≥ 0.95	≤ 0.05	≤ 0.08

Note. WRMR = weighted root-mean-square residual; NNFI = Bentler-Bonett Nonnormed Fit Index; CFI = comparative fit index; RMSEA = root mean square error of approximation; pclose = probability of RMSEA ≤ 0.05; 90% CI = 90% Confidence Intervals (lower value/upper value).

NORMS

Student participants in this normative sample were recruited from the undergraduate programs of eight government-funded universities in Hong Kong. As the lead institution, the research team at the Hong Kong Polytechnic University utilized the "mySurvey@PolyU" electronic survey system to prepare the online survey and shared the link to the coordinators of all other participating institutions. The coordinators then sent the prepared online survey link to students who were interested in taking part. All prospective respondents were well informed about the principles of voluntary participation, anonymity, and rights to withdraw from the study at any time prior to the start. As a token of appreciation, each respondent was entitled to a local supermarket voucher valued at HK$100 upon completion.

The data collection lasted from late March to early June in 2017. After excluding invalid cases such as repeated participation and participant ineligibility, a total of 4,486 sets of responses were included in the final sample for normative analysis. The participants were aged between 15 and 34 years ($M = 20.47$, $SD = 1.67$), comprised of 2,969 (66.18%) female students and 1,517 (33.82%) male students.

Table 8. Confirmatory factor analysis loadings

Items	Mean [a] (Standard Deviation)	Accuracy Rate [b]	Standardized factor loadings	R-squared	Residual variance	Corrected Item-total Correlations
SLK-01	0.391 (0.488)	39.12%	0.528	0.279	0.721	0.396
SLK-02	0.751 (0.433)	75.06%	0.545	0.297	0.703	0.396
SLK-03	0.830 (0.376)	83.01%	0.646	0.417	0.583	0.433
SLK-05	0.742 (0.438)	74.19%	0.537	0.289	0.711	0.391
SLK-06	0.439 (0.496)	43.87%	0.419	0.175	0.825	0.316
SLK-08	0.612 (0.487)	61.21%	0.570	0.325	0.675	0.444
SLK-10	0.447 (0.497)	44.72%	0.597	0.356	0.644	0.461
SLK-11	0.523 (0.500)	52.25%	0.522	0.272	0.728	0.399
SLK-12	0.607 (0.489)	60.65%	0.535	0.287	0.713	0.415
SLK-13	0.740 (0.439)	73.99%	0.831	0.690	0.310	0.621
SLK-14	0.592 (0.492)	59.16%	0.718	0.515	0.485	0.565
SLK-15	0.396 (0.489)	39.59%	0.676	0.456	0.544	0.509
SLK-16	0.604 (0.489)	60.43%	0.878	0.770	0.230	0.699
SLK-17	0.673 (0.469)	67.32%	0.869	0.755	0.245	0.682
SLK-18	0.597 (0.490)	59.74%	0.901	0.813	0.187	0.726
SLK-19	0.673 (0.469)	67.32%	0.558	0.311	0.689	0.422
SLK-20	0.624 (0.484)	62.44%	0.838	0.703	0.297	0.667
SLK-21	0.675 (0.468)	67.50%	0.570	0.324	0.676	0.433
SLK-22	0.685 (0.465)	68.46%	0.760	0.578	0.422	0.577
SLK-23	0.619 (0.486)	61.93%	0.819	0.672	0.328	0.652
SLK-24	0.542 (0.498)	54.19%	0.603	0.363	0.637	0.469
SLK-25	0.568 (0.495)	56.82%	0.755	0.570	0.430	0.598
SLK-26	0.594 (0.491)	59.38%	0.748	0.559	0.441	0.583
SLK-28	0.664 (0.472)	66.41%	0.316	0.100	0.900	0.653
SLK-30	0.672 (0.469)	67.23%	0.833	0.693	0.307	0.568
SLK-31	0.536 (0.499)	53.63%	0.731	0.534	0.466	0.573
SLK-32	0.552 (0.497)	55.19%	0.739	0.546	0.454	0.522
SLK-33	0.399 (0.490)	39.88%	0.662	0.438	0.562	0.494
SLK-34	0.536 (0.499)	53.59%	0.651	0.424	0.576	0.665
SLK-36	0.375 (0.484)	37.47%	0.820	0.673	0.327	0.462
SLK-38	0.429 (0.495)	42.93%	0.617	0.381	0.619	0.478
SLK-39	0.358 (0.480)	35.84%	0.618	0.382	0.618	0.318
SLK-41	0.608 (0.488)	60.81%	0.430	0.185	0.815	0.616
SLK-42	0.514 (0.500)	51.38%	0.772	0.596	0.404	0.580
SLK-44	0.343 (0.475)	34.26%	0.731	0.534	0.466	0.366
SLK-45	0.526 (0.499)	52.56%	0.497	0.247	0.753	0.591
SLK-46	0.649 (0.477)	64.87%	0.757	0.572	0.428	0.437
SLK-47	0.539 (0.499)	53.92%	0.563	0.317	0.683	0.343
SLK-48	0.363 (0.481)	36.31%	0.442	0.196	0.804	0.314
SLK-50	0.566 (0.496)	56.58%	0.421	0.177	0.823	0.575

Note. [a] Each correct (incorrect) response was coded "1" ("0"). [b] Accuracy Rate = (Number of correct responses)/(Total responses, i.e., 4,486) *100%. All standardized factor loadings and R^2 metrics were statistically significant at p <. 001 (two-tailed).

Table 9. Percentiles and related raw scores for Service Leadership Knowledge Scale (SLK-SF-40) by gender

Percentile (1-50)	Raw Score			Percentile (51-99)	Raw Score		
	Male (*N* = 1,517)	Female (*N* = 2,969)	Total sample (*N* = 4,486)		Male (*N* = 1,517)	Female (*N* = 2,969)	Total sample (*N* = 4,486)
1	≤ 4.00	≤ 5.00	≤ 5.00	51	18.00	27.00	24.00
2	5.00	6.00	6.00	52	19.00	27.00	25.00
3	6.00	7.00	6.00	53	19.00	27.00	25.00
4	6.00	7.00	6.00	54	20.00	28.00	26.00
5	6.00	7.00	7.00	55	20.00	28.00	26.00
6	6.00	8.00	7.00	56	21.00	28.00	27.00
7	7.00	8.00	7.00	57	22.00	29.00	27.00
8	7.00	9.00	8.00	58	23.00	29.00	28.00
9	7.00	9.00	8.00	59	23.00	29.00	28.00
10	7.00	9.00	8.00	60	24.00	30.00	28.00
11	7.00	10.00	9.00	61	24.00	30.00	29.00
12	8.00	10.00	9.00	62	25.00	30.00	29.00
13	8.00	10.00	9.00	63	26.00	30.00	29.00
14	8.00	10.00	9.00	64	26.00	31.00	30.00
15	8.00	11.00	10.00	65	27.00	31.00	30.00
16	8.00	11.00	10.00	66	27.00	31.00	30.00
17	9.00	11.00	10.00	67	28.00	31.00	30.00
18	9.00	12.00	10.00	68	28.00	31.00	31.00
19	9.00	12.00	11.00	69	28.42	32.00	31.00
20	9.00	12.00	11.00	70	29.00	32.00	31.00
21	9.00	13.00	11.00	71	29.00	32.00	31.00
22	9.96	13.00	12.00	72	30.00	32.00	32.00
23	10.00	13.00	12.00	73	30.00	32.00	32.00
24	10.00	14.00	12.00	74	30.00	33.00	32.00
25	10.00	14.00	12.00	75	31.00	33.00	32.00
26	10.00	14.00	13.00	76	31.00	33.00	33.00
27	10.00	15.00	13.00	77	31.00	33.00	33.00
28	11.00	15.00	13.00	78	32.00	33.60	33.00
29	11.00	16.00	14.00	79	32.00	34.00	33.00
30	11.00	16.00	14.00	80	32.00	34.00	33.00
31	12.00	17.00	14.00	81	32.00	34.00	34.00
32	12.00	17.00	15.00	82	33.00	34.00	34.00
33	12.00	18.00	15.00	83	33.00	34.00	34.00
34	12.00	18.00	15.00	84	33.00	35.00	34.00
35	13.00	19.00	16.00	85	34.00	35.00	35.00
36	13.00	19.00	16.00	86	34.00	35.00	35.00
37	13.00	20.00	17.00	87	34.00	35.00	35.00
38	13.00	20.00	17.00	88	35.00	35.00	35.00
39	13.00	21.00	18.00	89	35.00	36.00	35.00
40	14.00	21.00	18.00	90	35.00	36.00	36.00
41	14.00	22.00	19.00	91	35.00	36.00	36.00
42	14.00	23.00	19.00	92	36.00	36.00	36.00
43	15.00	23.00	20.00	93	36.00	36.00	36.00
44	15.00	23.00	20.00	94	36.00	37.00	36.00
45	15.00	24.00	21.00	95	36.00	37.00	37.00
46	16.00	24.00	22.00	96	37.00	37.00	37.00
47	16.00	25.00	22.00	97	37.00	38.00	37.00
48	16.64	25.00	23.00	98	38.00	38.00	38.00
49	17.00	26.00	23.00	99	38.82	39.00	39.00
50	17.00	26.00	24.00	100	39.00	40.00	40.00

Normative statistics

As the raw scores in the full normative sample and sub-groups (i.e., male and female groups) did not follow a normal distribution, instead of using z scores, percentile ranks were calculated. Norms of the total score of the full normative sample and sub-groups are presented in Table 9 (percentile ranks and corresponding raw scores) and Table 10 (raw scores and equivalent percentile ranks).

Table 10. Raw scores and related percentiles for Service Leadership Knowledge Scale (SLK-SF-40)

Raw score	Percentiles		
	Male (N = 1517)	Female (N = 2969)	Total sample (N = 4486)
1	0.0	0.0	0.0
2	0.0	0.0	0.0
3	0.0	0.0	0.0
4	1.0	0.0	0.0
5	2.0	1.0	1.0
6	5.0	2.0	3.0
7	9.0	4.0	6.0
8	14.0	6.0	9.0
9	19.0	9.0	12.0
10	25.0	12.0	17.0
11	29.0	16.0	20.0
12	33.0	19.0	24.0
13	37.0	22.0	27.0
14	41.0	25.0	30.0
15	44.0	27.0	33.0
16	47.0	30.0	35.0
17	49.0	32.0	38.0
18	51.0	34.0	40.0
19	53.0	36.0	41.0
20	55.0	37.0	43.0
21	56.0	39.0	45.0
22	57.0	41.0	47.0
23	59.0	43.0	48.0
24	60.0	45.0	50.0
25	62.0	48.0	52.0
26	64.0	50.0	54.0
27	66.0	52.0	57.0
28	68.0	55.0	59.0
29	70.0	58.0	62.0
30	73.0	62.0	66.0
31	76.0	66.0	70.0
32	80.0	71.0	74.0
33	83.0	76.0	78.0
34	86.0	81.0	83.0
35	90.0	86.0	87.0
36	94.0	91.0	92.0
37	97.0	95.0	96.0
38	98.0	98.0	98.0
39	100.0	99.0	99.0
40	100.0	100.0	100.0

Scoring and Interpretation

The SLK-SF-40 is consisted of 40 items, and each has a correct answer. Each participant's answer on each item was coded as "1" or "0" to indicate a correct or incorrect answer, respectively. A total score across the 40 items is computed as the Service Leadership knowledge score, with a maximum score of 40.

Handling missing items

Completion of all items in the present scale is important to ensure satisfactory reliability of the scale. Results have to be interpreted cautiously in the event of missing responses. The responses with missing value(s) should be excluded from data analysis or be imputed with appropriate method prior to further analysis.

Interpretation of test scores

The objective of SLK-SF-40 is to measure participants' mastery of key knowledge points in Service Leadership. Interpretation of SLK-SF-40 test score is based on the full scale. A higher total score (out of 40) is indicative of the acquisition of more key knowledge points a Service Leader is expected to have.

Table 9 shows percentile norms for the scores of SLK-SF-40. Percentile rank of a specific raw score represents the percentage of people in the normative sample whose score is the same or lower than the specific raw score for a particular measure. In other words, the percentile rank of an individual shows his/her standing in the relevant group. Taking a female student who gets score of 30 as an example, her received score has made her surpassed more than half (60%) of all female students.

As mentioned in earlier section, a higher total score indicates one has more understanding of key knowledge points on Service Leadership. There is no specific cut-off value to segregate "rich" from "inadequate" knowledge on Service Leadership. When interpreting test scores, scale users (i.e., researchers or program evaluators) are recommended to locate the score of the participant from the norm tables to gauge his/her relative position regarding Service Leadership knowledge. Scale users may utilize expressions such as "less as compared to the normative sample", "similar to the normative sample", or "more as compared to the normative sample" to describe participants' different levels on Service Leadership knowledge.

To evaluate the effectiveness of Service Leadership training program, it is recommended that the scale be administered by the program evaluators prior to and after completion of the program. Evaluators can compare participants' received score in pre and post-test, which means scores can be used without referring to the norm table.

ACKNOWLEDGMENTS

The validation project is financially supported by the Victor and William Fung Foundation. The preparation for this paper is supported by the Foundation and the Endowed Professorship in Service Leadership Education at The Hong Kong Polytechnic University.

REFERENCES

[1] Lanford M. Perceptions of higher education reform in Hong Kong: A glocalisation perspective. Int J Comp Educ Dev 2016;18(3):184–204.

[2] Shek DTL, Chung PPY, Leung H. Manufacturing economy vs. service economy: Implications for service leadership. Int J Disabil Hum Dev 2015;14(3):205–15.

[3] Shek DTL, Chung PPY, Lin L, Merrick J, eds. Service Leadership education for university students. New York: Nova Science, 2017.

[4] Information Services Department. Hong Kong: The Facts—Hong Kong as a service economy, 2016. URL: https://www.gov.hk/en/about/abouthk/factsheets/docs/service_economy.pdf.

[5] Chung PPY. Where there is no vision, the people will perish. In: Shek DTL, Chung PPY, eds. Promoting service leadership qualities in university students: The case of Hong Kong. Singapore: Springer, 2015: xv–xviii.

[6] Chung PPY, Elfassy R. The 12 dimensions of a service leader, 1st ed. New York: Lexingford, 2016.

[7] Shek DTL, Lin L. Validation of the Service Leadership Knowledge Scale: Criterion-Related validity. In: Shek DTL, Chung PPY, Lin L, Merrick J, eds. Service Leadership education for university students. New York: Nova Science, 2017:189–204.

[8] Johnson L. World mobility perspectives: 2016 global mobility trends. Relocate Global, 2016. URL: https://www.relocatemagazine.com/media/images/2016GlobalMobilityTrendsPerspectives-DigitalCWM1_7648.pdf.

[9] Towers Watson. The next high-stakes quest: Balancing employer and employee priorities— 2012-2013 global talent management and rewards study, 2012. URL: https://www.towerswatson.com/en-HK/Insights/IC-Types/Survey-ResearchResults/2012/09/2012-Global-Talent-Management-and-Rewards-Study.

[10] Hong Kong Institute of Service Leadership and Management Limited (HKI-SLAM). University level SLAM curriculum. URL: http://hki-slam.org/index.php?r=article&catid=3&aid=39.

[11] Shek DTL, Lin L. Core Beliefs in the Service Leadership model proposed by the Hong Kong Institute of Service Leadership and Management. Int J Disabil Hum Dev 2015;14:233–42.

[12] Chung PPY, Bell AH. 25 Principles of service leadership, 1st ed. New York: Lexingford, 2015.

[13] Shek DTL, Chung PPY, Lin L, Leung H, Ng ECW. Service Leadership under the Service Economy. In: Chin JL, Trimble JE, Garcia JE, eds. Global and culturally diverse leaders and leadership: New dimensions and challenges for business, education and society, 1st ed. Bingley, UK: Emerald 2018:143–61.

[14] Hong Kong Institute of Service Leadership and Management Limited (HKI-SLAM). HKI-SLAM's Core beliefs (CB 1-7) about service leadership and management. URL: http://hki-slam.org/index.php?r=article&catid=2&aid=22.

[15] Shek DTL, Chung PPY, Yu L, Merrick J, eds. Service Leadership curriculum and higher education reform in Hong Kong. Int J Disabil Hum Dev 2015;14(4):297–406.
[16] Kram KE. Mentoring at work: Developmental relationships in organizational life. Lanham, MD: University Press of America, 1988.
[17] McCrimmon M. Bottom-up leadership. Exec Dev 1995;8(5):6–12.
[18] Shek DTL, Ma LK, Yu L, Leung LMK. Validation of the Service Leadership Knowledge Scale: Factorial and convergent validity. Int J Child Adolesc Health, in press.
[19] Shek DTL, Ma LK, Ma CMS, Hoshmand AR. Convergent and factorial validation of the Service Leadership Behavior Scale. Int J Child Adolesc Health, in press.
[20] Briggs SR, Cheek JM. The role of factor analysis in the development and evaluation of personality scales. J Pers 1986;54:106–48.
[21] Diedenhofen B, Musch J. cocor: A comprehensive solution for the statistical comparison of correlations. PLoS One 2015;10:e0121945.
[22] Steiger JH. Tests for comparing elements of a correlation matrix. Psychol Bull 1980;87:245–51.
[23] Muthén LK, Muthén BO. Mplus user's guide, 6th ed. Los Angeles, CA: Muthén Muthén, 1998-2010.
[24] Hu L-T, Bentler PM. Cutoff criteria for fit indexes in covariance structure analysis: Conventional criteria versus new alternatives. Struct Equ Modeling 1999;6:1–55.

In: Service Leadership
Editors: Daniel TL Shek, Xiaoqin Zhu, Li Lin et al.
ISBN: 978-1-53614-852-7

Chapter 15

A USER MANUAL FOR SERVICE LEADERSHIP ATTITUDE SCALE

Daniel TL Shek[1-6,*], PhD, FHKPS, BBS, SBS, JP and Xiaoqin Zhu[1], PhD

[1]Department of Applied Social Sciences, The Hong Kong Polytechnic University, Hong Kong, PR China
[2]Centre for Innovative Programmes for Adolescents and Families, The Hong Kong Polytechnic University, Hong Kong, PR China
[3]Department of Social Work, East China Normal University, Shanghai, PR China
[4]Kiang Wu Nursing College of Macau, Macau, PR China
[5]Hong Kong Institute of Service Leadership and Management Limited, Hong Kong, PR China
[6]Division of Adolescent Medicine, Department of Pediatrics, Kentucky Children's Hospital, University of Kentucky School of Medicine, Lexington, Kentucky, US

ABSTRACT

As there are few objective measures of attitudes to leadership in the service economies, The Service Leadership Attitude Scale was developed to assess an individual's attitudes towards leadership and effective leadership in the service economies. The scale was based on the Service Leadership Theory proposed by Po Chung. With an initial item pool of 132

---

* Correspondence: Daniel TL Shek, PhD, FHKPS, BBS, SBS, JP, Associate Vice President (Undergraduate Programme), Chair Professor of Applied Social Sciences and Li and Fung Professor in Service Leadership Education, Department of Applied Social Sciences, The Hong Kong Polytechnic University, Hung Hom, Hong Kong, PR China. E-mail: daniel.shek@polyu.edu.hk. The authorship is equally shared by the first author and second author.

items, the final scale comprises 46 items which showed very good psychometric properties. In this chapter, the background of the development of this scale, validation process and the psychometric properties of the scale are presented. Reminders for administration of the scale and guides for interpretation of the scales are also outlined.

INTRODUCTION

Hong Kong has an economy heavily depending on traditional and creative service industries which contribute 92.2% to the total Gross Domestic Product (GDP) and 92.7% to the employment (1). To sustain the competitive advantage of Hong Kong's service industries in the Asian Pacific region and even in the whole world market, service leaders are expected to be people-oriented and care about individual human needs including not only one's own but also others' needs as well as wellness of group, environment and the society. To this end, Po Chung proposed a new concept of Service Leadership Theory, which regards leadership as "a service aims at ethically satisfying the needs of self, others, groups, communities, systems, and environments" and stresses on humanistic values, moral ethics, and care of a service leader (2).

Guided by the Service Leadership Theory, and financially supported by the Victor and William Fung Foundation, the "Fung Service Leadership Initiative" (FSI) was implemented in the eight government-funded universities in Hong Kong from 2012 to 2015, with an aim of spotting and nurturing future leaders with service mindset and key service leadership qualities. To evaluate service leadership attributes and the effectiveness of service leadership education, it is imperative to have validated assessment tools specifically designed based on Service Leadership Theory. Thus, three assessment tools including knowledge, attitude, and behavior scales were developed and validated. While this manual focuses on the attitude scale and its finalized 46-item version (i.e., SLA-SF-46), the other two scales are introduced in respective user manuals.

This manual was written for potential users of the SLA-SF-46, including university teachers, program evaluators, human resources trainers, and employers. There are five purposes of this manual. First, it provides the scale users a brief description of the conceptual framework of Service Leadership Attitude Scale. Second, it introduces how the different versions of the scale were developed. Third, it presents statistical evidence documenting the reliability and validity of the finalized scale as an effective measure of service leadership attitude. Fourth, the manual presents normative statistics for interpretation of raw scores. Finally, the manual provides users with other information they need to administer the test and interpret the results.

CONCEPTUAL FRAMEWORK

Service Leadership Theory is characterized by several unique features, such as the seven core beliefs (e.g., everyone can be a leader and three realms of leadership) (3) and the strong emphasis on service orientation and self-leadership (4, 5). Based on these propositions, attitude toward service leadership was conceptualized as one's beliefs and perceptions about the nature of leadership process and role of a leader with reference to the eight domains. These domains are briefly outlined below, and detailed elaborations can be found elsewhere (6).

The first domain pertains to service orientation. Service leaders should see leadership as a service rather than a tool merely for generating profits. Modern service leaders are expected to believe in the importance of contributing to improving service ecology without instant economic returns, which enhances wellbeing at the societal level and benefits all market participants in the long run.

The second domain is pertinent to the belief that "everyone can be (and is) a leader." It has been shown that leadership in the service sectors is a learned behavior rather than a natural gift (7, 8). When leaders establish the sense that leadership qualities are not innate but learned, they can better recognize and nurture followers' potential and maximize followers' personal contribution.

The third domain is seeing distributed leadership as a desirable leadership practice. Distributed leadership allows employees to extend their roles in implementing service improvement by initiating changes from the bottom (9). This process of shared decision making and empowerment entails employees to see themselves as part of the organization which increase job performance and commitment.

Fourth, service leaders believe that service leadership increases employability. Service leadership is built upon professional competence, moral character and caring disposition, which are fundamental leadership qualities demanded in modern service industries. Thus, belief is expected to be established among service leaders that service leadership increases the likelihood of being employed and being a service leader will enjoy monetary and spiritual benefits (3).

The fifth domain has to do with the belief of providing personalized service and being sensitive to people's diversified needs. With the rapid development of technologies, traditional notion of delivering "one-size-fits-all" service to customers is no longer an optimal choice in the modern service era (3). Instead, how to provide customized service that fits each individual's needs has become the key area of competition (11).

Sixth, service leaders believe that providing service is intrinsically enjoyable to the service providers. High-quality service provision is more likely to be invigorated in the organizations with enjoyable atmosphere, where leaders and followers are not motivated only by external rewards such as economic returns. Service leaders believe in the importance of service passion and cultivate service enthusiasm among subordinates.

Seventh, service leaders believe that good leaders should demonstrate competence, character, and care (3Cs). For competence, it is important to possess multiple intrapersonal and interpersonal skills, so as to fulfill one's duties. For character, service leaders must be aware of the importance of "doing the right thing" in right ways. Regarding the importance of care, it is well known that caring behaviors of a leader as a service-provider will breed trust, loyalty and commitment in the followers and service recipients (3).

The eighth domain is about commitment to continuous improvement. In addition to serving others, service leaders are also expected to realize the need of serving oneself by continuously improving oneself, in order to accumulate resources and capacities to serve and lead others more effectively.

DIFFERENT STAGES OF THE VALIDATION STUDY

To further support the development of service leadership education in Hong Kong, the Victor and William Fung Foundation provided additional funding for the eight universities which collaborated in developing and validating scales on the service leadership knowledge, attitude and behavior in 2015. As far as the development of the attitude scale is concerned, several stages were involved as follows:

Stage 1: With reference to the conceptual framework mentioned before, the original long-form Service Leadership Attitude Scale including 132 items (i.e., SLA-LF-132) was developed.

Stage 2: The SLA-LF-132 was initially validated through a content validation study involving three experts (6) and a quasi-experimental study. Based on the results of an exploratory factor analysis (EFA) which utilized the pre-test data collected in the quasi-experimental study, 73 items with a 5-factor structure were retained to form a short-form attitude scale (SLA-SF-73). The SLA-SF-73 demonstrated good reliability.

Stage 3: The SLA-SF-73 was subject to a large-scale validation study involving 4,468 undergraduates recruited from the eight public universities in Hong Kong. Based on EFA using a sub-sample ($N = 2{,}246$), 46 items with a 7-factor structure were retained to form a new short-form scale (i.e., SLA-SF-46E). The SLA-SF-46E showed excellent internal consistency and strong convergent validity (11).

Stage 4: The SLA-SF-46E was subject to confirmatory factor analysis (CFA) based on another sub-sample ($N = 2{,}240$), which informed a finalized 46-item scale with an 8-factor structure (i.e., SLA-SF-46). The finalized scale and its eight subscales showed good reliability and convergent validity, which will be reported in Section 5 of this manual.

DESIGN AND USE OF THE SCALE

The item contents of the attitude scale were derived from two sources. First, some items were modified from existing measures on attitude (12-14). Second, some items were specifically constructed with reference to the conceptual framework and related service leadership curriculum. In the finalized scale (i.e., SLA-SF-46), 46 items were structured into 8 factors. The names and sample items of these factors are listed below:

- Factor 1: Vision and competence (10 items). A hypothetical sample item is "good leaders do not give in easily when facing challenges."
- Factor 2: People orientation (8 items). A hypothetical sample item is "good leaders encourage subordinates to contribute their ideas."
- Factor 3: Caring disposition (7 items). A hypothetical sample item is "good leaders help followers develop their talents."
- Factor 4: Ethical role model (5 items). A hypothetical sample item is "leadership effectiveness is largely dependent on ethical beliefs of the leader."
- Factor 5: Social competence (4 items). A hypothetical sample item is "good leaders have good interpersonal skills."
- Factor 6: Self-understanding and self-reflection (5 items). A hypothetical sample item is "good leaders have much self-reflection."
- Factor 7: Positive views about human beings (2 items). A hypothetical sample item is "everyone has what it takes to be a leader."
- Factor 8: Unchangeable and dark human nature (5 items, reversed). A hypothetical sample item is "We have to closely monitor subordinates' work to make sure that they are not lazy" (reverse-item).

Target respondents

The SLA-SF-46 was designed for university students and employees who may receive training on service leadership. In principle, its target population is Chinese people who are or will be taking a leading role in service sectors in Hong Kong and other Chinese communities such as mainland China and Taiwan. When using the scale outside Hong Kong, it is necessary to construct local norms as the normative sample included in this manual was based on university students in Hong Kong.

Instructions

The SLA-SF-46 is administered in English. The questionnaire is normally completed in the self-administered manner. The scale should not be issued to respondents before they give formal consent to complete the scale. Before responding to scale items, participants should read through the instructions presented at the beginning of the questionnaire.

There is no specific time limit for respondents to complete the whole questionnaire. Generally speaking, the scale can be completed within 20-30 minutes. In principle, the questionnaire should be completed and collected in the administration venue and must not be taken away by the respondents.

Administration notes

Different users may adapt the instructions and response format by complying with the following principles:

1) The questionnaire should be completed by respondents alone. Participants are not allowed to discuss with each other about the items.
2) Field administrators may explain grammatical and expression issues raised by respondents who have difficulties in understanding the meaning of any specific words or phrases. However, respondents should respond to the items according to their own interpretations.
3) The scale can be adopted in terms of full scale or individual subscales. However, the items included in a specific subscale should be fully utilized without any deletion.
4) SLA-SF-46 uses a 6-point Likert scale ranging from 1 (Strongly disagree) to 6 (Strongly agree). Testers should use the same rating scale.
5) SLA-SF-46 can be administered in paper-and-pencil or computerized formats. If the questionnaire is completed in the paper-and-pencil form, the completed questionnaires must be submitted to field administrators immediately. The questionnaires are not allowed to be retained or taken away by participants.

RELIABILITY AND VALIDITY

The normative sample was obtained in the large-scale validation study mentioned above. The psychometric properties of SLA-SF-46 were examined based on the normative sample and following sections briefly describe related findings.

Internal consistency/reliability

Results showed that SLA-SF-46 and its eight factors demonstrated good internal consistency, as reflected by Cronbach's alphas ranging from .70 to .93 and mean inter-item correlations ranging between .28 and .56 (see Table 1).

Table 1. Internal Consistency of SLA-SF-46 and its subscales

Scale/subscale	No. of items	Cronbach's alpha	Mean Inter-Item Correlations
Vision and competence	10	.90	.46
People orientation	8	.87	.47
Caring disposition	7	.86	.47
Ethical role model	5	.85	.53
Social competence	4	.83	.56
Self-understanding and self-reflection	5	.82	.49
Positive view about human beings	2	.70	.54
Unchangeable and dark human nature	5	.79	.42
Full scale	46	.93	.28

Convergent validity

The convergent validity of SLA-SF-46 was supported by the correlations among its subscales (see Table 2) and their correlations with external criterion constructs (see Table 3), including service leadership knowledge, service leadership behavior, servant leadership, moral self-concept, leadership efficacy, interpersonal reactivity index, empathic concern, and perspective thinking.

Table 2. Inter-factor correlations of finalized attitude scale/subscales

	F1	F2	F3	F4	F5	F6	F7	F8
F1: Vision and competence	--							
F2: People orientation	$.77^{***}$	--						
F3: Caring disposition	$.63^{***}$	$.61^{***}$	--					
F4: Ethical role model	$.52^{***}$	$.47^{***}$	$.67^{***}$	--				
F5: Social competence	$.76^{***}$	$.73^{***}$	$.60^{***}$	$.47^{***}$	--			
F6: Self-understanding and reflection	$.65^{***}$	$.57^{***}$	$.57^{***}$	$.48^{***}$	$.60^{***}$	--		
F7: Positive view about human beings	$.24^{***}$	$.33^{***}$	$.35^{***}$	$.31^{***}$	$.24^{***}$	$.16^{***}$	--	
F8: Unchangeable and dark human nature	$-.05^{**}$	.02	$-.16^{***}$	$-.22^{***}$	$.04^{**}$	$-.15^{***}$	$.03^{*}$	--
Full scale	$.87^{***}$	$.86^{***}$	$.80^{***}$	$.68^{***}$	$.83^{***}$	$.72^{***}$	$.43^{***}$	$.12^{**}$

Note. F1 = Factor 1, F2 = Factor 2, F3 = Factor 3, F4 = Factor 4, F5 = Factor 5, F6 = Factor 6, F7 = Factor 7, F8 = Factor 8.
$*p < .05$, $** p < .01$, $*** p < .001$.

Table 3. Correlations between finalized attitude scale/subscales and external criterion constructs

	SLK-SF-40	SLB-SF-38	RSLP	MSC	LEF	IRI	IRI-EC	IRI-PT
SLA-SF-46	.38***	.57***	.57***	.57***	.25***	.46***	.39***	.42***
SLA-SF-46-F1	.32***	.51***	.49***	.49***	.20***	.36***	.29***	.34***
SLA-SF-46-F2	.34***	.48***	.48***	.50***	.21***	.39***	.33***	.36***
SLA-SF-46-F3	.16***	.50***	.52***	.44***	.19***	.33***	.26***	.31***
SLA-SF-46-F4	.06***	.41***	.45***	.36***	.17***	.24***	.19***	.24***
SLA-SF-46-F5	.37***	.48***	.47***	.50***	.18***	.40***	.34***	.37***
SLA-SF-46-F6	24***	.47***	.42***	.42***	.18***	.29***	.22***	.29***
SLA-SF-46-F7	.04*	.27***	.29***	.23***	.14***	.15***	.12***	.15***
SLA-SF-46-F8	.41***	-.06***	-.07***	.10***	.07***	.25***	.27***	.16***

Note. SLK-SF-40: Finalized Service Leadership Knowledge Scale (40 items); SLB-SF-38: Finalized Service Leadership Behavior Scale (38 items); SLA-SF-46: Finalized Service Leadership Attitude Scale (46 items); RSLP: Revised Servant Leadership Profile; MSC: Moral Self-Concept; LEF: Leadership Efficacy; IRI: Interpersonal Reactivity Index; EC: IRI- Empathic Concern; PT: IRI- Perspective Taking. SLA-SF-46-F1: Vision and competence; SLA-46-SF-F2: People orientation; SLA-SF-46-F3: Caring disposition; SLA-SF-46-F4: Ethical role model; SLA-SF-46-F5: Social competence; SLA-SF-46-F6: Self-Understanding and reflection; SLA-SF-46-F7: Positive view about human beings; SLA-SF-46-F8: Unchangeable and dark human nature. *p <.05, *** p <.001.

Factorial validity

Table 4. Confirmatory Factor Analysis loadings

Item	Factor loading	Item	Factor loading
Vision and competence 1	.67	Caring disposition 6	.67
Vision and competence 2	.66	Caring disposition 7	.69
Vision and competence 3	.70	Ethical role model 1	.71
Vision and competence 4	.74	Ethical role model 2	.80
Vision and competence 5	.74	Ethical role model 3	.76
Vision and competence 6	.62	Ethical role model 4	.67
Vision and competence 7	.67	Ethical role model 5	.66
Vision and competence 8	.72	Social competence 1	.73
Vision and competence 9	.68	Social competence 2	.74
Vision and competence 10	.61	Social competence 3	.76
People orientation 1	.61	Social competence 4	.73
People orientation 2	.63	Self-Understanding and reflection 1	.50
People orientation 3	.72	Self-Understanding and reflection 2	.71
People orientation 4	.69	Self-Understanding and reflection 3	.79
People orientation 5	.75	Self-Understanding and reflection 4	.76
People orientation 6	.68	Self-Understanding and reflection 5	.73
People orientation 7	.71	Positive view about human beings 1	.76
People orientation 8	.63	Positive view about human beings 2	.71
Caring disposition 1	.70	Unchangeable and dark human nature 1	.76
Caring disposition 2	.71	Unchangeable and dark human nature 2	.85
Caring disposition 3	.60	Unchangeable and dark human nature 3	.67
Caring disposition 4	.72	Unchangeable and dark human nature 4	.35
Caring disposition 5	.72	Unchangeable and dark human nature 5	.50

The 8-factor structure was shown to be the best solution fitting for the finalized 46-item attitude scale (i.e., SLA-SF-46). CFA based on the full normative sample (N = 4,486) yielded good fit indices of the 8-factor structure, with CFI = .92, TLI = .91, RMSEA = .044 (90% CI = [.043, .045]). As shown in Table 4, majority of factor loadings were above .60.

The related findings for the different validation studies can be seen in publications about background and development of the scale (15), content validation study (6), psychometric properties of the SLA-SF-46E obtained based on EFA (11), and a manuscript under preparation which aims to present findings of CFA using the normative sample and psychometric properties of the SLA-SF-46. In addition, norms and personal correlates of attitude to service leadership with reference to the full scale of SLA-SF-46 have also been reported by Shek and colleagues (16). Section below will further present norms of SLA-SF-46 based on its full scale and subscales as well.

NORMS

The snowball sampling approach was adopted to recruit undergraduate students from eight publically-funded universities in Hong Kong, including The Hong Kong Polytechnic University (PolyU), The University of Hong Kong (HKU), The Chinese University of Hong Kong (CUHK), Hong Kong Baptist University (HKBU), City University of Hong Kong (CityU), The Education University of Hong Kong (EdUHK), Lingnan University (LU), and Hong Kong University of Science and Technology (HKUST). With the assistance offered by the coordinator in each university, the link of online survey was issued to students who had shown willingness to join the study. Students were well informed of the principles of confidentiality and their rights to withdraw from this study at any time. A local supermarket voucher worth $HK100 was offered to each participant who completed the whole survey as an incentive.

The data were collected between late March and early June 2017. After excluding 6 students who refused to give a formal consent, 33 students who had a record of completing the survey for multiple times, and 30 students who reported they were postgraduates, the final sample consisted of 4,486 undergraduates whose data were used to perform normative analyses. The normative sample was aged between 15 and 34 years old (M = 20.47, SD = 1.67), comprised of 2,969 (66.18%) female students and 1,517 (33.82%) male students.

Normative statistics

Norms for full sample and subgroups (i.e., male and female groups) were calculated. Due to non-normalized distribution of the raw scores in the full sample and sub-groups, percentile ranks instead of standardized Z scores were provided. A total of 18 norm tables

(Tables 5-22) are presented in the manual. While Tables 5 and 6 demonstrate norms of total score of the full scale, Tables 7-22 are norm tables for the eight sub-scales. For both full sale and sub-scales, percentile ranks and corresponding raw scores (Tables 5, 7, 9, 11, 13, 15, 17, 19, 21) as well as each raw score and its equivalent percentile rank (Tables 6, 8, 10, 12, 14, 16, 18, 20, 22) are presented, for the full sample and the two sub-groups.

Table 5. Percentiles and related raw scores for SLA-SF-46 (full scale) by gender

Percentile	Raw Score				Percentile	Raw Score		
(1-50)	Male	Female	Full sample		(51-99)	Male	Female	Full sample
1	≤ 136.00	≤ 164.00	≤ 155.00		51	214.00	218.00	216.37
2	155.00	173.40	165.74		52	214.00	218.00	217.00
3	161.54	179.00	172.00		53	215.00	219.00	217.00
4	167.00	182.00	176.48		54	215.00	219.00	218.00
5	172.00	185.00	179.00		55	215.00	219.00	218.00
6	174.00	187.00	182.00		56	215.00	220.00	218.00
7	176.00	190.00	184.00		57	216.00	220.00	219.00
8	178.00	191.00	186.00		58	216.00	220.00	219.00
9	179.00	193.00	188.00		59	217.00	221.00	220.00
10	181.00	194.00	190.00		60	217.00	221.00	220.00
11	182.00	195.70	191.00		61	218.00	221.00	220.00
12	184.00	197.00	192.00		62	218.00	222.00	221.00
13	186.00	198.00	194.00		63	219.00	222.00	221.00
14	187.00	199.00	195.00		64	219.00	223.00	222.00
15	188.00	200.00	196.00		65	220.00	223.00	222.00
16	190.00	201.00	197.00		66	220.00	224.00	222.00
17	191.00	202.00	198.00		67	221.00	224.00	223.00
18	192.00	203.00	199.00		68	221.00	225.00	223.00
19	193.00	203.00	200.00		69	222.00	225.00	224.00
20	194.00	204.00	201.00		70	222.00	226.00	224.00
21	195.00	205.00	202.00		71	223.00	226.00	225.00
22	196.00	206.00	203.00		72	223.00	227.00	226.00
23	197.00	207.00	203.00		73	224.00	227.00	226.00
24	197.32	207.00	204.00		74	224.00	228.00	227.00
25	198.00	207.00	205.00		75	225.00	228.00	227.00
26	199.00	208.00	205.00		76	226.00	229.00	228.00
27	200.00	209.00	206.00		77	226.00	229.00	228.00
28	201.00	209.00	207.00		78	227.00	230.00	229.00
29	202.00	210.00	207.00		79	228.00	231.00	230.00
30	203.00	210.00	208.00		80	228.00	231.00	230.00
31	203.00	210.00	209.00		81	229.00	232.00	231.00
32	204.00	211.00	209.00		82	229.00	233.00	232.00
33	204.00	211.00	209.00		83	230.00	233.00	232.00
34	205.00	212.00	210.00		84	231.00	234.00	233.00
35	206.00	212.00	210.45		85	232.00	235.00	234.00
36	206.00	213.00	211.00		86	234.00	236.00	235.00
37	207.00	213.00	211.00		87	235.00	237.00	236.00
38	207.00	213.00	212.00		88	236.00	239.00	237.56
39	208.00	214.00	212.00		89	237.00	240.00	239.00
40	209.00	214.00	213.00		90	238.00	242.00	240.00

Percentile (1-50)	Raw Score				Percentile (51-99)	Raw Score		
	Male	Female	Full sample			Male	Female	Full sample
41	209.00	214.00	213.00		91	239.00	243.70	242.00
42	210.00	215.00	213.00		92	241.00	246.00	244.00
43	211.00	215.00	214.00		93	243.00	247.00	246.00
44	211.00	215.00	214.00		94	245.00	248.80	248.00
45	212.00	215.00	214.00		95	247.10	250.00	249.00
46	212.00	216.00	215.00		96	251.00	252.00	251.00
47	212.00	216.00	215.00		97	252.00	254.00	253.00
48	213.00	217.00	215.00		98	255.00	257.00	256.00
49	213.00	217.00	216.00		99	259.00	261.00	261.00
50	214.00	217.00	216.00		100	≥ 271.00	≥ 272.00	≥ 272.00

Note. N = 1,517 for male sample, N = 2,969 for female sample, N = 4,486 for full sample.

Table 6. Raw scores and related percentiles for SLA-SF-46 (full scale) by gender

Raw score (≤ 182)	Percentiles Male	Female	Full sample	Raw score (183-229)	Percentiles Male	Female	Full sample	Raw score (230-276)	Percentiles Male	Female	Full sample
≤ 136	1.0	1.0	1.0	183	12.0	5.0	7.0	230	83.0	78.0	80.0
137	2.0	1.0	1.0	184	12.0	5.0	7.0	231	84.0	80.0	81.0
138	2.0	1.0	1.0	185	13.0	5.0	8.0	232	85.0	81.0	83.0
139	2.0	1.0	1.0	186	13.0	6.0	8.0	233	86.0	83.0	84.0
140	2.0	1.0	1.0	187	14.0	6.0	9.0	234	86.0	84.0	85.0
141	2.0	1.0	1.0	188	15.0	7.0	9.0	235	87.0	85.0	86.0
142	2.0	1.0	1.0	189	16.0	7.0	10.0	236	88.0	86.0	87.0
143	2.0	1.0	1.0	190	16.0	7.0	10.0	237	89.0	87.0	88.0
144	2.0	1.0	1.0	191	17.0	8.0	11.0	238	90.0	88.0	88.0
145	2.0	1.0	1.0	192	18.0	9.0	12.0	239	91.0	88.0	89.0
146	2.0	1.0	1.0	193	19.0	9.0	13.0	240	92.0	89.0	90.0
147	2.0	1.0	1.0	194	20.0	10.0	13.0	241	92.0	90.0	91.0
148	2.0	1.0	1.0	195	21.0	11.0	14.0	242	93.0	90.0	91.0
149	2.0	1.0	1.0	196	22.0	11.0	15.0	243	93.0	91.0	92.0
150	2.0	1.0	1.0	197	24.0	12.0	16.0	244	94.0	91.0	92.0
151	2.0	1.0	1.0	198	25.0	13.0	17.0	245	94.0	92.0	93.0
152	2.0	1.0	1.0	199	26.0	14.0	18.0	246	95.0	92.0	93.0
153	2.0	1.0	1.0	200	27.0	15.0	19.0	247	95.0	93.0	94.0
154	2.0	1.0	1.0	201	28.0	16.0	20.0	248	96.0	94.0	94.0
155	2.0	1.0	1.0	202	29.0	17.0	21.0	249	96.0	94.0	95.0
156	3.0	1.0	2.0	203	31.0	19.0	23.0	250	96.0	95.0	96.0
157	3.0	1.0	2.0	204	33.0	20.0	24.0	251	96.0	96.0	96.0
158	3.0	1.0	2.0	205	34.0	21.0	26.0	252	97.0	96.0	97.0
159	3.0	1.0	2.0	206	36.0	22.0	27.0	253	98.0	97.0	97.0
160	3.0	1.0	2.0	207	38.0	24.0	29.0	254	98.0	97.0	98.0
161	3.0	1.0	2.0	208	39.0	26.0	30.0	255	98.0	98.0	98.0
162	4.0	1.0	2.0	209	41.0	28.0	32.0	256	99.0	98.0	98.0
163	4.0	1.0	2.0	210	42.0	30.0	35.0	257	99.0	98.0	99.0
164	4.0	1.0	2.0	211	44.0	33.0	37.0	258	99.0	99.0	99.0
165	4.0	2.0	2.0	212	46.0	35.0	39.0	259	99.0	99.0	99.0
166	4.0	2.0	2.0	213	49.0	37.0	41.0	260	99.0	99.0	99.0
167	4.0	2.0	3.0	214	51.0	40.0	44.0	261	99.0	99.0	99.0

Table 6. (Continued)

Raw score (≤ 182)	Percentiles			Raw score (183-229)	Percentiles			Raw score (230-276)	Percentiles		
	Male	Female	Full sample		Male	Female	Full sample		Male	Female	Full sample
168	5.0	2.0	3.0	215	55.0	44.0	47.0	262	99.0	99.0	99.0
169	5.0	2.0	3.0	216	58.0	47.0	50.0	263	99.0	99.0	99.0
170	5.0	2.0	3.0	217	60.0	49.0	53.0	264	99.0	99.0	99.0
171	5.0	2.0	3.0	218	62.0	52.0	55.0	265	99.0	99.0	99.0
172	5.0	2.0	3.0	219	64.0	54.0	58.0	266	99.0	99.0	99.0
173	6.0	2.0	4.0	220	66.0	57.0	60.0	267	99.0	99.0	99.0
174	6.0	3.0	4.0	221	68.0	60.0	63.0	268	99.0	99.0	99.0
175	7.0	3.0	4.0	222	70.0	63.0	65.0	269	99.0	99.0	99.0
176	7.0	3.0	4.0	223	72.0	65.0	68.0	270	99.0	99.0	99.0
177	8.0	3.0	5.0	224	74.0	67.0	70.0	271	100.0	99.0	100.0
178	8.0	3.0	5.0	225	75.0	69.0	71.0	272	100.0	100.0	100.0
179	9.0	3.0	5.0	226	77.0	71.0	73.0	273	100.0	100.0	100.0
180	10.0	4.0	6.0	227	78.0	73.0	75.0	274	100.0	100.0	100.0
181	10.0	4.0	6.0	228	80.0	75.0	77.0	275	100.0	100.0	100.0
182	11.0	4.0	6.0	229	82.0	77.0	78.0	276	100.0	100.0	100.0

Note. N = 1,517 for male sample, N = 2,969 for female sample, N = 4,486 for full sample.

Table 7. Raw scores and related percentiles for SLA-SF-46 (Factor 1) by gender

Percentile (1-50)	Raw Score				Percentile (51-100)	Raw Score		
	Male	Female	Full sample			Male	Female	Full sample
1	≤ 26.00	≤ 35.00	≤ 31.00		51	50.00	50.00	50.00
2	31.00	38.00	36.00		52	50.00	50.00	50.00
3	35.00	40.00	38.00		53	50.00	50.00	50.00
4	36.00	40.00	39.00		54	50.00	50.00	50.00
5	37.00	41.00	40.00		55	50.00	50.00	50.00
6	38.00	42.00	40.00		56	50.00	50.00	50.00
7	39.00	43.00	41.00		57	50.00	51.00	50.00
8	40.00	43.00	42.00		58	50.00	51.00	50.46
9	40.00	44.00	42.00		59	50.00	51.00	51.00
10	40.00	44.00	43.00		60	50.00	51.00	51.00
11	41.00	45.00	43.00		61	51.00	51.00	51.00
12	41.00	45.00	44.00		62	51.00	51.00	51.00
13	42.00	45.00	44.00		63	51.00	51.00	51.00
14	42.00	46.00	45.00		64	51.00	51.00	51.00
15	43.00	46.00	45.00		65	51.00	52.00	51.00
16	43.00	46.00	45.00		66	51.00	52.00	52.00
17	44.00	46.00	46.00		67	51.00	52.00	52.00
18	44.00	47.00	46.00		68	51.00	52.00	52.00
19	44.00	47.00	46.00		69	52.00	52.00	52.00
20	44.00	47.00	46.00		70	52.00	52.00	52.00
21	45.00	47.00	46.00		71	52.00	52.00	52.00
22	45.00	47.00	47.00		72	52.00	53.00	52.00
23	45.00	48.00	47.00		73	52.00	53.00	53.00
24	45.00	48.00	47.00		74	52.00	53.00	53.00
25	46.00	48.00	47.00		75	53.00	53.00	53.00

Percentile (1-50)	Raw Score			Percentile (51-100)	Raw Score		
	Male	Female	Full sample		Male	Female	Full sample
26	46.00	48.00	47.00	76	53.00	53.00	53.00
27	46.00	48.00	48.00	77	53.00	53.00	53.00
28	46.00	48.00	48.00	78	53.00	54.00	53.00
29	47.00	48.00	48.00	79	53.00	54.00	54.00
30	47.00	49.00	48.00	80	53.00	54.00	54.00
31	47.00	49.00	48.00	81	54.00	54.00	54.00
32	47.00	49.00	48.00	82	54.00	54.00	54.00
33	47.00	49.00	48.00	83	54.00	55.00	54.00
34	48.00	49.00	49.00	84	54.00	55.00	55.00
35	48.00	49.00	49.00	85	55.00	55.00	55.00
36	48.00	49.00	49.00	86	55.00	56.00	55.00
37	48.00	49.00	49.00	87	55.00	56.00	56.00
38	48.00	49.00	49.00	88	56.00	56.00	56.00
39	48.00	49.00	49.00	89	56.00	56.00	56.00
40	48.00	50.00	49.00	90	56.00	57.00	57.00
41	48.00	50.00	49.00	91	57.00	57.00	57.00
42	49.00	50.00	50.00	92	57.00	58.00	57.00
43	49.00	50.00	50.00	93	57.00	58.00	58.00
44	49.00	50.00	50.00	94	58.00	58.00	58.00
45	49.00	50.00	50.00	95	59.00	59.00	59.00
46	49.00	50.00	50.00	96	59.00	59.00	59.00
47	49.00	50.00	50.00	97	60.00	60.00	60.00
48	50.00	50.00	50.00	98	60.00	60.00	60.00
49	50.00	50.00	50.00	99	60.00	60.00	60.00
50	50.00	50.00	50.00	100	60.00	60.00	60.00

Note. $N = 1{,}517$ for male sample, $N = 2{,}969$ for female sample, $N = 4{,}486$ for full sample.

Table 8. Raw scores and related percentiles for SLA-SF-46 (Factor 1) by gender

Raw score (≤ 37)	Percentiles			Raw score (38-49)	Percentiles			Raw score (50-60)	Percentiles		
	Male	Female	Full sample		Male	Female	Full sample		Male	Female	Full sample
≤ 26	1.0	1.0	1.0	38	6.0	2.0	3.0	50	54.0	48.0	50.0
27	2.0	1.0	1.0	39	7.0	4.0	4.0	51	65.0	61.0	62.0
28	2.0	1.0	1.0	40	9.0	4.0	6.0	52	72.0	68.0	69.0
29	2.0	1.0	1.0	41	12.0	5.0	7.0	53	78.0	75.0	76.0
30	2.0	1.0	1.0	42	14.0	6.0	9.0	54	83.0	80.0	81.0
31	2.0	1.0	1.0	43	16.0	8.0	11.0	55	86.0	84.0	85.0
32	3.0	1.0	2.0	44	19.0	10.0	13.0	56	89.0	88.0	88.0
33	3.0	1.0	2.0	45	23.0	12.0	15.0	57	92.0	91.0	91.0
34	3.0	1.0	2.0	46	27.0	16.0	19.0	58	94.0	93.0	94.0
35	3.0	1.0	2.0	47	31.0	20.0	24.0	59	96.0	96.0	96.0
36	4.0	2.0	2.0	48	38.0	26.0	30.0	60	100.0	100.0	100.0
37	5.0	2.0	3.0	49	45.0	35.0	38.0				

Note. $N = 1{,}517$ for male sample, $N = 2{,}969$ for female sample, $N = 4{,}486$ for full sample.

Table 9. Raw scores and related percentiles for SLA-SF-46 (Factor 2) by gender

Percentile (1-50)	Raw Score Male	Raw Score Female	Raw Score Full sample		Percentile (51-100)	Raw Score Male	Raw Score Female	Raw Score Full sample
1	≤ 20	≤ 28.00	≤ 25.00		51	40.00	40.00	40.00
2	25.00	30.00	28.00		52	40.00	40.00	40.00
3	27.00	31.00	29.00		53	40.00	40.00	40.00
4	28.00	32.00	31.00		54	40.00	41.00	41.00
5	29.00	32.00	32.00		55	40.00	41.00	41.00
6	30.00	33.00	32.00		56	40.00	41.00	41.00
7	30.00	34.00	32.00		57	40.00	41.00	41.00
8	31.00	34.00	33.00		58	40.00	41.00	41.00
9	32.00	35.00	33.00		59	40.00	41.00	41.00
10	32.00	35.00	34.00		60	40.00	41.00	41.00
11	32.00	36.00	34.00		61	40.00	41.00	41.00
12	33.00	36.00	35.00		62	41.00	41.00	41.00
13	33.00	36.00	35.00		63	41.00	41.00	41.00
14	34.00	36.00	35.00		64	41.00	42.00	42.00
15	34.00	37.00	36.00		65	41.00	42.00	42.00
16	34.00	37.00	36.00		66	41.00	42.00	42.00
17	35.00	37.00	36.00		67	41.00	42.00	42.00
18	35.00	37.00	36.00		68	41.00	42.00	42.00
19	35.00	38.00	37.00		69	41.00	42.00	42.00
20	35.00	38.00	37.00		70	41.00	42.00	42.00
21	36.00	38.00	37.00		71	42.00	42.00	42.00
22	36.00	38.00	37.00		72	42.00	42.00	42.00
23	36.00	38.00	38.00		73	42.00	43.00	43.00
24	36.00	38.00	38.00		74	42.00	43.00	43.00
25	36.00	39.00	38.00		75	42.00	43.00	43.00
26	37.00	39.00	38.00		76	42.00	43.00	43.00
27	37.00	39.00	38.00		77	42.00	43.00	43.00
28	37.00	39.00	38.00		78	43.00	43.00	43.00
29	37.00	39.00	39.00		79	43.00	43.00	43.00
30	37.00	39.00	39.00		80	43.00	44.00	44.00
31	38.00	39.00	39.00		81	43.00	44.00	44.00
32	38.00	39.00	39.00		82	43.00	44.00	44.00
33	38.00	39.00	39.00		83	43.00	44.00	44.00
34	38.00	39.00	39.00		84	44.00	44.00	44.00
35	38.00	40.00	39.00		85	44.00	45.00	45.00
36	38.00	40.00	39.00		86	44.00	45.00	45.00
37	38.00	40.00	39.00		87	44.00	45.00	45.00
38	39.00	40.00	39.00		88	44.00	45.00	45.00
39	39.00	40.00	40.00		89	45.00	46.00	46.00
40	39.00	40.00	40.00		90	45.00	46.00	46.00
41	39.00	40.00	40.00		91	45.00	46.00	46.00
42	39.00	40.00	40.00		92	46.00	46.00	46.00
43	39.00	40.00	40.00		93	46.00	47.00	47.00
44	39.00	40.00	40.00		94	46.00	47.00	47.00
45	39.00	40.00	40.00		95	47.00	47.00	47.00
46	39.00	40.00	40.00		96	47.00	48.00	48.00

Percentile (1-50)	Raw Score				Percentile (51-100)	Raw Score		
	Male	Female	Full sample			Male	Female	Full sample
47	40.00	40.00	40.00		97	48.00	48.00	48.00
48	40.00	40.00	40.00		98	48.00	48.00	48.00
49	40.00	40.00	40.00		99	48.00	48.00	48.00
50	40.00	40.00	40.00		100	48.00	48.00	48.00

Note. N = 1,517 for male sample, N = 2,969 for female sample, N = 4,486 for full sample.

Table 10. Raw scores and related percentiles for SLA-SF-46 (Factor 2) by gender

Raw score (≤ 29)	Percentiles			Raw score (30-39)	Percentiles			Raw score (40-48)	Percentiles		
	Male	Female	Full sample		Male	Female	Full sample		Male	Female	Full sample
≤ 20	1.0	1.0	1.0	30	7.0	2.0	4.0	40	54.0	44.0	46.0
21	2.0	1.0	1.0	31	8.0	3.0	4.0	41	66.0	59.0	59.0
22	2.0	1.0	1.0	32	10.0	5.0	5.0	42	74.0	68.0	68.0
23	2.0	1.0	1.0	33	13.0	6.0	9.0	43	81.0	76.0	76.0
24	2.0	1.0	1.0	34	15.0	8.0	11.0	44	86.0	82.0	83.0
25	2.0	1.0	1.0	35	19.0	10.0	13.0	45	90.0	87.0	87.0
26	3.0	1.0	2.0	36	23.0	13.0	17.0	46	93.0	91.0	91.0
27	3.0	1.0	2.0	37	28.0	17.0	21.0	47	96.0	94.0	94.0
28	4.0	1.0	2.0	38	34.0	22.0	26.0	48	100.0	100.0	100.0
29	5.0	2.0	3.0	39	42.0	30.0	34.0				

Note. N = 1,517 for male sample, N = 2,969 for female sample, N = 4,486 for full sample.

Table 11. Raw scores and related percentiles for SLA-SF-46 (Factor 3) by gender

Percentile (1-50)	Raw Score				Percentile (51-100)	Raw Score		
	Male	Female	Full sample			Male	Female	Full sample
1	≤ 18.00	≤ 22.00	≤ 20.00		51	34.00	34.00	34.00
2	21.00	24.00	22.74		52	34.00	34.00	34.00
3	22.00	24.10	24.00		53	34.00	34.00	34.00
4	23.00	25.00	24.00		54	34.00	34.00	34.00
5	24.00	26.00	25.00		55	34.00	34.00	34.00
6	24.08	26.00	26.00		56	34.00	35.00	34.00
7	25.00	27.00	26.00		57	34.00	35.00	34.00
8	26.00	27.00	27.00		58	34.00	35.00	35.00
9	26.00	28.00	27.00		59	34.00	35.00	35.00
10	26.00	28.00	27.00		60	34.00	35.00	35.00
11	27.00	28.00	28.00		61	34.98	35.00	35.00
12	27.00	28.00	28.00		62	35.00	35.00	35.00
13	27.00	29.00	28.00		63	35.00	35.00	35.00
14	27.00	29.00	28.00		64	35.00	35.00	35.00
15	28.00	29.00	28.00		65	35.00	35.00	35.00
16	28.00	29.00	29.00		66	35.00	35.00	35.00
17	28.00	29.00	29.00		67	35.00	35.00	35.00
18	28.00	30.00	29.00		68	35.00	35.00	35.00
19	28.00	30.00	30.00		69	35.00	35.00	35.00
20	29.00	30.00	30.00		70	35.00	35.00	35.00
21	29.00	30.00	30.00		71	35.00	35.00	35.00
22	29.00	30.00	30.00		72	35.00	35.00	35.00

Table 11. (Continued)

Percentile (1-50)	Raw Score				Percentile (51-100)	Raw Score		
	Male	Female	Full sample			Male	Female	Full sample
23	30.00	31.00	30.00		73	35.00	35.00	35.00
24	30.00	31.00	30.00		74	35.00	35.00	35.00
25	30.00	31.00	31.00		75	35.00	36.00	36.00
26	30.00	31.00	31.00		76	36.00	36.00	36.00
27	30.00	31.00	31.00		77	36.00	36.00	36.00
28	30.00	31.00	31.00		78	36.00	36.00	36.00
29	31.00	32.00	31.00		79	36.00	36.00	36.00
30	31.00	32.00	31.00		80	36.00	36.00	36.00
31	31.00	32.00	32.00		81	36.00	36.00	36.00
32	31.00	32.00	32.00		82	37.00	37.00	37.00
33	31.00	32.00	32.00		83	37.00	37.00	37.00
34	31.00	32.00	32.00		84	37.00	37.00	37.00
35	32.00	32.00	32.00		85	37.00	37.00	37.00
36	32.00	33.00	32.00		86	37.00	38.00	37.00
37	32.00	33.00	32.00		87	38.00	38.00	38.00
38	32.00	33.00	33.00		88	38.00	38.00	38.00
39	32.00	33.00	33.00		89	38.00	38.00	38.00
40	32.00	33.00	33.00		90	38.20	38.00	38.00
41	32.00	33.00	33.00		91	39.00	39.00	39.00
42	33.00	33.00	33.00		92	39.00	39.00	39.00
43	33.00	33.00	33.00		93	39.00	40.00	40.00
44	33.00	33.00	33.00		94	40.00	40.00	40.00
45	33.00	34.00	33.00		95	41.00	41.00	41.00
46	33.00	34.00	33.00		96	41.00	41.00	41.00
47	33.00	34.00	34.00		97	42.00	42.00	42.00
48	33.00	34.00	34.00		98	42.00	42.00	42.00
49	33.00	34.00	34.00		99	42.00	42.00	42.00
50	33.00	34.00	34.00		100	42.00	42.00	42.00

Note. N = 1,517 for male sample, N = 2,969 for female sample, N = 4,486 for full sample.

Table 12. Raw scores and related percentiles for SLA-SF-46 (Factor 3) by gender

Raw score (≤ 26)	Percentiles			Raw score (27-35)	Percentiles			Raw score (36-42)	Percentiles		
	Male	Female	Full sample		Male	Female	Full sample		Male	Female	Full sample
≤ 18	1.0	1.0	1.0	27	13.0	8.0	9.0	36	79.0	78.0	78.0
19	2.0	1.0	1.0	28	17.0	11.0	13.0	37	84.0	84.0	84.0
20	2.0	1.0	1.0	29	21.0	15.0	17.0	38	89.0	88.0	89.0
21	2.0	1.0	1.0	30	26.0	20.0	22.0	39	92.0	92.0	92.0
22	3.0	1.0	1.0	31	32.0	26.0	28.0	40	94.0	94.0	94.0
23	4.0	2.0	2.0	32	38.0	32.0	34.0	41	96.0	96.0	96.0
24	6.0	2.0	4.0	33	46.0	40.0	42.0	42	100.0	100.0	100.0
25	7.0	4.0	5.0	34	56.0	50.0	52.0				
26	9.0	6.0	7.0	35	68.0	65.0	66.0				

Note. *N* = 1,517 for male sample, *N* = 2,969 for female sample, *N* = 4,486 for full sample.

Table 13. Raw scores and related percentiles for SLA-SF-46 (Factor 4) by gender

Percentile	Raw Score			Percentile	Raw Score		
(1-50)	Male	Female	Full sample	(51-100)	Male	Female	Full sample
1	≤ 10.00	≤ 12.00	≤ 11.00	51	24.00	24.00	24.00
2	12.00	14.00	13.00	52	24.00	24.00	24.00
3	14.00	15.00	15.00	53	24.00	24.00	24.00
4	15.00	16.00	16.00	54	24.00	24.00	24.00
5	16.00	16.00	16.00	55	24.00	24.00	24.00
6	16.00	17.00	17.00	56	24.00	25.00	24.00
7	17.00	18.00	17.00	57	24.00	25.00	24.00
8	17.00	18.00	18.00	58	24.00	25.00	25.00
9	18.00	18.00	18.00	59	24.00	25.00	25.00
10	18.00	19.00	18.00	60	24.00	25.00	25.00
11	18.00	19.00	19.00	61	24.00	25.00	25.00
12	18.00	19.00	19.00	62	25.00	25.00	25.00
13	19.00	19.00	19.00	63	25.00	25.00	25.00
14	19.00	20.00	19.00	64	25.00	25.00	25.00
15	19.00	20.00	20.00	65	25.00	25.00	25.00
16	19.00	20.00	20.00	66	25.00	25.00	25.00
17	19.00	20.00	20.00	67	25.00	25.00	25.00
18	20.00	20.00	20.00	68	25.00	25.00	25.00
19	20.00	20.00	20.00	69	25.00	25.00	25.00
20	20.00	21.00	20.00	70	25.00	25.00	25.00
21	20.00	21.00	20.00	71	25.00	25.00	25.00
22	20.00	21.00	21.00	72	25.00	25.00	25.00
23	20.00	21.00	21.00	73	25.00	25.00	25.00
24	20.00	21.00	21.00	74	25.00	25.00	25.00
25	21.00	21.00	21.00	75	25.00	25.00	25.00
26	21.00	22.00	21.00	76	25.00	25.00	25.00
27	21.00	22.00	21.00	77	25.00	26.00	25.00
28	21.00	22.00	21.00	78	25.00	26.00	26.00
29	21.00	22.00	22.00	79	26.00	26.00	26.00
30	21.00	22.00	22.00	80	26.00	26.00	26.00
31	21.00	22.00	22.00	81	26.00	26.00	26.00
32	21.00	22.00	22.00	82	26.00	26.00	26.00
33	21.00	22.00	22.00	83	26.00	26.00	26.00
34	22.00	23.00	22.00	84	26.00	27.00	26.00
35	22.00	23.00	22.00	85	26.00	27.00	27.00
36	22.00	23.00	22.00	86	27.00	27.00	27.00
37	22.00	23.00	23.00	87	27.00	27.00	27.00
38	22.00	23.00	23.00	88	27.00	27.00	27.00
39	22.00	23.00	23.00	89	27.00	28.00	28.00
40	22.00	23.00	23.00	90	28.00	28.00	28.00
41	22.00	23.00	23.00	91	28.00	28.00	28.00
42	23.00	23.00	23.00	92	28.00	28.00	28.00
43	23.00	23.00	23.00	93	28.00	29.00	29.00
44	23.00	23.00	23.00	94	29.00	29.00	29.00
45	23.00	24.00	23.00	95	29.00	29.00	29.00
46	23.00	24.00	23.00	96	30.00	30.00	30.00

Table 13. (Continued)

Percentile (1-50)	Raw Score				Percentile (51-100)	Raw Score		
	Male	Female	Full sample			Male	Female	Full sample
47	23.00	24.00	24.00		97	30.00	30.00	30.00
48	23.00	24.00	24.00		98	30.00	30.00	30.00
49	23.00	24.00	24.00		99	30.00	30.00	30.00
50	23.00	24.00	24.00		100	30.00	30.00	30.00

Note. N = 1,517 for male sample, N = 2,969 for female sample, N = 4,486 for full sample.

Table 14. Raw scores and related percentiles for SLA-SF-46 (Factor 4) by gender

Raw score (≤ 17)	Percentiles			Raw score (18-25)	Percentiles			Raw score (26-30)	Percentiles		
	Male	Female	Full sample		Male	Female	Full sample		Male	Female	Full sample
10	1.0	1.0	1.0	18	11.0	8.0	9.0	26	82.0	80.0	81.0
11	2.0	1.0	1.0	19	15.0	12.0	13.0	27	88.0	86.0	87.0
12	2.0	1.0	2.0	20	21.0	17.0	18.0	28	92.0	91.0	91.0
13	3.0	2.0	2.0	21	29.0	23.0	25.0	29	95.0	94.0	94.0
14	3.0	2.0	3.0	22	38.0	30.0	33.0	30	100.0	100.0	100.0
15	4.0	3.0	3.0	23	46.0	39.0	42.0				
16	6.0	5.0	5.0	24	56.0	50.0	52.0				
17	8.0	6.0	7.0	25	70.0	66.0	68.0				

Note. N = 1,517 for male sample, N = 2,969 for female sample, N = 4,486 for full sample.

Table 15. Raw scores and related percentiles for SLA-SF-46 (Factor 5) by gender

Percentile (1-50)	Raw Score				Percentile (51-100)	Raw Score		
	Male	Female	Full sample			Male	Female	Full sample
1	≤ 10.00	≤ 13.00	≤ 12.00		51	20.00	21.00	20.00
2	12.00	15.00	14.00		52	20.00	21.00	20.00
3	13.00	16.00	15.00		53	20.00	21.00	20.00
4	14.00	16.00	16.00		54	20.00	21.00	20.00
5	15.00	16.00	16.00		55	20.00	21.00	21.00
6	15.00	17.00	16.00		56	20.00	21.00	21.00
7	16.00	17.00	16.00		57	20.00	21.00	21.00
8	16.00	17.00	17.00		58	20.00	21.00	21.00
9	16.00	17.00	17.00		59	20.00	21.00	21.00
10	16.00	18.00	17.00		60	20.80	21.00	21.00
11	16.00	18.00	17.00		61	21.00	21.00	21.00
12	17.00	18.00	18.00		62	21.00	21.00	21.00
13	17.00	18.00	18.00		63	21.00	21.00	21.00
14	17.00	19.00	18.00		64	21.00	21.00	21.00
15	17.00	19.00	18.00		65	21.00	22.00	21.00
16	17.00	19.00	18.00		66	21.00	22.00	21.00
17	18.00	19.00	18.00		67	21.00	22.00	21.00
18	18.00	19.00	19.00		68	21.00	22.00	22.00
19	18.00	19.00	19.00		69	21.00	22.00	22.00
20	18.00	19.00	19.00		70	21.00	22.00	22.00
21	18.00	20.00	19.00		71	21.00	22.00	22.00

Percentile	Raw Score				Percentile	Raw Score		
(1-50)	Male	Female	Full sample		(51-100)	Male	Female	Full sample
22	18.00	20.00	19.00		72	22.00	22.00	22.00
23	18.00	20.00	19.00		73	22.00	22.00	22.00
24	18.00	20.00	19.00		74	22.00	22.00	22.00
25	19.00	20.00	19.00		75	22.00	22.00	22.00
26	19.00	20.00	20.00		76	22.00	22.00	22.00
27	19.00	20.00	20.00		77	22.00	23.00	22.00
28	19.00	20.00	20.00		78	22.00	23.00	22.00
29	19.00	20.00	20.00		79	22.00	23.00	23.00
30	19.00	20.00	20.00		80	22.00	23.00	23.00
31	19.00	20.00	20.00		81	22.00	23.00	23.00
32	19.00	20.00	20.00		82	22.00	23.00	23.00
33	19.00	20.00	20.00		83	23.00	23.00	23.00
34	19.00	20.00	20.00		84	23.00	23.00	23.00
35	19.00	20.00	20.00		85	23.00	23.00	23.00
36	20.00	20.00	20.00		86	23.00	23.00	23.00
37	20.00	20.00	20.00		87	23.00	23.00	23.00
38	20.00	20.00	20.00		88	23.00	24.00	23.00
39	20.00	20.00	20.00		89	23.00	24.00	24.00
40	20.00	20.00	20.00		90	23.00	24.00	24.00
41	20.00	20.00	20.00		91	24.00	24.00	24.00
42	20.00	20.00	20.00		92	24.00	24.00	24.00
43	20.00	20.00	20.00		93	24.00	24.00	24.00
44	20.00	20.00	20.00		94	24.00	24.00	24.00
45	20.00	20.00	20.00		95	24.00	24.00	24.00
46	20.00	20.00	20.00		96	24.00	24.00	24.00
47	20.00	20.00	20.00		97	24.00	24.00	24.00
48	20.00	20.00	20.00		98	24.00	24.00	24.00
49	20.00	20.00	20.00		99	24.00	24.00	24.00
50	20.00	20.00	20.00		100	24.00	24.00	24.00

Note. N = 1,517 for male sample, N = 2,969 for female sample, N = 4,486 for full sample.

Table 16. Raw scores and related percentiles for SLA-SF-46 (Factor 5) by gender

Raw score	Percentiles			Raw	Percentiles			Raw	Percentiles		
(≤ 15)	Male	Female	Full sample	score (16-21)	Male	Female	Full sample	score (22-24)	Male	Female	Full sample
10	1.0	1.0	1.0	16	9.0	4.0	6.0	22	77.0	71.0	73.0
11	2.0	1.0	1.0	17	14.0	8.0	10.0	23	87.0	82.0	84.0
12	2.0	1.0	1.0	18	21.0	12.0	15.0	24	100.0	100.0	100.0
13	3.0	1.0	2.0	19	30.0	17.0	22.0				
14	4.0	2.0	2.0	20	47.0	36.0	40.0				
15	6.0	2.0	3.0	21	66.0	58.0	61.0				

Note. N = 1,517 for male sample, N = 2,969 for female sample, N = 4,486 for full sample.

Table 17. Raw scores and related percentiles for SLA-SF-46 (Factor 6) by gender

Percentile (1-50)	Raw Score				Percentile (51-100)	Raw Score		
	Male	Female	Full sample			Male	Female	Full sample
1	≤ 12.00	≤ 16.00	≤ 14.00		51	25.00	25.00	25.00
2	15.36	17.40	17.00		52	25.00	25.00	25.00
3	17.00	18.00	18.00		53	25.00	25.00	25.00
4	18.00	19.00	18.00		54	25.00	25.00	25.00
5	18.00	19.00	19.00		55	25.00	25.00	25.00
6	19.00	20.00	19.00		56	25.00	25.00	25.00
7	19.00	20.00	20.00		57	25.00	25.00	25.00
8	19.00	20.00	20.00		58	25.00	25.00	25.00
9	20.00	20.00	20.00		59	25.00	25.00	25.00
10	20.00	21.00	20.00		60	25.00	25.00	25.00
11	20.00	21.00	20.00		61	25.00	25.00	25.00
12	20.00	21.00	21.00		62	25.00	25.00	25.00
13	20.00	21.00	21.00		63	25.00	25.00	25.00
14	20.00	21.00	21.00		64	25.00	25.00	25.00
15	20.00	22.00	21.00		65	25.00	25.00	25.00
16	21.00	22.00	21.00		66	25.00	25.00	25.00
17	21.00	22.00	22.00		67	25.00	25.00	25.00
18	21.00	22.00	22.00		68	25.00	25.60	25.00
19	21.00	22.00	22.00		69	25.00	26.00	26.00
20	21.00	22.00	22.00		70	26.00	26.00	26.00
21	22.00	23.00	22.00		71	26.00	26.00	26.00
22	22.00	23.00	22.00		72	26.00	26.00	26.00
23	22.00	23.00	23.00		73	26.00	26.00	26.00
24	22.00	23.00	23.00		74	26.00	26.00	26.00
25	22.00	23.00	23.00		75	26.00	26.00	26.00
26	22.00	23.00	23.00		76	26.00	26.00	26.00
27	22.00	23.00	23.00		77	26.00	26.00	26.00
28	23.00	23.00	23.00		78	26.00	27.00	26.00
29	23.00	23.00	23.00		79	26.00	27.00	27.00
30	23.00	23.00	23.00		80	27.00	27.00	27.00
31	23.00	24.00	23.00		81	27.00	27.00	27.00
32	23.00	24.00	23.00		82	27.00	27.00	27.00
33	23.00	24.00	24.00		83	27.00	27.00	27.00
34	23.00	24.00	24.00		84	27.00	27.00	27.00
35	23.00	24.00	24.00		85	27.00	28.00	27.00
36	23.00	24.00	24.00		86	27.00	28.00	28.00
37	24.00	24.00	24.00		87	28.00	28.00	28.00
38	24.00	24.00	24.00		88	28.00	28.00	28.00
39	24.00	24.00	24.00		89	28.00	28.00	28.00
40	24.00	24.00	24.00		90	28.00	28.00	28.00
41	24.00	24.00	24.00		91	28.00	29.00	28.00
42	24.00	24.00	24.00		92	29.00	29.00	29.00
43	24.00	24.00	24.00		93	29.00	29.00	29.00
44	24.00	24.00	24.00		94	29.00	29.00	29.00
45	24.00	24.50	24.00		95	29.00	29.00	29.00
46	24.00	25.00	24.00		96	30.00	30.00	30.00
47	24.00	25.00	25.00		97	30.00	30.00	30.00
48	24.00	25.00	25.00		98	30.00	30.00	30.00

Percentile	Raw Score				Percentile	Raw Score		
(1-50)	Male	Female	Full sample		(51-100)	Male	Female	Full sample
49	24.00	25.00	25.00		99	30.00	30.00	30.00
50	25.00	25.00	25.00		100	30.00	30.00	30.00

Note. N = 1,517 for male sample, N = 2,969 for female sample, N = 4,486 for full sample.

Table 18. Raw scores and related percentiles for SLA-SF-46 (Factor 6) by gender

Raw score	Percentiles			Raw	Percentiles			Raw	Percentiles		
(≤ 18)	Male	Female	Full sample	score (19-25)	Male	Female	Full sample	score (26-30)	Male	Female	Full sample
12	1.0	1.0	1.0	19	7.0	5.0	6.0	26	75.0	73.0	74.0
13	2.0	1.0	1.0	20	12.0	8.0	9.0	27	83.0	81.0	82.0
14	2.0	1.0	1.0	21	18.0	12.0	14.0	28	89.0	88.0	89.0
15	2.0	1.0	2.0	22	24.0	18.0	20.0	29	94.0	93.0	94.0
16	3.0	1.0	2.0	23	32.0	26.0	28.0	30	100.0	100.0	100.0
17	3.0	2.0	2.0	24	44.0	38.0	40.0				
18	5.0	3.0	4.0	25	60.0	56.0	58.0				

Note. N = 1,517 for male sample, N = 2,969 for female sample, N = 4,486 for full sample.

Table 19. Raw scores and related percentiles for SLA-SF-46 (Factor 7) by gender

Percentile	Raw Score				Percentile	Raw Score		
(1-50)	Male	Female	Full sample		(51-100)	Male	Female	Full sample
1	≤ 2.00	≤ 3.00	≤ 3.00		51	9.00	9.00	9.00
2	3.00	4.00	4.00		52	9.00	9.00	9.00
3	3.00	4.10	4.00		53	9.00	9.00	9.00
4	4.00	5.00	4.00		54	9.00	9.00	9.00
5	4.00	5.00	5.00		55	9.00	9.00	9.00
6	4.00	5.00	5.00		56	9.00	9.00	9.00
7	4.00	6.00	5.00		57	9.00	9.00	9.00
8	5.00	6.00	5.00		58	9.00	10.00	9.00
9	5.00	6.00	6.00		59	9.00	10.00	9.00
10	5.00	6.00	6.00		60	9.00	10.00	10.00
11	5.00	6.00	6.00		61	9.00	10.00	10.00
12	6.00	6.00	6.00		62	9.00	10.00	10.00
13	6.00	6.00	6.00		63	9.00	10.00	10.00
14	6.00	6.00	6.00		64	10.00	10.00	10.00
15	6.00	7.00	6.00		65	10.00	10.00	10.00
16	6.00	7.00	6.00		66	10.00	10.00	10.00
17	6.00	7.00	7.00		67	10.00	10.00	10.00
18	6.00	7.00	7.00		68	10.00	10.00	10.00
19	6.00	7.00	7.00		69	10.00	10.00	10.00
20	7.00	7.00	7.00		70	10.00	10.00	10.00
21	7.00	7.00	7.00		71	10.00	10.00	10.00
22	7.00	7.00	7.00		72	10.00	10.00	10.00
23	7.00	7.00	7.00		73	10.00	10.00	10.00
24	7.00	7.00	7.00		74	10.00	10.00	10.00
25	7.00	8.00	7.00		75	10.00	10.00	10.00
26	7.00	8.00	7.00		76	10.00	10.00	10.00

Table 19. (Continued)

Percentile (1-50)	Raw Score				Percentile (51-100)	Raw Score		
	Male	Female	Full sample			Male	Female	Full sample
27	7.00	8.00	8.00		77	10.00	10.00	10.00
28	7.00	8.00	8.00		78	10.00	10.00	10.00
29	7.00	8.00	8.00		79	10.00	10.00	10.00
30	8.00	8.00	8.00		80	10.00	10.00	10.00
31	8.00	8.00	8.00		81	10.00	10.00	10.00
32	8.00	8.00	8.00		82	10.00	10.00	10.00
33	8.00	8.00	8.00		83	10.00	10.00	10.00
34	8.00	8.00	8.00		84	10.00	11.00	10.00
35	8.00	8.00	8.00		85	10.00	11.00	11.00
36	8.00	8.00	8.00		86	10.00	11.00	11.00
37	8.00	8.00	8.00		87	11.00	11.00	11.00
38	8.00	8.00	8.00		88	11.00	11.00	11.00
39	8.00	8.00	8.00		89	11.00	11.00	11.00
40	8.00	8.00	8.00		90	11.00	11.00	11.00
41	8.00	8.00	8.00		91	11.00	11.00	11.00
42	8.00	9.00	8.00		92	11.00	11.00	11.00
43	8.00	9.00	8.00		93	11.00	12.00	12.00
44	8.00	9.00	9.00		94	12.00	12.00	12.00
45	8.00	9.00	9.00		95	12.00	12.00	12.00
46	8.00	9.00	9.00		96	12.00	12.00	12.00
47	8.00	9.00	9.00		97	12.00	12.00	12.00
48	9.00	9.00	9.00		98	12.00	12.00	12.00
49	9.00	9.00	9.00		99	12.00	12.00	12.00
50	9.00	9.00	9.00		100	12.00	12.00	12.00

Note. N = 1,517 for male sample, N = 2,969 for female sample, N = 4,486 for full sample.

Table 20. Raw scores and related percentiles for SLA-SF-46 (Factor 7) by gender

Raw score (≤ 5)	Percentiles			Raw score (6-9)	Percentiles			Raw score (10-12)	Percentiles		
	Male	Female	Full sample		Male	Female	Full sample		Male	Female	Full sample
2	1.0	1.0	1.0	6	16.0	11.0	13.0	10	75.0	71.0	72.0
3	3.0	1.0	1.0	7	25.0	20.0	22.0	11	90.0	88.0	89.0
4	6.0	3.0	3.0	8	39.0	33.0	35.0	12	100.0	100.0	100.0
5	10.0	5.0	7.0	9	56.0	50.0	52.0				

Note. N = 1,517 for male sample, N = 2,969 for female sample, N = 4,486 for full sample.

Table 21. Raw scores and related percentiles for SLA-SF-46 (Factor 8) by gender

Percentile (1-50)	Raw Score				Percentile (51-100)	Raw Score		
	Male	Female	Full sample			Male	Female	Full sample
1	≤ 5.00	≤ 6.00	≤ 6.00		51	16.00	16.00	16.00
2	7.00	8.00	7.00		52	16.00	16.00	16.00
3	8.00	9.00	8.00		53	16.00	16.00	16.00
4	8.00	9.00	9.00		54	16.00	17.00	16.00
5	9.00	9.00	9.00		55	16.00	17.00	16.00

Percentile	Raw Score				Percentile	Raw Score		
(1-50)	Male	Female	Full sample		(51-100)	Male	Female	Full sample
6	9.00	10.00	9.00		56	16.00	17.00	17.00
7	9.00	10.00	10.00		57	16.00	17.00	17.00
8	9.00	10.00	10.00		58	17.00	17.00	17.00
9	10.00	10.00	10.00		59	17.00	17.00	17.00
10	10.00	10.00	10.00		60	17.00	17.00	17.00
11	10.00	10.00	10.00		61	17.00	18.00	17.00
12	10.00	10.00	10.00		62	17.00	18.00	17.00
13	10.00	11.00	10.00		63	17.00	18.00	18.00
14	10.00	11.00	11.00		64	17.00	18.00	18.00
15	10.00	11.00	11.00		65	18.00	18.00	18.00
16	10.00	11.00	11.00		66	18.00	18.00	18.00
17	11.00	11.00	11.00		67	18.00	18.00	18.00
18	11.00	11.00	11.00		68	18.00	18.00	18.00
19	11.00	12.00	11.00		69	18.00	19.00	18.00
20	11.00	12.00	12.00		70	18.00	19.00	19.00
21	11.00	12.00	12.00		71	18.00	19.00	19.00
22	11.00	12.00	12.00		72	19.00	19.00	19.00
23	11.00	12.00	12.00		73	19.00	19.00	19.00
24	12.00	13.00	12.00		74	19.00	19.00	19.00
25	12.00	13.00	12.00		75	19.00	19.00	19.00
26	12.00	13.00	13.00		76	19.00	20.00	19.00
27	12.00	13.00	13.00		77	19.00	20.00	20.00
28	12.00	13.00	13.00		78	19.00	20.00	20.00
29	12.00	13.00	13.00		79	20.00	20.00	20.00
30	12.40	13.00	13.00		80	20.00	20.00	20.00
31	13.00	14.00	13.00		81	20.00	20.00	20.00
32	13.00	14.00	13.00		82	20.00	21.00	20.00
33	13.00	14.00	14.00		83	20.00	21.00	21.00
34	13.00	14.00	14.00		84	20.00	21.00	21.00
35	13.30	14.00	14.00		85	21.00	21.00	21.00
36	14.00	14.00	14.00		86	21.00	21.00	21.00
37	14.00	14.00	14.00		87	21.00	21.00	21.00
38	14.00	15.00	14.00		88	21.00	22.00	21.56
39	14.00	15.00	14.00		89	21.00	22.00	22.00
40	14.00	15.00	15.00		90	22.00	22.00	22.00
41	14.00	15.00	15.00		91	22.00	22.00	22.00
42	15.00	15.00	15.00		92	22.00	23.00	23.00
43	15.00	15.00	15.00		93	22.74	23.00	23.00
44	15.00	15.00	15.00		94	23.00	23.00	23.00
45	15.00	15.00	15.00		95	24.00	24.00	24.00
46	15.00	15.00	15.00		96	24.00	24.00	24.00
47	15.00	16.00	15.00		97	25.00	25.00	25.00
48	15.00	16.00	16.00		98	25.00	25.00	25.00
49	15.00	16.00	16.00		99	27.00	26.00	27.00
50	15.00	16.00	16.00		100	30.00	30.00	30.00

Note. N = 1,517 for male sample, N = 2,969 for female sample, N = 4,486 for full sample.

Table 22. Raw scores and related percentiles for SLA-SF-46 (Factor 8) by gender

Raw score (≤ 13)	Percentiles			Raw score (14-22)	Percentiles			Raw score (23-30)	Percentiles		
	Male	Female	Full sample		Male	Female	Full sample		Male	Female	Full sample
5	1.0	1.0	1.0	14	39.0	34.0	36.0	23	94.0	93.0	93.0
6	2.0	1.0	1.0	15	46.0	42.0	44.0	24	96.0	96.0	96.0
7	2.0	2.0	2.0	16	54.0	50.0	52.0	25	98.0	98.0	98.0
8	4.0	2.0	3.0	17	61.0	57.0	59.0	26	99.0	99.0	99.0
9	7.0	4.0	5.0	18	68.0	65.0	66.0	27	99.0	99.0	99.0
10	13.0	9.0	10.0	19	75.0	72.0	73.0	28	99.0	99.0	99.0
11	20.0	16.0	17.0	20	82.0	79.0	80.0	29	99.0	99.0	99.0
12	27.0	21.0	23.0	21	87.0	85.0	85.0	30	100.0	100.0	100.0
13	33.0	28.0	29.0	22	91.0	90.0	90.0				

Note. N = 1,517 for male sample, N = 2,969 for female sample, N = 4,486 for full sample.

SCORING AND INTERPRETATION

The SLA-SF-46 has 46 items operating on eight content specific subscales. The score of each subscale is calculated by summing up the scores of respective items. The total score of service leadership attitude is calculated by summing up the scores of all eight subscales. It has the property of having a minimum score of 46 and a maximum score of 276.

Handling of missing items

The satisfactory internal consistency is conditioned on that all items in a subscale or full scale have been completed. When there are missing values in any subscale, the responses should be interpreted with caution. The responses with missing value(s) should not be adopted for analysis or appropriate methods should be used for computing missing value(s) before doing further analyses.

Interpretation of test scores

Interpretation of SLA-SF-46 test scores can be based on the score of full scale or each subscale. The score of full scale shows how favorable the core value of contemporary service leadership is viewed by participant, while the score of each subscale reflects his/her perception of specific service leadership quality. For example, a high score of "ethical role model" subscale indicates a strong belief that a service leader must take a leading role in setting ethical standards.

As mentioned before, Tables 5-22 present percentile norms for the score of full scale and each subscale. Percentile rank scores represent the percentage of people in the normative sample (full sample or sub-samples) who scored at or below a particular raw score for a particular measure (full scale or subscales). In other words, a percentile rank score informs the relative position of one's score in relation to his/her relevant group. For example, if a male college student wants to surpass 20% of his male peers in developing positive service leadership attitude, he needs to get at least 194 points (see Table 5). Likewise, if a male college student gets 214 points for full scale, he has already surpassed half of all male students (see Table 6).

When interpreting test scores, we do not intend to define a cut-off value for determining positive versus negative attitude toward service leadership. Thus, "positive attitude" and "negative attitude" are not suggested to be adopted to differentiate people with different attitude. Researchers or program evaluators may locate the score of a student into the norm tables to determine his/her comparative position regarding service leadership attitude, and use "less positive than the normative sample," "similar to the normative sample," or "more positive than the normative sample" to conclude different levels of service leadership attitude. Furthermore, when evaluating the effectiveness of a specific service leadership education program, evaluators are suggested to compare participants' attitude scores obtained before and after they receive the program. In this case, mean scores could be used without making reference to the norm tables.

ACKNOWLEDGMENTS

The validation project is financially supported by the Victor and William Fung Foundation. The preparation for this chapter is supported by the Foundation and the Endowed Professorship in Service Leadership Education at The Hong Kong Polytechnic University.

REFERENCES

[1] Census and Statistics Department. Hong Kong Annual Digest of Statistics. Hong Kong: Hong Kong Government Printer, 2017.

[2] Hong Kong Institute of Service Leadership and Management. Service leadership definitions. Hong Kong: Hong Kong Institute of Service Leadership and Management Limited, 2013. URL: http://hki-slam.org/index.php?r=article&catid=1&aid=11.

[3] Shek DTL, Lin L. Core beliefs in the service leadership model proposed by the Hong Kong Institute of Service Leadership and Management. Int J Disabil Hum Dev 2015;14(3):233-42.

[4] Chung PPY, Elfassy R. The 12 dimensions of a service leader. New York: Lexingford; 2016.

[5] Shek DTL, Ma CMS, Liu TT, Siu AMH. The role of self-leadership in service leadership. Int J Disabil Hum Dev 2015;14:343-50.

[6] Shek DTL, Lin L, Leung H, Yu L, Ma CMS, Li X. Content validation of the service leadership attitude scale [Reprint]. In: Shek DTL, Chung PPY, Lin L, Merrick J, eds. Service leadership education for university students. New York: Nova Science, 2017: 205–26.

[7] Claar V, Jackson L, TenHaken V. Are servant leaders born or made? Servant Leadersh Theory Pract 2016;1(1):46-52.

[8] Pandya T, Dirks R, Kwok A. Leaders are made, not born: A leadership development curriculum for general surgery residents. J Am Coll Surg 2017;225(4):e154-5.

[9] Fitzgerald L, Ferlie E, McGivern G, Buchanan D. Distributed leadership patterns and service improvement: Evidence and argument from English healthcare. Leadersh Q 2013;24(1):227-239.

[10] Chuang SH, Lin HN. Co-creating e-service innovations: Theory, practice, and impact on firm performance. Int J Inf Manag 2015;35(3):277-91.

[11] Shek DTL, Zhu AYF, Ma LK, Lin L. Validation of the Service Leadership Attitude Scale in Hong Kong. Int J Child Adolesc health, in press.

[12] Wong CS, Law KS. The effects of leader and follower emotional intelligence on performance and attitude: An exploratory study. Leadersh Q 2002;13: 243-274.

[13] Wang H, Tsui AS, Xin KR. CEO leadership behaviors, organizational performance, and employees' attitudes. Leadersh Q 2011;22(1):92-105.

[14] Page D, Wong PTP. A conceptual framework for measuring servant-leadership. In: Adjibolosoo S, ed. The human factor in shaping the course of history and development. New York: University Press of America, 2000:69-109.

[15] Ma CMS, Shek DTL. Development of the attitude to service leadership scale in Hong Kong. Int J Child Adolesc health, in press.

[16] Shek DTL, Wu J, Chan BYB. The Service Leadership Attitude Scale: Normative data and personal correlates in Chinese university students. Int J Child Adolesc health, in press.

In: Service Leadership
Editors: Daniel TL Shek, Xiaoqin Zhu, Li Lin et al.
ISBN: 978-1-53614-852-7

Chapter 16

A USER MANUAL FOR THE SERVICE LEADERSHIP BEHAVIOR SCALE

Daniel TL Shek[1-6,*], PhD, FHKPS, BBS, SBS, JP, Xiaoqin Zhu[1], PhD and Diya Dou[1], PhD

[1]Department of Applied Social Sciences,
The Hong Kong Polytechnic University, Hong Kong, PR China
[2]Centre for Innovative Programmes for Adolescents and Families,
The Hong Kong Polytechnic University, Hong Kong, PR China
[3]Department of Social Work, East China Normal University, Shanghai, PR China
[4]Kiang Wu Nursing College of Macau, Macau, PR China
[5]Hong Kong Institute of Service Leadership and Management Limited,
Hong Kong, PR China
[6]Division of Adolescent Medicine, Department of Pediatrics,
Kentucky Children's Hospital, University of Kentucky School of Medicine,
Lexington, Kentucky, US

ABSTRACT

The rapid development of service economies calls for validated tools measuring service leadership qualities. In view of the dearth of measures of leadership behaviors in the service economies, the Service Leadership Behavior Scale was developed to assess service leaders' leadership skills and practices based on the Service Leadership Theory, which defines effective leadership behavior in service economies. With an initial item pool of 97 items,

[*] Correspondence: Daniel TL Shek, PhD, FHKPS, BBS, SBS, JP, Associate Vice President (Undergraduate Programme), Chair Professor of Applied Social Sciences and Li and Fung Professor in Service Leadership Education, Department of Applied Social Sciences, The Hong Kong Polytechnic University, Hung Hom, Hong Kong, PR China. E-mail: daniel.shek@polyu.edu.hk.

the final scale was trimmed to 38 items after several validation studies, which demonstrated very good psychometric properties. In this chapter, we briefly introduce the background of the development of the Service Leadership Behavior Scale and its related conceptual framework. In addition, validation process, reliability and validity of the scale, norm statistics, and guidelines for administrating the scale and interpreting scores are outlined as well.

INTRODUCTION

In recent decades, there is rapid development of the service sector in industrialized economies worldwide (1). Service economy has become the leading contributor to local GDP in many countries and areas. For example, Hong Kong is regarded as a highly developed service economy with a significant portion of service sector contributing to the local economic development. It is argued that the prosperity of Hong Kong fundamentally relies on the success of the service sector (2).

The growth of service economy calls for strong leadership to adjust organization to respond to turbulent and complex environments. Among the various leadership models, service leadership has attracted increasing attention in response to a call for more ethical and people-focused leadership style associated with the rise of the service economy. According to Service Leadership Theory proposed by Po Chung (3), service leadership is about "satisfying needs by consistently providing quality personal service to everyone one comes into contact with, including one's self, others, groups, communities, systems, and environments." Service Leadership Theory is unique because it integrates three key attributes of effective leadership required by service economy: competence, moral character, and caring disposition.

To develop future leaders and citizens with service mindset and attributes qualities, the Victor and William Fung Foundation funded the Service Leadership Initiative in eight government-funded universities in Hong Kong from 2012 to 2015. To strengthen the assessment component of the service leadership education initiative, assessment tools have subsequently been developed and validated to evaluate service leadership attributes and the impact of service leadership education. In particular, three scales were developed to evaluate the attitude, knowledge, and behavior of students' service leadership.

This manual introduces the development, validation, and usage of the finalized 38-item version of behavior scale (i.e., SLB-SF-38). It is useful for academics, practitioners, and researchers who are concerned about the evaluation of leadership behavior and the effectiveness of training programme aiming at promoting desired leadership behavior. This manual also provides evidence showing that the Service Leadership Behavior Scale is a reliable and valid tool. Normative data can be used for interpreting raw scores and group comparison. Some suggestions and directions of interpretation of the results are also discussed.

CONCEPTUAL FRAMEWORK

Based on the Service Leadership Theory and its unique propositions such as the emphasis on character and caring behaviors (i.e., not just leadership skills), the Service Leadership Behavior Scale was developed with reference to four fundamental areas as briefly outlined in the following paragraphs. Detailed elaborations can be found elsewhere (4, 5).

The first area is "service provision" describing an individual's people- and service-oriented mindset of providing high-quality and personalized services. Effective service leaders are expected to be sensitive to others' needs and be willing to transcend one's own interests to satisfy the needs of others and society.

The second area is pertinent to key skills intrinsic for an effective service leader. In particular, effective service leaders possess not only "competence" but also "character" and "care" (i.e., the 3Cs). Competence includes both intrapersonal and interpersonal competence (6, 7). Intrapersonal competence covers a wide range of human intellectual abilities related to processing information and understanding and managing oneself and others. Shek and Lin (6) highlighted four types of intelligence particularly reflecting intrapersonal competence, which include intelligence quotient (IQ), emotional quotient (EQ), adversity quotient (AQ), and spiritual quotient (SQ). In addition to intrapersonal competence, effective service leaders should also be capable of forming and maintaining positive relationships, collaborating and communicating effectively with people, and being assertive and solving conflicts in a constructive way. All these skills are considered interpersonal competence. Regarding the second C (i.e., character), a good service leader is expected to lead oneself and others with moral values that are universally upheld, such as integrity, humility, and fairness (8). For the third C (i.e., care), it is argued that a good service leader should be a caring leader who cares about others' interests and wellness in terms of showing empathy and compassion, loving others, being supportive, and helping others to have better development (9).

The third area is related to continuous improvement. Service Leadership Theory stresses that one should continuously improve oneself for better providing services to others and systems. To improve one's competence and willingness to serve, an effective service leader should promote self-leadership through active self-reflection and life-long learning.

The last area highlights the importance of distributed leadership. First, a good service leader maintains shared decision-making by encouraging every teammate to voice out and take initiatives. Second, a quality service leader also respects their followers' views and recognizes their contributions. Third, a good service leader is expected to trust his or her followers' abilities and help them to maximize their potentials and grow to good service leaders as well.

DIFFERENT STAGES OF THE VALIDATION PROCESS

The Service Leadership Behavior Scale is one of the three assessment tools evaluating service leadership education and related leadership qualities. With the financial support from the Victor and William Fung Foundation, The Hong Kong Polytechnic University (PolyU) led the collaboration with other seven government-funded universities in Hong Kong for carrying out validation studies on the attitude, knowledge, and behavior scales of service leadership. To develop the behavior scale, several stages were involved in the process:

Stage 1: The original 97-item Long-Form Service Leadership Behavior Scale (SLB-LF-97) was developed with reference to the conceptual framework of the Service Leadership Theory.

Stage 2: A study investigating the content validity of SLB-LF-97 was first conducted (4). Ratings from three experts suggested that the SLB-LF-97 has good content validity indexed by clarity, relevance, and representativeness of each item.

Stage 3: The SLB-LF-97 was further validated and streamlined through an initial validation study involving 231 university students (10). According to the results of exploratory factor analysis (EFA), 65 of the original 97 items were retained to form a short-form behavior scale (i.e., SLB-SF-65), which had a 12-dimension structure. The SLB-SF-65 demonstrated good reliability and convergent validity.

Stage 4: To further refine the behavior scale, a large-scale validation study ($N = 4{,}486$) was jointly carried out in the eight government-funded universities in Hong Kong. EFA based on a half-dataset ($N = 2{,}246$) suggested a new 48-item short form (SLB-SF-48) which consisted of six subscales (11).

Stage 5: Based on the other half-dataset ($N = 2{,}240$), a confirmatory factor analysis (CFA) was used to finalize the SLB-SF-48. Informed by CFA, 38 items were kept in the finalized behavior scale (SLB-SF-38), which also possessed a 6-factor structure. This finalized behavior scale and its six subscales showed good internal consistency and convergent validity. Detailed information is summarized in Section 5 of this manual.

DESIGN AND USE OF THE SCALE

Some items of the Service Leadership Behavior Scale were modified from existing scale items related to leadership behaviors (12, 13). Other items were developed by the research team based on the conceptual framework and propositions related to Service Leadership Theory (14). The six factors of the finalized behavior scale (i.e., SLB-SF-38) are described below:

- Factor 1: Self-improvement and self-reflection (9 items). A hypothetical sample item is "I have a habit of reflecting my work and life."
- Factor 2: People and principles orientation (9 items). A hypothetical sample item is "I allow others to decide how to get things done."
- Factor 3: Resilience (7 items). A hypothetical sample item is "I usually become stronger instead of weaker when facing adversity such as failures and setbacks."
- Factor 4: Social competence (5 items). A hypothetical sample item is "I can maintain positive relationships with others."
- Factor 5: Problem-solving (5 items). A hypothetical sample item is "I am good at independent thinking."
- Factor 6: Mentorship (3 items). A hypothetical sample item is "I can facilitate other's growth by mentoring them."

Target respondents

The SLB-SF-38 can be used to assess the service leadership behavior of university students or employees in different Chinese communities (e.g., Hong Kong, Taiwan, and mainland China). Noteworthy, local norms need to be constructed when the scale is used in a context other than Hong Kong, because the normative data reported in this manual were derived from a university student sample in Hong Kong.

Instructions

The SLB-SF-38 is administrated in a self-report manual in English. Formal written consent should be obtained from respondents. Instructions are outlined at the beginning of the questionnaire for participants to follow.

In general, respondents can complete the whole questionnaire without a specific time limit. On average, a respondent can complete the scale within 15-20 minutes. In principle, participants should return the completed questionnaire to test administrator. Taking the questionnaire out of the administration venue is not normally allowed.

Administration guidelines

The test administrator should observe the following principles:

1) Respondents should complete the questionnaire independently. Discussion and communication on scale items among participants are not allowed.
2) Field administrators can give explanations on grammars or meaning of scale items if respondents have difficulties in understanding any specific words or phrases. However, respondents need to complete all times based on their own understanding.
3) In addition to full-scale, subscale(s) can be used independently if all items of the subscale(s) are included without any omission.
4) The same rating scale (i.e., 6-point Likert scale) should be used.
5) SLB-SF-38 can be administered using paper-and-pencil or online questionnaire. If paper-and-pencil administration is applied, the completed questionnaire should be collected by testers on-site in a confidential manner.

RELIABILITY AND VALIDITY

The reliability and validity of SLB-SF-38 were investigated in the aforementioned large-scale validation study using a normative sample (*N* = 4,486) (11, 15). Related findings are briefly outlined below.

Internal consistency/reliability

SLB-SF-38 and its six subscales demonstrated good internal consistency. Cronbach's alphas of the full-scale and subscales ranged from .85 to .96. The mean inter-item correlations across scale/subscales ranged between .38 and .65 (see Table 1).

Table 1. Internal consistency of SLB-SF-38 and its subscales

Scale/subscale	No. of items	Cronbach's alpha	Mean Inter-Item Correlations
Self-improvement and self-reflection	9	.91	.53
People and principles orientation	9	.87	.42
Resilience	7	.87	.50
Social competence	5	.86	.55
Problem-solving	5	.87	.56
Mentorship	3	.85	.65
Full scale	38	.96	.38

Convergent validity

SLB-SF-38 showed good convergent validity. First, the full-scale and its six subscales significantly correlated with each other (see Table 2). Second, as shown in Table 3, there were significant correlations between full-scale/subscales and the eight external criterion scales (e.g., the knowledge and attitude to service leadership, moral self-concept, and leadership efficacy).

Table 2. Inter-factor correlations of finalized behavior scale/subscales

	F1	F2	F3	F4	F5	F6
F1: Self-improvement and self-reflection	--					
F2: People and principles orientation	.70***	--				
F3: Resilience	.61***	.57***	--			
F4: Social competence	.61***	.69***	.62***	--		
F5: Problem-solving	.58***	.50***	.60***	.50***	--	
F6: Mentorship	.56***	.58***	.50***	.48***	.43***	--
Full scale	.87***	.86***	.82***	.80***	.74***	.70***

Note. F1 = Factor 1, F2 = Factor 2, F3 = Factor 3, F4 = Factor 4, F5 = Factor 5, F6 = Factor 6. *** $p < .001$.

Table 3. Correlations between finalized behavior scale/subscales and external criterion constructs

	SLK-SF-40	SLA-SF-46	RSLP	MSC	LEF	IRI	IRI-EC	IRI-PT
SLB-SF-38	.18***	.57***	.79***	.65***	.52***	.42***	.30***	.45***
SLB-SF-38-F1	.23***	.51***	.69***	.58***	.43***	.37***	.26***	.39***
SLB-SF-38-F2	.27***	.62***	.77***	.69***	.37***	.54***	.43***	.52***
SLB-SF-38-F3	.05**	.37***	.57***	.43***	.44***	.22***	.11***	.29***
SLB-SF-38-F4	.21***	.50***	.63***	.59***	.46***	.41***	.32***	.40***
SLB-SF-38-F5	.12***	.37***	.49***	.37***	.45***	.19***	.10***	.25***
SLB-SF-38-F6	-.10***	.32***	.63***	.43***	.40***	.25***	.16***	.28***

Note. SLK-SF-40: Finalized Service Leadership Knowledge Scale (40 items); SLB-SF-38: Finalized Service Leadership Behavior Scale (38 items); SLA-SF-46: Finalized Service Leadership Attitude Scale (46 items). RSLP: Revised Servant Leadership Profile; MSC: Moral Self-Concept; LEF: Leadership Efficacy; IRI: Interpersonal Reactivity Index; EC: IRI- Empathic Concern; PT: IRI- Perspective Taking. SLB-38-F1: Self-improvement and self-reflection; SLB-38-F2: People and principles orientation; SLB-38-F3: Resilience; SLB-38-F4: Social competence; SLB-38-F5: Problem-solving; SLB-38-F6: Mentorship. **$p < .01$, *** $p < .001$.

Factorial validity

Results of CFA based on the normative sample ($N = 4{,}486$) suggested a good fit of the 6-factor structure of SLB-SF-38 (CFI = .91, TLI = .90, RMSEA = .055, 90% CI = [.054, .056]). As shown in Table 4, factor loadings were between .51 and .86.

More detailed findings of different validation studies aforementioned can be found in publications on the background and conceptual model of the scale (5), content valuation (4), the initial validation study (10), factorial and convergent validity of SLB-SF-48 based on EFA (11) and a manuscript in preparation which attempts to report findings of CFA and psychometric properties of the finalized behavior scale (SLB-SF-38). Additionally, percentile norms and personal correlates of service leadership behavior regarding the full scale of SLB-SF-38 have also been presented by Shek and collaborators (15). Norms of SLB-SF-38 with reference to the full scale and its subscales will be outlined in the following section.

Table 4. Confirmatory Factor Analysis loadings

Item	Factor loading	Item	Factor loading
Self-improvement and self-reflection 1	.73	Resilience 2	.71
Self-improvement and self-reflection 2	.67	Resilience 3	.76
Self-improvement and self-reflection 3	.65	Resilience 4	.77
Self-improvement and self-reflection 4	.76	Resilience 5	.78
Self-improvement and self-reflection 5	.75	Resilience 6	.69
Self-improvement and self-reflection 6	.73	Resilience 7	.69
Self-improvement and self-reflection 7	.75	Social competence 1	.79
Self-improvement and self-reflection 8	.80	Social competence 2	.83
Self-improvement and self-reflection 9	.71	Social competence 3	.81
People and principles orientation 1	.51	Social competence 4	.72
People and principles orientation 2	.71	Social competence 5	.64
People and principles orientation 3	.73	Problem-solving 1	.70
People and principles orientation 4	.62	Problem-solving 2	.70
People and principles orientation 5	.63	Problem-solving 3	.77
People and principles orientation 6	.70	Problem-solving 4	.77
People and principles orientation 7	.69	Problem-solving 5	.73
People and principles orientation 8	.63	Mentorship 1	.75
People and principles orientation 9	.65	Mentorship 2	.86
Resilience 1	.62	Mentorship 3	.82

NORMS

The normative sample involved in this manual was obtained through a snowball sampling strategy in the aforementioned large-scale validation study. First, PolyU initially set up an online survey and distributed the link to the coordinators in other seven participating universities in Hong Kong. Second, the coordinator in each university invited undergraduate students to respond to the online survey. Student participants were well informed of several important principles, such as confidentiality, anonymity, and freedom to withdraw. After completing the questionnaire, each participant was given a local supermarket voucher worth HK$100 as an incentive.

The final normative sample of 4,486 undergraduate students was recruited from late March to early June 2017. The age of participants ranged between 15 and 34 years (M = 20.47, SD = 1.67). Among these participants, 2,969 (66.18%) were female students and 1,517 (33.82%) were male students.

Normative statistics

The raw scores of full-scale and sub-scales obtained from full sample and gender-specific samples were non-normative. Therefore, norms of percentile rank of the score of full- and sub-scales instead of standardized Z scores were calculated for full sample and gender-specific samples. Related norm tables are presented in Tables 5-18. While Tables 5 and 6 show norms of total score, Tables 7-18 demonstrate norms of the six subscales in SLB-SF-38. For both total score and scores of subscales, percentile ranks (1-100) and corresponding raw scores are summarized in Tables 5, 7, 9, 11, 13, 15, and 17. Raw scores and related equivalent percentile ranks are outlined in Tables 6, 8, 10, 12, 14, 16, and 18.

Table 5. Percentiles and corresponding raw scores of Service Leadership Behavior Scale (SLB-SF-38) by gender

Percentile (1-50)	Raw Score				Percentile (51-99)	Raw Score		
	Male (N = 1,517)	Female (N = 2,969)	Total sample (N = 4,486)			Male (N = 1,517)	Female (N = 2,969)	Total sample (N = 4,486)
1	≤ 94.36	≤ 112.70	≤ 107.00		51	173.00	174.00	174.00
2	112.36	123.00	119.74		52	173.00	175.00	174.00
3	121.00	131.00	128.00		53	174.00	175.00	175.00
4	126.00	135.00	131.00		54	175.00	176.00	175.00
5	129.00	137.00	134.00		55	175.00	176.00	176.00
6	131.00	139.00	136.00		56	176.00	177.00	177.00
7	133.00	142.00	138.00		57	177.00	177.00	177.00
8	135.00	143.00	141.00		58	177.00	178.00	178.00
9	137.00	145.00	142.00		59	178.00	178.00	178.00
10	139.00	146.00	144.00		60	178.00	179.00	179.00
11	141.00	147.00	145.00		61	179.00	179.00	179.00
12	142.00	148.00	146.00		62	180.00	180.00	180.00
13	143.00	149.00	147.00		63	180.34	180.00	180.00
14	144.00	150.00	148.00		64	181.00	181.00	181.00
15	146.00	151.00	149.00		65	182.00	181.00	181.00
16	147.00	152.00	150.00		66	182.00	182.00	182.00
17	148.00	152.00	151.00		67	183.00	182.00	183.00
18	149.00	152.60	152.00		68	183.00	183.00	183.00
19	150.00	154.00	152.00		69	184.00	183.00	183.00
20	151.00	154.00	153.00		70	184.00	184.00	184.00
21	152.00	155.00	154.00		71	185.00	184.00	185.00
22	152.00	156.00	154.00		72	186.00	185.00	185.00
23	152.00	156.00	155.00		73	186.00	185.00	186.00

Table 5. (Continued)

Percentile (1-50)	Raw Score				Percentile (51-99)	Raw Score		
	Male (*N* = 1,517)	Female (*N* = 2,969)	Total sample (*N* = 4,486)			Male (*N* = 1,517)	Female (*N* = 2,969)	Total sample (*N* = 4,486)
24	153.00	157.00	156.00		74	187.00	186.00	186.00
25	154.00	158.00	157.00		75	188.00	186.00	187.00
26	155.00	159.00	157.00		76	188.00	187.00	187.00
27	155.00	160.00	158.00		77	189.00	187.00	188.00
28	156.00	160.00	159.00		78	190.00	188.00	188.00
29	157.00	161.00	160.00		79	190.00	188.00	189.00
30	158.00	162.00	160.10		80	190.00	189.00	189.00
31	158.00	162.70	161.00		81	190.00	189.00	190.00
32	159.00	163.00	162.00		82	191.00	190.00	190.00
33	160.00	164.00	163.00		83	191.00	190.00	191.00
34	161.00	165.00	163.00		84	192.00	191.00	191.00
35	162.00	165.00	164.00		85	193.00	191.50	192.00
36	162.00	166.00	165.00		86	194.00	192.00	193.00
37	163.00	167.00	165.00		87	195.00	193.00	194.00
38	164.00	167.00	166.00		88	196.00	194.00	195.00
39	164.00	168.00	167.00		89	197.00	195.00	196.00
40	165.00	168.00	167.00		90	198.00	197.00	197.00
41	165.00	169.00	168.00		91	199.00	198.00	199.00
42	166.00	169.00	168.00		92	201.00	200.00	200.00
43	167.00	170.00	169.00		93	202.00	201.00	201.00
44	167.00	171.00	170.00		94	204.00	202.00	203.00
45	168.00	171.00	170.00		95	207.00	205.00	205.00
46	169.00	172.00	171.00		96	208.00	207.20	208.00
47	169.00	172.00	171.00		97	212.00	211.00	212.00
48	171.00	173.00	172.00		98	217.00	215.00	216.00
49	171.00	173.00	173.00		99	222.82	221.30	222.00
50	172.00	174.00	173.00		100	≥ 228.00	≥ 228.00	≥ 228.00

Table 6. Raw scores and corresponding percentiles of Service Leadership Behavior Scale (SLB-SF-38)

Raw score	Percentiles			Raw score	Percentiles			Raw score	Percentiles		
	Male	Female	Total sample		Male	Female	Total sample		Male	Female	Total sample
≤ 94	1.0	1.0	1.0	134	8.0	4.0	5.0	174	53.0	51.0	52.0
95	2.0	1.0	1.0	135	8.0	4.0	6.0	175	54.0	53.0	54.0
96	2.0	1.0	1.0	136	9.0	5.0	6.0	176	56.0	55.0	55.0
97	2.0	1.0	1.0	137	9.0	5.0	7.0	177	58.0	57.0	57.0
98	2.0	1.0	1.0	138	10.0	6.0	7.0	178	60.0	59.0	59.0
99	2.0	1.0	1.0	139	10.0	6.0	8.0	179	61.0	61.0	61.0
100	2.0	1.0	1.0	140	11.0	7.0	8.0	180	62.0	63.0	63.0
101	2.0	1.0	1.0	141	11.0	7.0	8.0	181	64.0	65.0	65.0
102	2.0	1.0	1.0	142	12.0	7.0	9.0	182	66.0	67.0	66.0
103	2.0	1.0	1.0	143	13.0	8.0	10.0	183	68.0	69.0	68.0
104	2.0	1.0	1.0	144	14.0	9.0	10.0	184	70.0	71.0	70.0
105	2.0	1.0	1.0	145	15.0	9.0	11.0	185	71.0	73.0	72.0

Raw score	Percentiles			Raw score	Percentiles			Raw score	Percentiles		
	Male	Female	Total sample		Male	Female	Total sample		Male	Female	Total sample
105	2.0	1.0	1.0	145	15.0	9.0	11.0	185	71.0	73.0	72.0
106	2.0	1.0	1.0	146	15.0	10.0	12.0	186	73.0	75.0	74.0
107	2.0	1.0	1.0	147	16.0	11.0	13.0	187	74.0	77.0	76.0
108	2.0	1.0	2.0	148	17.0	12.0	14.0	188	76.0	79.0	78.0
109	2.0	1.0	2.0	149	18.0	13.0	15.0	189	77.0	81.0	80.0
110	2.0	1.0	2.0	150	19.0	14.0	16.0	190	80.0	83.0	82.0
111	2.0	1.0	2.0	151	20.0	15.0	17.0	191	83.0	84.0	84.0
112	2.0	1.0	2.0	152	22.0	17.0	19.0	192	84.0	86.0	85.0
113	3.0	2.0	2.0	153	24.0	19.0	20.0	193	85.0	87.0	86.0
114	3.0	2.0	2.0	154	25.0	20.0	22.0	194	86.0	88.0	87.0
115	3.0	2.0	2.0	155	27.0	21.0	23.0	195	87.0	89.0	88.0
116	3.0	2.0	2.0	156	28.0	23.0	24.0	196	88.0	90.0	89.0
117	3.0	2.0	2.0	157	29.0	24.0	26.0	197	89.0	90.0	90.0
118	3.0	2.0	2.0	158	31.0	25.0	27.0	198	90.0	91.0	91.0
119	3.0	2.0	2.0	159	32.0	26.0	28.0	199	91.0	92.0	91.0
120	3.0	2.0	3.0	160	33.0	28.0	29.0	200	92.0	92.0	92.0
121	3.0	2.0	3.0	161	34.0	29.0	31.0	201	92.0	93.0	93.0
122	4.0	2.0	3.0	162	36.0	30.0	32.0	202	93.0	94.0	94.0
123	4.0	2.0	3.0	163	37.0	32.0	34.0	203	94.0	95.0	94.0
124	4.0	3.0	3.0	164	39.0	33.0	35.0	204	94.0	95.0	95.0
125	4.0	3.0	3.0	165	41.0	35.0	37.0	205	95.0	95.0	95.0
126	4.0	3.0	3.0	166	42.0	36.0	38.0	206	95.0	96.0	96.0
127	5.0	3.0	3.0	167	44.0	38.0	40.0	207	95.0	96.0	96.0
128	5.0	3.0	3.0	168	45.0	40.0	42.0	208	96.0	97.0	96.0
129	5.0	3.0	4.0	169	47.0	42.0	43.0	209	96.0	97.0	97.0
130	5.0	3.0	4.0	170	48.0	43.0	45.0	210	96.0	97.0	97.0
131	6.0	3.0	4.0	171	49.0	45.0	47.0	211	96.0	97.0	97.0
132	7.0	4.0	5.0	172	50.0	47.0	48.0	212	97.0	98.0	97.0
133	7.0	4.0	5.0	173	52.0	49.0	49.0	213	98.0	98.0	98.0
214	98.0	98.0	98.0	219	99.0	99.0	99.0	224	100.0	100.0	100.0
215	98.0	98.0	98.0	220	100.0	99.0	99.0	225	100.0	100.0	100.0
216	98.0	99.0	98.0	221	100.0	99.0	99.0	226	100.0	100.0	100.0
217	98.0	99.0	99.0	222	100.0	100.0	99.0	227	100.0	100.0	100.0
218	99.0	99.0	99.0	223	100.0	100.0	100.0	228	100.0	100.0	100.0

Note. $N = 1{,}517$ for male sample, $N = 2{,}969$ for female sample, $N = 4{,}486$ for full sample.

Table 7. Percentiles and corresponding raw scores of Service Leadership Behavior Scale (Factor 1) by gender

Percentile (1-50)	Raw Score				Percentile (51-99)	Raw Score		
	Male	Female	Total sample			Male	Female	Total sample
1	≤ 20.00	≤ 24.00	≤ 22.00		51	42.00	43.00	42.00
2	24.00	27.40	27.00		52	42.00	43.00	43.00
3	27.00	29.00	28.00		53	42.00	43.00	43.00
4	28.00	30.00	30.00		54	42.00	43.00	43.00
5	29.00	31.00	30.00		55	42.90	43.00	43.00
6	30.00	32.00	31.00		56	43.00	43.00	43.00
7	30.00	33.00	32.00		57	43.00	44.00	43.00

Table 7. (Continued)

Percentile	Raw Score				Percentile	Raw Score		
(1-50)	Male	Female	Total sample		(51-99)	Male	Female	Total sample
8	31.00	33.00	32.00		58	43.00	44.00	43.00
9	31.00	33.00	33.00		59	43.00	44.00	44.00
10	32.00	34.00	33.00		60	43.00	44.00	44.00
11	32.00	34.00	34.00		61	43.00	44.00	44.00
12	33.00	35.00	34.00		62	44.00	44.00	44.00
13	33.00	35.00	34.00		63	44.00	44.00	44.00
14	34.00	35.00	35.00		64	44.00	44.00	44.00
15	34.00	36.00	35.00		65	44.00	45.00	44.00
16	34.00	36.00	35.00		66	44.00	45.00	45.00
17	35.00	36.00	36.00		67	44.00	45.00	45.00
18	35.00	36.00	36.00		68	45.00	45.00	45.00
19	35.00	36.00	36.00		69	45.00	45.00	45.00
20	36.00	36.00	36.00		70	45.00	45.00	45.00
21	36.00	36.00	36.00		71	45.00	45.00	45.00
22	36.00	37.00	36.00		72	45.00	45.00	45.00
23	36.00	37.00	37.00		73	45.00	45.00	45.00
24	36.00	37.00	37.00		74	45.00	45.00	45.00
25	36.00	38.00	37.00		75	45.00	45.00	45.00
26	36.00	38.00	37.00		76	45.00	45.00	45.00
27	37.00	38.00	38.00		77	46.00	46.00	46.00
28	37.00	38.00	38.00		78	46.00	46.00	46.00
29	37.00	39.00	38.00		79	46.00	46.00	46.00
30	37.00	39.00	38.00		80	46.00	46.00	46.00
31	37.58	39.00	39.00		81	47.00	47.00	47.00
32	38.00	39.00	39.00		82	47.00	47.00	47.00
33	38.00	39.00	39.00		83	47.00	47.00	47.00
34	38.00	40.00	39.00		84	47.00	47.00	47.00
35	39.00	40.00	39.00		85	48.00	48.00	48.00
36	39.00	40.00	40.00		86	48.00	48.00	48.00
37	39.00	40.00	40.00		87	48.00	48.00	48.00
38	39.00	40.00	40.00		88	48.00	48.60	48.00
39	40.00	41.00	40.00		89	49.00	49.00	49.00
40	40.00	41.00	40.00		90	49.00	49.00	49.00
41	40.00	41.00	41.00		91	50.00	50.00	50.00
42	40.00	41.00	41.00		92	50.00	50.00	50.00
43	40.00	41.00	41.00		93	50.00	51.00	51.00
44	41.00	42.00	41.00		94	51.00	51.00	51.00
45	41.00	42.00	41.00		95	52.00	52.00	52.00
46	41.00	42.00	42.00		96	52.28	53.00	53.00
47	41.00	42.00	42.00		97	53.00	53.00	53.00
48	41.00	42.00	42.00		98	54.00	54.00	54.00
49	41.00	42.00	42.00		99	54.00	54.00	54.00
50	42.00	42.00	42.00		100	54.00	54.00	54.00

Note. N = 1,517 for male sample, N = 2,969 for female sample, N = 4,486 for full sample.

Table 8. Raw scores and corresponding percentiles of Service Leadership Behavior Scale (Factor 1)

Raw score	Percentiles			Raw score	Percentiles			Raw score	Percentiles		
	Male	Female	Total sample		Male	Female	Total sample		Male	Female	Total sample
20	1.0	1.0	1.0	32	11.0	6.0	8.0	44	65.0	61.0	62.0
21	2.0	1.0	1.0	33	13.0	8.0	10.0	45	72.0	71.0	71.0
22	2.0	1.0	1.0	34	16.0	11.0	12.0	46	79.0	79.0	79.0
23	2.0	1.0	2.0	35	18.0	13.0	15.0	47	83.0	83.0	83.0
24	2.0	1.0	2.0	36	23.0	18.0	20.0	48	87.0	86.0	87.0
25	3.0	2.0	2.0	37	29.0	23.0	25.0	49	90.0	90.0	90.0
26	3.0	2.0	2.0	38	33.0	27.0	29.0	50	92.0	92.0	92.0
27	3.0	2.0	2.0	39	37.0	31.0	33.0	51	94.0	94.0	94.0
28	4.0	3.0	3.0	40	41.0	36.0	38.0	52	95.0	95.0	95.0
29	5.0	3.0	4.0	41	47.0	41.0	43.0	53	97.0	97.0	97.0
30	7.0	4.0	5.0	42	52.0	47.0	49.0	54	100.0	100.0	100.0
31	9.0	5.0	6.0	43	59.0	54.0	55.0				

Note. N = 1,517 for male sample, N = 2,969 for female sample, N = 4,486 for full sample.

Table 9. Percentiles and corresponding raw scores of Service Leadership Behavior Scale (Factor 2) by gender

Percentile (1-50)	Raw Score				Percentile (51-99)	Raw Score		
	Male	Female	Total sample			Male	Female	Total sample
1	≤ 22.00	≤ 27.00	≤ 25.00		51	42.00	43.00	42.00
2	25.00	30.00	29.00		52	42.00	43.00	43.00
3	28.54	32.00	31.00		53	42.00	43.00	43.00
4	30.00	33.00	32.00		54	42.00	43.00	43.00
5	31.00	34.00	32.00		55	42.00	43.00	43.00
6	31.00	34.00	33.00		56	42.00	44.00	43.00
7	32.00	35.00	34.00		57	42.00	44.00	43.00
8	32.00	35.00	34.00		58	42.00	44.00	43.00
9	33.00	36.00	34.00		59	43.00	44.00	44.00
10	33.00	36.00	35.00		60	43.00	44.00	44.00
11	33.00	36.00	35.00		61	43.00	44.00	44.00
12	34.00	36.00	36.00		62	43.00	44.00	44.00
13	34.00	36.00	36.00		63	43.00	44.00	44.00
14	35.00	36.00	36.00		64	43.00	44.00	44.00
15	35.00	37.00	36.00		65	44.00	44.00	44.00
16	35.00	37.00	36.00		66	44.00	45.00	44.00
17	35.00	37.00	36.00		67	44.00	45.00	44.00
18	36.00	37.00	37.00		68	44.00	45.00	45.00
19	36.00	38.00	37.00		69	44.00	45.00	45.00
20	36.00	38.00	37.00		70	44.00	45.00	45.00
21	36.00	38.00	37.00		71	44.00	45.00	45.00
22	36.00	38.00	38.00		72	45.00	45.00	45.00
23	36.00	39.00	38.00		73	45.00	45.00	45.00
24	36.00	39.00	38.00		74	45.00	45.00	45.00
25	37.00	39.00	38.00		75	45.00	45.00	45.00

Table 9. (Continued)

Percentile (1-50)	Raw Score				Percentile (51-99)	Raw Score		
	Male	Female	Total sample			Male	Female	Total sample
26	37.00	39.00	38.00		76	45.00	45.00	45.00
27	37.00	39.00	39.00		77	45.00	46.00	45.00
28	37.00	39.00	39.00		78	45.00	46.00	46.00
29	38.00	40.00	39.00		79	45.22	46.00	46.00
30	38.00	40.00	39.00		80	46.00	46.00	46.00
31	38.00	40.00	39.00		81	46.00	46.00	46.00
32	38.00	40.00	40.00		82	46.00	47.00	46.00
33	38.00	40.00	40.00		83	46.00	47.00	47.00
34	39.00	41.00	40.00		84	47.00	47.00	47.00
35	39.00	41.00	40.00		85	47.00	47.00	47.00
36	39.00	41.00	40.00		86	47.00	47.00	47.00
37	39.00	41.00	41.00		87	47.00	48.00	48.00
38	39.00	41.00	41.00		88	47.00	48.00	48.00
39	40.00	41.00	41.00		89	48.00	48.00	48.00
40	40.00	41.00	41.00		90	48.00	49.00	48.00
41	40.00	42.00	41.00		91	49.00	49.00	49.00
42	40.00	42.00	41.00		92	49.00	49.00	49.00
43	40.00	42.00	41.00		93	49.00	50.00	49.00
44	41.00	42.00	42.00		94	50.00	50.00	50.00
45	41.00	42.00	42.00		95	50.00	50.00	50.00
46	41.00	42.00	42.00		96	51.00	51.00	51.00
47	41.00	42.00	42.00		97	52.00	52.00	52.00
48	41.00	43.00	42.00		98	53.00	52.00	53.00
49	41.00	43.00	42.00		99	53.82	54.00	54.00
50	41.00	43.00	42.00		100	54.00	54.00	54.00

Note. N = 1,517 for male sample, N = 2,969 for female sample, N = 4,486 for full sample.

Table 10. Raw scores and corresponding percentiles of Service Leadership Behavior Scale (Factor 2)

Raw score	Percentiles			Raw score	Percentiles			Raw score	Percentiles		
	Male	Female	Total sample		Male	Female	Total sample		Male	Female	Total sample
22	1.0	1.0	1.0	34	13.0	6.0	8.0	46	82.0	79.0	80.0
23	2.0	1.0	1.0	35	16.0	8.0	11.0	47	86.0	84.0	85.0
24	2.0	1.0	1.0	36	21.0	12.0	15.0	48	90.0	88.0	89.0
25	2.0	1.0	1.0	37	27.0	17.0	20.0	49	92.0	91.0	92.0
26	3.0	1.0	2.0	38	31.0	21.0	24.0	50	95.0	94.0	95.0
27	3.0	1.0	2.0	39	36.0	26.0	29.0	51	96.0	96.0	96.0
28	3.0	2.0	2.0	40	41.0	31.0	34.0	52	97.0	99.0	97.0
29	4.0	2.0	2.0	41	47.0	37.0	40.0	53	98.0	99.0	98.0
30	4.0	2.0	3.0	42	55.0	44.0	48.0	54	100.0	100.0	100.0
31	6.0	3.0	3.0	43	62.0	52.0	55.0				
32	8.0	3.0	5.0	44	68.0	61.0	63.0				
33	10.0	4.0	6.0	45	75.0	71.0	73.0				

Note. N = 1,517 for male sample, N = 2,969 for female sample, N = 4,486 for full sample.

Table 11. Percentiles and corresponding raw scores of Service Leadership Behavior Scale (Factor 3) by gender

Percentile	Raw Score				Percentile	Raw Score		
(1-50)	Male	Female	Total sample		(51-99)	Male	Female	Total sample
1	≤ 15.00	≤ 15.00	≤ 15.00		51	31.00	30.00	31.00
2	18.00	18.00	18.00		52	31.00	31.00	31.00
3	19.00	19.00	19.00		53	32.00	31.00	31.00
4	20.00	20.00	20.00		54	32.00	31.00	31.00
5	21.00	21.00	21.00		55	32.00	31.00	31.00
6	21.00	22.00	22.00		56	32.00	31.00	32.00
7	22.00	22.00	22.00		57	32.00	31.00	32.00
8	22.00	23.00	23.00		58	32.00	32.00	32.00
9	23.00	23.00	23.00		59	32.00	32.00	32.00
10	23.00	23.00	23.00		60	32.00	32.00	32.00
11	24.00	24.00	24.00		61	33.00	32.00	32.00
12	24.00	24.00	24.00		62	33.00	32.00	32.00
13	25.00	24.00	24.00		63	33.00	32.00	33.00
14	25.00	25.00	25.00		64	33.00	33.00	33.00
15	25.00	25.00	25.00		65	33.00	33.00	33.00
16	25.00	25.00	25.00		66	33.00	33.00	33.00
17	26.00	25.00	25.79		67	33.00	33.00	33.00
18	26.00	26.00	26.00		68	34.00	33.00	33.00
19	26.00	26.00	26.00		69	34.00	33.00	33.00
20	26.00	26.00	26.00		70	34.00	33.00	34.00
21	26.00	26.00	26.00		71	34.00	34.00	34.00
22	27.00	26.00	26.00		72	34.00	34.00	34.00
23	27.00	27.00	27.00		73	34.00	34.00	34.00
24	27.00	27.00	27.00		74	35.00	34.00	34.00
25	27.00	27.00	27.00		75	35.00	34.00	34.00
26	27.00	27.00	27.00		76	35.00	34.00	34.00
27	27.00	27.00	27.00		77	35.00	34.00	35.00
28	28.00	27.00	27.36		78	35.00	35.00	35.00
29	28.00	28.00	28.00		79	35.00	35.00	35.00
30	28.00	28.00	28.00		80	35.00	35.00	35.00
31	28.00	28.00	28.00		81	35.00	35.00	35.00
32	28.00	28.00	28.00		82	35.00	35.00	35.00
33	28.00	28.00	28.00		83	35.00	35.00	35.00
34	28.00	28.00	28.00		84	35.00	35.00	35.00
35	28.00	28.00	28.00		85	36.00	35.00	35.00
36	28.00	28.00	28.00		86	36.00	35.00	35.00
37	29.00	28.00	28.00		87	36.00	35.00	36.00
38	29.00	28.60	29.00		88	36.00	36.00	36.00
39	29.00	29.00	29.00		89	36.02	36.00	36.00
40	29.00	29.00	29.00		90	37.00	36.00	37.00
41	29.00	29.00	29.00		91	37.00	37.00	37.00
42	30.00	29.00	29.00		92	38.00	37.00	37.00
43	30.00	29.00	29.00		93	38.00	37.00	38.00
44	30.00	29.00	30.00		94	38.00	38.00	38.00
45	30.00	30.00	30.00		95	39.00	38.00	38.00
46	30.00	30.00	30.00		96	39.00	39.00	39.00

Table 11. (Continued)

Percentile (1-50)	Raw Score				Percentile (51-99)	Raw Score		
	Male	Female	Total sample			Male	Female	Total sample
47	30.00	30.00	30.00		97	40.00	39.90	40.00
48	31.00	30.00	30.00		98	41.00	40.00	41.00
49	31.00	30.00	30.00		99	42.00	42.00	42.00
50	31.00	30.00	31.00		100	42.00	42.00	42.00

Note. N = 1,517 for male sample, N = 2,969 for female sample, N = 4,486 for full sample.

Table 12. Raw scores and corresponding percentiles of Service Leadership Behavior Scale (Factor 3)

Raw score	Percentiles			Raw score	Percentiles			Raw score	Percentiles		
	Male	Female	Total sample		Male	Female	Total sample		Male	Female	Total sample
15	1.0	1.0	1.0	25	15.0	16.0	15.0	35	79.0	83.0	82.0
16	2.0	2.0	2.0	26	19.0	20.0	20.0	36	87.0	89.0	88.0
17	2.0	2.0	2.0	27	25.0	26.0	25.0	37	91.0	92.0	91.0
18	2.0	2.0	2.0	28	32.0	33.0	33.0	38	93.0	95.0	94.0
19	3.0	3.0	3.0	29	39.0	42.0	41.0	39	96.0	96.0	96.0
20	4.0	4.0	4.0	30	45.0	48.0	47.0	40	97.0	98.0	97.0
21	6.0	5.0	5.0	31	50.0	55.0	53.0	41	98.0	99.0	98.0
22	8.0	7.0	7.0	32	57.0	61.0	59.0	42	100.0	100.0	100.0
23	10.0	9.0	9.0	33	64.0	67.0	66.0				
24	12.0	12.0	12.0	34	71.0	74.0	73.0				

Note. N = 1,517 for male sample, N = 2,969 for female sample, N = 4,486 for full sample.

Table 13. Percentiles and corresponding raw scores of Service Leadership Behavior Scale (Factor 4) by gender

Percentile (1-50)	Raw Score				Percentile (51-99)	Raw Score		
	Male	Female	Total sample			Male	Female	Total sample
1	≤ 10.00	≤ 13.00	≤ 12.00		51	23.00	24.00	24.00
2	13.00	15.00	14.00		52	23.00	24.00	24.00
3	14.00	16.00	15.00		53	23.00	24.00	24.00
4	15.00	17.00	16.00		54	23.00	24.00	24.00
5	15.00	17.00	17.00		55	23.00	24.00	24.00
6	16.00	18.00	17.00		56	23.00	24.00	24.00
7	17.00	18.00	18.00		57	23.00	24.00	24.00
8	17.00	18.00	18.00		58	24.00	24.00	24.00
9	17.00	19.00	18.00		59	24.00	24.00	24.00
10	18.00	19.00	18.00		60	24.00	25.00	24.00
11	18.00	19.00	19.00		61	24.00	25.00	24.00
12	18.00	19.00	19.00		62	24.00	25.00	24.00
13	18.00	20.00	19.00		63	24.00	25.00	25.00
14	18.00	20.00	19.00		64	24.00	25.00	25.00
15	19.00	20.00	20.00		65	24.00	25.00	25.00
16	19.00	20.00	20.00		66	24.00	25.00	25.00

Percentile (1-50)	Raw Score				Percentile (51-99)	Raw Score		
	Male	Female	Total sample			Male	Female	Total sample
17	19.00	20.00	20.00		67	24.00	25.00	25.00
18	19.00	20.00	20.00		68	25.00	25.00	25.00
19	19.00	20.00	20.00		69	25.00	25.00	25.00
20	19.60	20.00	20.00		70	25.00	25.00	25.00
21	20.00	20.00	20.00		71	25.00	25.00	25.00
22	20.00	21.00	20.00		72	25.00	25.00	25.00
23	20.00	21.00	20.00		73	25.00	25.00	25.00
24	20.00	21.00	20.00		74	25.00	25.00	25.00
25	20.00	21.00	21.00		75	25.00	25.00	25.00
26	20.00	21.00	21.00		76	25.00	25.00	25.00
27	20.00	21.00	21.00		77	25.00	25.00	25.00
28	20.00	21.00	21.00		78	25.00	25.00	25.00
29	20.00	21.00	21.00		79	25.00	26.00	25.00
30	20.00	22.00	21.00		80	25.00	26.00	26.00
31	20.00	22.00	21.00		81	25.00	26.00	26.00
32	21.00	22.00	21.00		82	25.00	26.00	26.00
33	21.00	22.00	22.00		83	26.00	26.00	26.00
34	21.00	22.00	22.00		84	26.00	26.00	26.00
35	21.00	22.00	22.00		85	26.00	26.00	26.00
36	21.00	22.00	22.00		86	26.00	27.00	26.00
37	21.00	23.00	22.00		87	26.00	27.00	27.00
38	21.00	23.00	22.00		88	27.00	27.00	27.00
39	21.00	23.00	22.00		89	27.00	27.00	27.00
40	21.00	23.00	22.00		90	27.00	28.00	27.00
41	22.00	23.00	23.00		91	27.00	28.00	28.00
42	22.00	23.00	23.00		92	28.00	28.00	28.00
43	22.00	23.00	23.00		93	28.00	28.00	28.00
44	22.00	23.00	23.00		94	28.00	28.80	28.00
45	22.00	23.00	23.00		95	29.00	29.00	29.00
46	22.00	23.00	23.00		96	29.00	29.00	29.00
47	22.00	24.00	23.00		97	30.00	29.90	30.00
48	22.00	24.00	23.00		98	30.00	30.00	30.00
49	23.00	24.00	23.00		99	30.00	30.00	30.00
50	23.00	24.00	23.50		100	30.00	30.00	30.00

Note. N = 1,517 for male sample, N = 2,969 for female sample, N = 4,486 for full sample.

Table 14. Raw scores and corresponding percentiles of Service Leadership Behavior Scale (Factor 4)

Raw score	Percentiles			Raw score	Percentiles			Raw score	Percentiles		
	Male	Female	Total sample		Male	Female	Total sample		Male	Female	Total sample
10	1.0	1.0	1.0	17	8.0	5.0	6.0	24	63.0	53.0	57.0
11	2.0	1.0	1.0	18	12.0	7.0	9.0	25	75.0	69.0	71.0
12	2.0	1.0	1.0	19	17.0	11.0	13.0	26	85.0	82.0	83.0
13	2.0	1.0	2.0	20	26.0	17.0	20.0	27	90.0	88.0	89.0
14	3.0	2.0	2.0	21	36.0	26.0	29.0	28	93.0	92.0	93.0
15	5.0	2.0	3.0	22	45.0	33.0	37.0	29	96.0	96.0	96.0
16	6.0	3.0	4.0	23	53.0	42.0	45.0	30	100.0	100.0	100.0

Note. N = 1,517 for male sample, N = 2,969 for female sample, N = 4,486 for full sample.

Table 15. Percentiles and corresponding raw scores of Service Leadership Behavior Scale (Factor 5) by gender

Percentile	Raw Score				Percentile	Raw Score		
(1-50)	Male	Female	Total sample		(51-99)	Male	Female	Total sample
1	≤ 11.00	≤ 11.00	≤ 11.00		51	23.00	22.00	23.00
2	13.00	13.00	13.00		52	23.00	22.00	23.00
3	14.00	14.00	14.00		53	23.00	23.00	23.00
4	15.00	15.00	15.00		54	23.00	23.00	23.00
5	16.00	15.00	15.00		55	24.00	23.00	23.00
6	16.00	16.00	16.00		56	24.00	23.00	23.00
7	17.00	16.00	16.00		57	24.00	23.00	23.00
8	17.00	17.00	17.00		58	24.00	23.00	23.00
9	17.00	17.00	17.00		59	24.00	23.00	23.00
10	18.00	17.00	17.00		60	24.00	23.00	24.00
11	18.00	17.00	18.00		61	24.00	23.00	24.00
12	18.00	18.00	18.00		62	24.00	24.00	24.00
13	18.00	18.00	18.00		63	24.00	24.00	24.00
14	19.00	18.00	18.00		64	24.00	24.00	24.00
15	19.00	18.00	18.00		65	24.00	24.00	24.00
16	19.00	18.00	19.00		66	25.00	24.00	24.00
17	19.00	18.00	19.00		67	25.00	24.00	24.00
18	19.00	19.00	19.00		68	25.00	24.00	24.00
19	19.00	19.00	19.00		69	25.00	24.00	24.00
20	20.00	19.00	19.00		70	25.00	24.00	25.00
21	20.00	19.00	19.00		71	25.00	24.00	25.00
22	20.00	19.00	19.00		72	25.00	25.00	25.00
23	20.00	19.00	20.00		73	25.00	25.00	25.00
24	20.00	20.00	20.00		74	25.00	25.00	25.00
25	20.00	20.00	20.00		75	25.00	25.00	25.00
26	20.00	20.00	20.00		76	25.00	25.00	25.00
27	20.00	20.00	20.00		77	25.00	25.00	25.00
28	20.00	20.00	20.00		78	25.00	25.00	25.00
29	20.00	20.00	20.00		79	25.00	25.00	25.00
30	20.00	20.00	20.00		80	26.00	25.00	25.00
31	21.00	20.00	20.00		81	26.00	25.00	25.00
32	21.00	20.00	20.00		82	26.00	25.00	25.00
33	21.00	20.00	20.00		83	26.00	25.00	25.00
34	21.00	20.00	21.00		84	26.00	25.00	26.00
35	21.00	21.00	21.00		85	27.00	25.00	26.00
36	21.00	21.00	21.00		86	27.00	26.00	26.00
37	21.00	21.00	21.00		87	27.00	26.00	26.00
38	22.00	21.00	21.00		88	27.00	26.00	26.56
39	22.00	21.00	21.00		89	28.00	26.00	27.00
40	22.00	21.00	21.00		90	28.00	27.00	27.00
41	22.00	21.00	21.00		91	28.00	27.00	27.00
42	22.00	21.00	22.00		92	28.00	27.00	28.00
43	22.00	21.00	22.00		93	28.00	27.00	28.00
44	22.00	22.00	22.00		94	29.00	28.00	28.00
45	23.00	22.00	22.00		95	29.00	28.00	29.00
46	23.00	22.00	22.00		96	29.00	29.00	29.00

Percentile (1-50)	Raw Score				Percentile (51-99)	Raw Score		
	Male	Female	Total sample			Male	Female	Total sample
47	23.00	22.00	22.00		97	30.00	29.00	29.00
48	23.00	22.00	22.00		98	30.00	30.00	30.00
49	23.00	22.00	22.00		99	30.00	30.00	30.00
50	23.00	22.00	23.00		100	30.00	30.00	30.00

Note. N = 1,517 for male sample, N = 2,969 for female sample, N = 4,486 for full sample.

Table 16. Raw scores and corresponding percentiles of Service Leadership Behavior Scale (Factor 5)

Raw score	Percentiles			Raw score	Percentiles			Raw score	Percentiles		
	Male	Female	Total sample		Male	Female	Total sample		Male	Female	Total sample
11	1.0	1.0	1.0	18	12.0	15.0	13.0	25	73.0	79.0	77.0
12	2.0	2.0	2.0	19	17.0	21.0	19.0	26	82.0	88.0	86.0
13	2.0	2.0	2.0	20	25.0	29.0	28.0	27	87.0	92.0	90.0
14	3.0	3.0	3.0	21	34.0	39.0	38.0	28	91.0	95.0	93.0
15	4.0	5.0	5.0	22	41.0	48.0	46.0	29	95.0	97.0	96.0
16	6.0	7.0	7.0	23	50.0	57.0	55.0	30	100.0	100.0	100.0
17	8.0	10.0	9.0	24	60.0	67.0	65.0				

Note. N = 1,517 for male sample, N = 2,969 for female sample, N = 4,486 for full sample.

Table 17. Percentiles and corresponding raw scores of Service Leadership Behavior Scale (Factor 6) by gender

Percentile (1-50)	Raw Score				Percentile (51-99)	Raw Score		
	Male	Female	Total sample			Male	Female	Total sample
1	≤ 5.00	≤ 6.00	≤ 6.00		51	13.00	13.00	13.00
2	6.00	6.00	6.00		52	13.00	13.00	13.00
3	7.00	7.00	7.00		53	13.00	13.00	13.00
4	7.00	7.00	7.00		54	13.00	13.00	13.00
5	8.00	8.00	8.00		55	13.00	13.00	13.00
6	8.00	8.00	8.00		56	13.00	13.00	13.00
7	9.00	9.00	9.00		57	13.00	13.00	13.00
8	9.00	9.00	9.00		58	14.00	13.00	13.00
9	9.00	9.00	9.00		59	14.00	14.00	14.00
10	9.00	9.00	9.00		60	14.00	14.00	14.00
11	9.00	9.00	9.00		61	14.00	14.00	14.00
12	9.00	9.00	9.00		62	14.00	14.00	14.00
13	10.00	10.00	10.00		63	14.00	14.00	14.00
14	10.00	10.00	10.00		64	14.00	14.00	14.00
15	10.00	10.00	10.00		65	14.00	14.00	14.00
16	10.00	10.00	10.00		66	14.00	14.00	14.00
17	10.00	10.00	10.00		67	14.00	14.00	14.00
18	10.00	10.00	10.00		68	14.00	14.00	14.00
19	10.00	11.00	10.00		69	14.00	14.00	14.00
20	11.00	11.00	11.00		70	15.00	14.00	14.00
21	11.00	11.00	11.00		71	15.00	15.00	15.00
22	11.00	11.00	11.00		72	15.00	15.00	15.00

Table 17. (Continued)

Percentile (1-50)	Raw Score				Percentile (51-99)	Raw Score		
	Male	Female	Total sample			Male	Female	Total sample
23	11.00	11.00	11.00		73	15.00	15.00	15.00
24	11.00	11.00	11.00		74	15.00	15.00	15.00
25	11.00	11.00	11.00		75	15.00	15.00	15.00
26	11.00	11.00	11.00		76	15.00	15.00	15.00
27	11.00	12.00	11.00		77	15.00	15.00	15.00
28	11.00	12.00	12.00		78	15.00	15.00	15.00
29	12.00	12.00	12.00		79	15.00	15.00	15.00
30	12.00	12.00	12.00		80	15.00	15.00	15.00
31	12.00	12.00	12.00		81	15.00	15.00	15.00
32	12.00	12.00	12.00		82	15.00	15.00	15.00
33	12.00	12.00	12.00		83	15.00	15.00	15.00
34	12.00	12.00	12.00		84	15.00	15.00	15.00
35	12.00	12.00	12.00		85	15.00	15.00	15.00
36	12.00	12.00	12.00		86	15.00	15.00	15.00
37	12.00	12.00	12.00		87	15.00	15.00	15.00
38	12.00	12.00	12.00		88	16.00	15.00	15.00
39	12.00	12.00	12.00		89	16.00	15.00	15.00
40	12.00	12.00	12.00		90	16.00	16.00	16.00
41	12.00	12.00	12.00		91	16.00	16.00	16.00
42	12.00	12.00	12.00		92	16.00	16.00	16.00
43	12.00	12.00	12.00		93	16.00	16.00	16.00
44	12.00	12.00	12.00		94	17.00	17.00	17.00
45	12.00	12.00	12.00		95	17.00	17.00	17.00
46	13.00	13.00	13.00		96	17.00	17.00	17.00
47	13.00	13.00	13.00		97	18.00	18.00	18.00
48	13.00	13.00	13.00		98	18.00	18.00	18.00
49	13.00	13.00	13.00		99	18.00	18.00	18.00
50	13.00	13.00	13.00		100	18.00	18.00	18.00

Note. N = 1,517 for male sample, N = 2,969 for female sample, N = 4,486 for full sample.

Table 18. Raw scores and corresponding percentiles of Service Leadership Behavior Scale (Factor 5)

Raw score	Percentiles			Raw score	Percentiles			Raw score	Percentiles		
	Male	Female	Total sample		Male	Female	Total sample		Male	Female	Total sample
5	1.0	1.0	1.0	10	16.0	16.0	16.0	15	79.0	80.0	80.0
6	2.0	1.0	2.0	11	24.0	23.0	24.0	16	91.0	92.0	92.0
7	4.0	4.0	4.0	12	37.0	36.0	37.0	17	95.0	95.0	95.0
8	6.0	6.0	6.0	13	52.0	52.0	52.0	18	100.0	100.0	99.0
9	10.0	10.0	10.0	14	64.0	65.0	65.0				

Note. N = 1,517 for male sample, N = 2,969 for female sample, N = 4,486 for full sample.

SCORING AND INTERPRETATION

The SLB-SF-38 includes 38 items grouped into six subscales. The score of each subscale is calculated on the sum of each item of the subscale. The total score of service leadership behavior is calculated by adding up the scores of all 38 items. Theoretically, the total score ranges between 38 and 228.

Handling of missing items

Satisfactory reliability of the scale/subscales largely depends on participants' responses to all items included in the scale/subscales. If there is missing value in any item, the results should be interpreted with cautions. Cases with missing value(s) should be excluded from data analysis or handled by appropriate missing value imputation methods before conducting data analysis.

Interpretation of test scores

Test scores of SLB-SF-38 can be interpreted in terms of a total score of full scale or test score(s) of subscale(s). The total score represents an individual's overall behavioral characteristics with reference to service leadership. The score of an individual subscale shows one's leadership practice and related skills in one specific area. For example, a high score of "Resilience" reflects one's capability of using effective strategies to overcome adversity and bounce back.

Tables 5-18 show norms of percentile ranks for the scores of full scale and the subscales. The percentile rank of a particular raw score represents the percentage of people in the normative sample scored no higher than this raw score. In other words, a percentile rank can be interpreted as one's relative standing in the relevant group according to the score. For instance, if a female university student wishes to surpass 50% of her female peers in demonstrating resilience, she has to get at least 30 points (see Table 11). Similarly, if a university student, regardless of gender, gets 31 points for subscale of resilience (i.e., Subscale 3), he/she has already surpassed 53% of all university students (see Table 12).

There is no specific cut-off value to define effective/good versus ineffective/bad service leadership behaviors. Therefore, testers are not recommended to describe people with different service leadership behaviors using objectives such as "effective," "good," "ineffective" or "bad," although norm-referenced descriptors may be used. For instance, scale users are suggested to locate a participant's test score in the norm tables to determine his/her relative position regarding service leadership behavior. Descriptions like "less effective than the normative sample," "similar to the normative sample," or "more effective than the normative sample" can be adopted to differentiate people with different service leadership behaviors.

In addition, when using the scale/subscales to examine the effectiveness of service leadership training programmes, evaluators are suggested to monitor the improvement through the comparison between pre- and post-test. In this case, using mean scores provides more meaningful information than referring to the norm tables does.

Acknowledgments

The validation project is financially supported by the Victor and William Fung Foundation. The preparation for this chapter is supported by the Foundation and the Endowed Professorship in Service Leadership Education at The Hong Kong Polytechnic University.

References

[1] Buera FJ, Kaboski JP. The rise of the service economy. Am Econ Rev 2012;102(6):2540-69. doi:10.1257/aer.102.6.2540.

[2] Chung PPY, Bell AH. Service reborn: The knowledge, skills and attitudes of service companies. New York: Lexingford, 2012.

[3] Chung PPY. (2010). Distinguishing characteristics of service leadership and management education. The Hong Kong Institute of Service Leadership & Management, 2010. URL: http://hki-slam.org/index.php?r=article&catid=2&aid=29.

[4] Shek DTL, Wu J, Lin L, Li X. Content validation of a Service Leadership Behavior Scale in Hong Kong. Int J Child Adolesc Health, in press.

[5] Shek DTL, Zhu X, Chan KM. Development of Service Leadership Behavior Scale: Background and conceptual model. Int J Child Adolesc Health, in press.

[6] Shek DTL, Lin L. Intrapersonal competencies and service leadership. Int J Disabil Hum Dev 2015;14(3):255-63. doi: 10.1515/ijdhd-2015-0406.

[7] Shek DTL, Yu L, Siu AMH. Interpersonal competence and service leadership. Int J Disabil Hum Dev 2015;14(3):265-74. doi: 10.1515/ijdhd-2015-0407.

[8] Shek DTL, Yu L. Character strengths and service leadership. Int J Disabil Hum Dev 2015;14(4):299-307. doi: 10.1515/ijdhd-2015-0451.

[9] Shek DTL, Li X. The role of a caring disposition in service leadership. Int J Disabil Hum Dev 2015;14(4):319-32. doi: 10.1515/ijdhd-2015-0453.

[10] Shek DTL, Ma LK, Lin L, Leung H. Psychometric properties of the Service Leadership Behavior Scale: Preliminary findings. Int J Child Adolesc Health, in press.

[11] Shek DTL, Ma LK, Ma CMS, Hoshmand AR. Convergent and factorial validation of the Service Leadership Behavior Scale. Int J Child Adolesc Health, in press.

[12] Amram Y, Dryer DC. The Integrated Spiritual Intelligence Scale (ISIS): Development and preliminary validation. Paper presented at the 116th Annual Conference of the American Psychological Association, 2008.

[13] Hwang KK, Chang J. Self-cultivation: Culturally sensitive psychotherapies in Confucian societies. Couns Psychol, 2009;37(7):1010-32.

[14] Chung PPY, Bell AH. The 25 Principles of Service Leadership. New York: Lexingford, 2015.

[15] Shek DTL, Dou D, Snell RS. The Service Leadership Behavior Scale: Norms and personal correlates. Int J Child Adolesc Health, in press.

SECTION FOUR: ACKNOWLEDGMENTS

In: Service Leadership
Editors: Daniel TL Shek, Xiaoqin Zhu, Li Lin et al.
ISBN: 978-1-53614-852-7

Chapter 17

About the Editors

Daniel TL Shek, PhD, FHKPS, BBS, SBS, JP, is Associate Vice President (undergraduate Programme), Chair Professor of Applied Social Sciences, and Li and Fung Professor in Service Leadership Education, The Hong Kong Polytechnic University, Hung Hom, Hong Kong, PRC, Advisory Professor of East China Normal University, Honorary Professor of Kiang Wu Nursing College of Macau and Adjunct Professor, Division of Adolescent Medicine, Department of Pediatrics, University of Kentucky College of Medicine, Lexington, United States. He is Chief Editor of *Journal of Youth Studies* and *Applied Research in Quality of Life*, past Consulting Editor of *Journal of Clinical Psychology*, and editorial board member of *Social Indicators Research, International Journal of Adolescent Medicine and Health, Asian Journal of Counseling, International Journal of Disability and Human Development,* and *International Journal of Adolescent Medicine and Health.* He has served in many government advisory bodies, including the Action Committee against Narcotics, Commission on Youth, Fight Crime Committee and Family Council. He has published numerous books, book chapters and more than 500 scientific articles in international refereed journals. Email: daniel.shek@polyu.edu.hk

Xiaoqin Zhu, PhD, is an instructor in the Department of Applied Social Sciences of The Hong Kong Polytechnic University, Hong Kong. She received her PhD degree in Psychology from The Chinese University of Hong Kong. Her research interests lie in the areas of child and adolescent development and leadership education, such as parent-child relationship, adolescent risk behavior, positive youth development program and its evaluation, service leadership education and evaluation. Her work appears in *Frontiers in Psychology, Applied Research in Quality of Life, Research on Social Work Practice, International Journal of Child and Adolescent Health, and International Journal on Disability* and other book chapters about positive youth development and service leadership. Email: xiaoqin.zhu@polyu.edu.hk.

Li Lin, PhD, is a Research Assistant Professor in the Department of Social Sciences of The Hong Kong Polytechnic University, Hong Kong. She received her PhD degree in psychology from The Chinese University of Hong Kong. She teaches leadership course for university students. Her research interests largely involve development of adolescence and emerging adulthood, particularly positive youth development, adolescent risk behavior, parent-child relationship, and sociocultural influence. She has published several articles in peer-referred journals such as *Social Indicators Research, Journal of Adolescent Health, and Journal of Youth and Adolescence,* and other book chapters about positive youth development and service leadership. Email: jocelyn.lin@polyu.edu.hk

Joav Merrick, MD, MMedSci, DMSc, born and educated in Denmark is professor of pediatrics, Division of Pediatrics, Hadassah Hebrew University Medical Center, Mt Scopus Campus, Jerusalem, Israel and Kentucky Children's Hospital, University of Kentucky, Lexington, Kentucky United States and professor of public health at the Center for Healthy Development, School of Public Health, Georgia State University, Atlanta, United States, the former medical director of the Health Services, Division for Intellectual and Developmental Disabilities, Ministry of Social Affairs and Social Services, Jerusalem, the founder and director of the National Institute of Child Health and Human Development in Israel. Numerous publications in the field of pediatrics, child health and human development, rehabilitation, intellectual disability, disability, health, welfare, abuse, advocacy, quality of life and prevention. Received the Peter Sabroe Child Award for outstanding work on behalf of Danish Children in 1985 and the International LEGO-Prize ("The Children's Nobel Prize") for an extraordinary contribution towards improvement in child welfare and well-being in 1987. In 2017 appointed a Kentucky Colonel by the Commonwealth of Kentucky, the highest honor the governor can bestow to a person. Email: jmerrick@zahav.net.il

In: Service Leadership
Editors: Daniel TL Shek, Xiaoqin Zhu, Li Lin et al.
ISBN: 978-1-53614-852-7

Chapter 18

About the Department of Applied Social Sciences, The Hong Kong Polytechnic University, Hung Hom, Hong Kong

The Department of Applied Social Sciences (APSS) of the Hong Kong Polytechnic University began as the Institute of Social Work Training in 1973 before it became the School of Social Work in the Hong Kong Polytechnic in 1977. In 1986, the department was renamed as the Department of Applied Social Sciences. It is now one of the largest social science departments in the Asia-Pacific region with a strong tradition of researching on and working with socially vulnerable groups through education, research and service in diverse areas incorporating social work, social policy and administration, psychology, sociology and philosophy.

Education

In education, we strive to nurture human service professionals who are knowledgeable, resourceful, caring, worldly but reflexive, and possess a strong commitment to social justice and responsibility. We also see them as practitioners and researchers who are able to integrate theory and practice, and develop appropriate indigenous knowledge that can meet the challenges of rapid social change in Chinese societies.

Research

In research, to respond to the constantly changing global socio-economic order and addressing the subsequently emerged local problems, the strategic foci of our research and social investigation have also been expanded to include migration and mobilities, family and life-span development, social economy, online communities/social media, disaster and risks reduction, applied philosophy and social work practices.

Community service

In community service, we continue to collaborate with community partners to allow our students to understand better the different lifeworlds of our society, design programmes and supportive services that are innovative, relevant and socially responsible.

Students

As students in our department, we see it necessary for them to develop a global outlook while firmly grounded in Hong Kong. To this end, in recent years more than 200 full-time and part-time students as well as alumni have participated in the various study tours and exchange programmes we held in the Chinese Mainland and overseas, including the University of Nottingham, United Kingdom; University of Queensland, Australia; University of California at Berkeley, United States; Washington University at St. Louis, United States; York University, Canada; Peking University and Yunnan University in China.

Faculty and teaching

In the 2017/18 academic year, the Department has more than 200 members, including academic staff, part-time fieldwork instructors, research and project staff and administrative and supporting technical staff. The APSS offers many undergraduate and coursework and research postgraduate programmes. Over the years, more than 14,000 students have graduated.

In: Service Leadership
Editors: Daniel TL Shek, Xiaoqin Zhu, Li Lin et al.
ISBN: 978-1-53614-852-7

Chapter 19

About the National Institute of Child Health and Human Development in Israel

The National Institute of Child Health and Human Development (NICHD) in Israel was established in 1998 as a virtual institute under the auspices of the Medical Director, Ministry of Social Affairs and Social Services in order to function as the research arm for the Office of the Medical Director. In 1998 the National Council for Child Health and Pediatrics, Ministry of Health and in 1999 the Director General and Deputy Director General of the Ministry of Health endorsed the establishment of the NICHD.

Mission

The mission of a National Institute for Child Health and Human Development in Israel is to provide an academic focal point for the scholarly interdisciplinary study of child life, health, public health, welfare, disability, rehabilitation, intellectual disability and related aspects of human development. This mission includes research, teaching, clinical work, information and public service activities in the field of child health and human development.

Service and academic activities

Over the years many activities became focused in the south of Israel due to collaboration with various professionals at the Faculty of Health Sciences (FOHS) at the Ben Gurion University of the Negev (BGU). Since 2000 an affiliation with the Zusman Child Development Center at the Pediatric Division of Soroka University Medical Center has resulted in collaboration around the establishment of the Down Syndrome Clinic at that center. In 2002 a full course on "Disability" was established at the Recanati School for Allied Professions in the Community, FOHS, BGU and in 2005 collaboration was started with the Primary Care Unit of the faculty and disability became part of the master of public health course on "Children and society". In the academic year 2005-2006 a one semester course on "Aging with disability" was started as part of the master of science program in gerontology in our collaboration with the Center for Multidisciplinary Research in Aging. In 2010 collaborations with the Division of Pediatrics, Hadassah Hebrew University Medical Center, Jerusalem, Israel around the National Down Syndrome Center and teaching students and residents about intellectual and developmental disabilities as part of their training at this campus.

Research activities

The affiliated staff have over the years published work from projects and research activities in this national and international collaboration. In the year 2000 the International Journal of Adolescent Medicine and Health and in 2005 the International Journal on Disability and Human Development of De Gruyter Publishing House (Berlin and New York) were affiliated with the National Institute of Child Health and Human Development. From 2008 also the International Journal of Child Health and Human Development (Nova Science, New York), the International Journal of Child and Adolescent Health (Nova Science) and the Journal of Pain Management (Nova Science) affiliated and from 2009 the International Public Health Journal (Nova Science) and Journal of Alternative Medicine Research (Nova Science). All peer-reviewed international journals.

National collaborations

Nationally the NICHD works in collaboration with the Faculty of Health Sciences, Ben Gurion University of the Negev; Department of Physical Therapy, Sackler School of Medicine, Tel Aviv University; Autism Center, Assaf HaRofeh Medical Center; National Rett and PKU Centers at Chaim Sheba Medical Center, Tel HaShomer; Department of Physiotherapy, Haifa University; Department of Education, Bar Ilan University, Ramat Gan, Faculty of Social Sciences and Health Sciences; College of Judea and Samaria in Ariel and in 2011 affiliation with Center for Pediatric Chronic Diseases and National Center for Down Syndrome, Department of Pediatrics, Hadassah Hebrew University Medical Center, Mount Scopus Campus, Jerusalem.

International collaborations

Internationally with the Department of Disability and Human Development, College of Applied Health Sciences, University of Illinois at Chicago; Strong Center for Developmental Disabilities, Golisano Children's Hospital at Strong, University of Rochester School of Medicine and Dentistry, New York; Centre on Intellectual Disabilities, University of Albany, New York; Centre for Chronic Disease Prevention and Control, Health Canada, Ottawa; Chandler Medical Center and Children's Hospital, Kentucky Children's Hospital, Section of Adolescent Medicine, University of Kentucky, Lexington; Chronic Disease Prevention and Control Research Center, Baylor College of Medicine, Houston, Texas; Division of Neuroscience, Department of Psychiatry, Columbia University, New York; Institute for the Study of Disadvantage and Disability, Atlanta; Center for Autism and Related Disorders, Department Psychiatry, Children's Hospital Boston, Boston; Department of Pediatric and Adolescent Medicine, Western Michigan University Homer Stryker MD School of Medicine, Kalamazoo, Michigan, United States; Department of Paediatrics, Child Health and Adolescent Medicine, Children's Hospital at Westmead, Westmead, Australia; International Centre for the Study of Occupational and Mental Health, Düsseldorf, Germany; Centre for Advanced Studies in Nursing, Department of General Practice and Primary Care, University of Aberdeen, Aberdeen, United Kingdom; Quality of Life Research Center, Copenhagen, Denmark; Nordic School of Public Health, Gottenburg, Sweden, Scandinavian Institute of Quality of Working Life, Oslo, Norway; The Department of Applied Social Sciences (APSS) of The Hong Kong Polytechnic University Hong Kong.

Targets

Our focus is on research, international collaborations, clinical work, teaching and policy in health, disability and human development and to establish the NICHD as a permanent institute in Israel in order to conduct model research and policy.

Contact

Professor Joav Merrick, MD, MMedSci, DMSc
Director, National Institute of Child Health and Human Development, Jerusalem, Israel.
E-mail: jmerrick@zahav.net.il

In: Service Leadership
Editors: Daniel TL Shek, Xiaoqin Zhu, Li Lin et al.
ISBN: 978-1-53614-852-7

Chapter 20

ABOUT THE BOOK SERIES "PUBLIC HEALTH: PRACTICES, METHODS AND POLICIES"

Public health is a book series with publications from a multidisciplinary group of researchers, practitioners and clinicians for an international professional forum interested in the broad spectrum of public health issues. Books already published:

- Rubin IL, Merrick J, eds. Environment and public health: Environmental health, law and international perspectives. New York: Nova Science, 2014.
- Shek DTL, Siu AMH, Merrick J, eds. Tomorrow's leaders: Service leadership and holistic development in Chinese university students. New York: Nova Science, 2015.
- Siziya S, Mazaba ML, Merrick J, eds. Arbovirus: Public health experience from Zambia. New York: Nova Science, 2015.
- Obeng C, Obeng SG, Merrick J, eds. Health issues in diverse cultures. New York: Nova Science, 2015.
- Friedman BD, Merrick J, eds. Public health, social work and health inequalities. New York: Nova Science, 2015.
- Rubin IL, Merrick J, eds. Environmental health disparities: Costs and benefits of breaking the cycle. New York: Nova Science, 2016.
- Mazaba ML, Siziya S, Merrick J, eds. Smoking and adolescence: International public health experiences. New York: Nova Science, 2016.
- Merrick J, ed. Public health: Some international perspectives. New York: Nova Science, 2016.
- Greydanus DE, Merrick J. Medical history: Some perspectives. New York: Nova Science, 2016.

- Rubin IL, Merrick J, eds. Public health: International aspects on environment and health. New York: Nova Science, 2016.
- Shek DTL, Ma C, Lin L, Merrick J, eds. Education in Hong Kong: Service leadership for university students. New York: Nova Science, 2016.
- Shek DTL, Siu AMH, Leung H, Merrick J, eds. Higher education in Hong Kong: Nurturing students to be caring service leaders. New York: Nova Science, 2016.
- Marufu T, Siziya S, Mazaba ML, Merrick J, eds. Measles: Epidemiology and control of measles in the Gweru urban district in Zimbabwe. New York: Nova Science, 2016.
- Hegamin-Younger C, Merrick J, eds. Caribbean adolescents: Misuse and abuse of alcohol. New York: Nova Science, 2016.
- Greydanus DE, Merrick J. Diabetes mellitus: A medical history journey. New York: Nova Science, 2016.
- Rubin IL, Merrick J, eds. Public health: An ecological framework for child environmental health interventions. New York: Nova Science, 2017.
- Shek DTL, Chung P, Lin L, Merrick J, eds. Service leadership education for university students. New York: Nova Science, 2017.
- Shek DTL, Ma C, Merrick J, eds. Leadership: Promoting leadership and intrapersonal development in university students. New York: Nova Science, 2017.
- Shek DTL, Yu L, Merrick J, eds. University students: Promoting of holistic development in Hong Kong. New York: Nova Science, 2017.
- Chow R, Hollenberg D, Borean M, Merrick J, eds. Alzheimer's disease: Awareness among young adults. New York: Nova Science, 2017.
- Rubin IL, Merrick J, eds. Resilience and health: A potent dynamic. New York: Nova Science, 2018.
- Greydanus DE, Merrick J. Medical history: Some new perspectives, Second edition. New York: Nova Science, 2018.

Contact

Professor Joav Merrick, MD, MMedSci, DMSc
Director, National Institute of Child Health and Human Development, Jerusalem, Israel
E-mail: jmerrick@zahav.net.il

SECTION FIVE: INDEX

INDEX

A

B

C

D

E

F

G

H

I

K

L

M

N

O

P

R

S

T

U

V

Medical History: Some Perspectives. Second Edition

Authors: Donald E. Greydanus, M.D. and Joav Merrick, M.D.

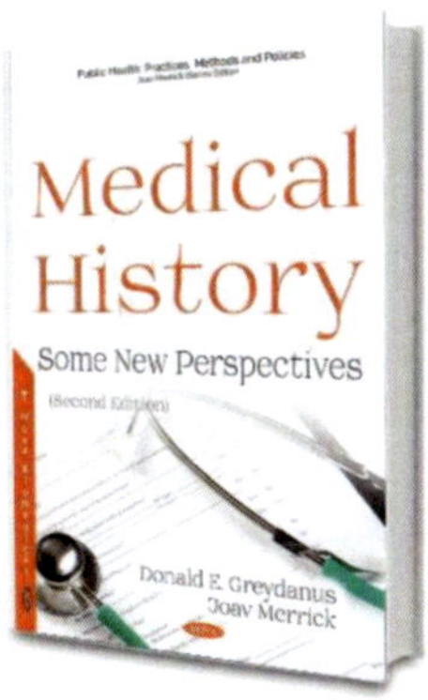

Series: Public Health: Practices, Methods and Policies

Book Description: A variety of topics are presented in this book that seek to reflect on medical history before and after the golden age of the Medical Renaissance.

Hardcover ISBN: 978-1-53613-319-6
Retail Price: $230

Resilience and Health: A Potent Dynamic

Editors: I. Leslie Rubin, M.D. and Joav Merrick, M.D.

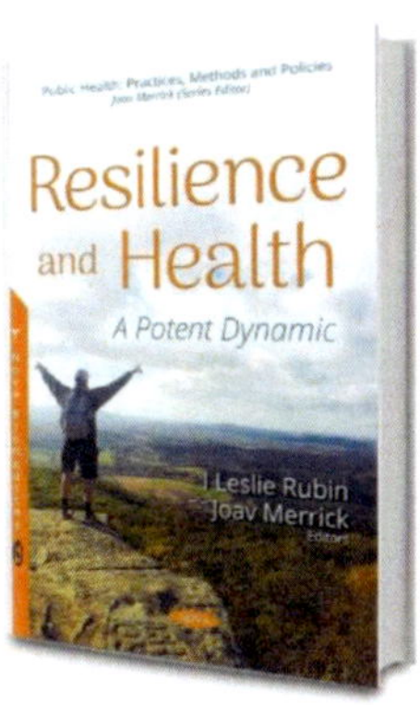

Series: Public Health: Practices, Methods and Policies

Book Description: Break the Cycle of Children's Environmental Health Disparities (or simply, Break the Cycle) is an annual collaborative interdisciplinary research and training program involving university students in academic tracks that focus on the impact of adverse social, economic, and environmental factors on children's health, development, and education.

Hardcover ISBN: 978-1-53613-412-4
Retail Price: $160

Public Health Yearbook 2017

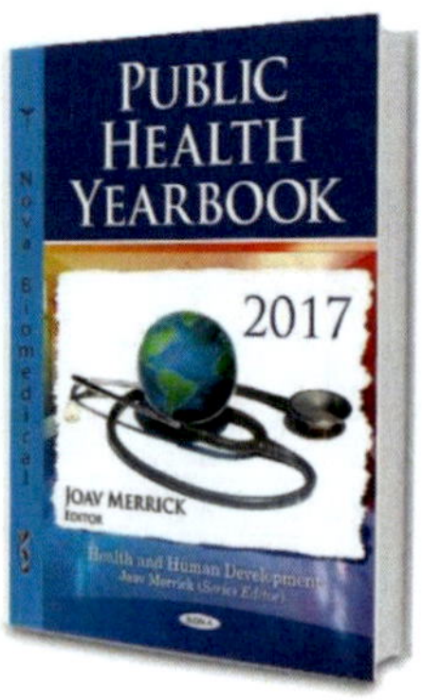

Editor: Joav Merrick, M.D.

Series: Public Health: Practices, Methods and Policies

Book Description: Public Health Yearbook 2017 present research on: adolescent alcohol use in the Caribbean region; discussion about how to break the cycle of child and adolescent environmental health disparities affecting development; serious debate about parental refusal of childhood vaccinations; food security; social and health issues surrounding Chinese adolescents; and a world tour of suicide ideation in school-age teenagers. We hope this Yearbook and the research will be of interest to our readers.

Hardcover ISBN: 978-1-53613-792-7
Retail Price: $270

Alzheimer's Disease: Awareness among Young Adults

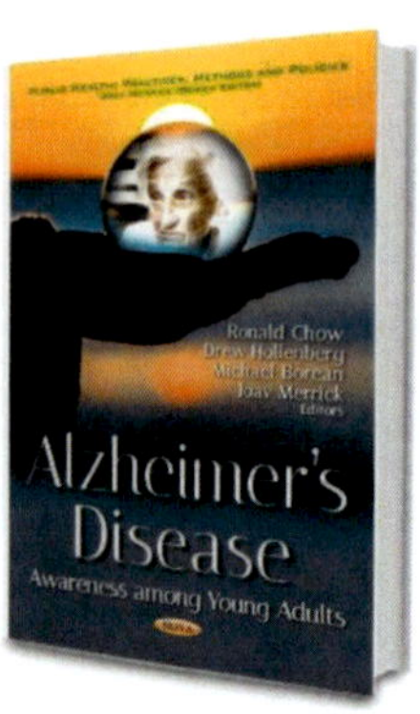

Editors: Ronald Chow, Drew Hollenberg, Michael Borean, and Joav Merrick, M.D., MMedSci, DMSc

Series: Public Health: Practices, Methods and Policies

Book Description: Alzheimer's disease will become more prevalent in the upcoming decades. In this book, we present studies that looked into the awareness level of young adults by geographical location, age, sex, and familial ties to the disease.

Hardcover ISBN: 978-1-53612-456-9
Retail Price: $195